COPING WITH
PHYSICAL ILLNESS

Current Topics in Mental Health

Series Editors: **Paul I. Ahmed**
Southeastern University

and
Stanley C. Plog
Plog Research, Inc.

COPING WITH PHYSICAL ILLNESS

Edited by
Rudolf H. Moos
Stanford University Medical Center
and
Veterans Administration Hospital
Palo Alto, California

In collaboration with
Vivien Davis Tsu

PLENUM MEDICAL BOOK COMPANY
New York and London

Library of Congress Cataloging in Publication Data

Main Entry under title:

Coping with physical illness.

(Current topics in mental health)
Includes bibliographies and index.
1. Crisis intervention (Psychiatry) 2. Sick—Psychology. 3. Medicine and psychology. I. Moos, Rudolf H., 1934-   II. Tsu, Vivien Davis. [DNLM: 1. Adaptation, Psychological. 2. Attitude to health. 3. Stress, Psychological. BF335 C783]
RC480.6.C66   616.08   76-26175
ISBN 0-306-30936-X

© 1977 Plenum Publishing Corporation
227 West 17th Street, New York, N. Y. 10011

Plenum Medical Book Company is an imprint of Plenum Publishing Corporation

Printed in the United States of America

Preface

This book discusses how human beings cope with serious physical illness and injury. A conceptual model for understanding the process of coping with the crisis of illness is provided, and basic adaptive tasks and types of coping skills are identified.

The major portion of the book is organized around various types of physical illness. These physical illnesses, which almost all people face either in themselves or their family members, raise common relevant coping issues. The last few sections cover "the crisis of treatment," emphasizing the importance of unusual hospital environments and radical new medical treatments, of stresses on professional staff, and of issues related to death and the fear of dying. The material highlights the fact that people can successfully cope with life crises such as major illness and injury, rather than the fact that severe symptoms and/or breakdowns sometimes occur. The importance of support from professional care-givers, such as physicians, nurses, and social workers, and from family, friends, and other sources of help in the community, is emphasized. Many of the selections include case examples which serve to illustrate the material.

Coping with Physical Illness has been broadly conceived to meet the needs of a diverse audience. There is substantial information about how human beings cope with illness and physical disability, but this material has never been collected in one place. The material is relevant in selected courses in schools of nursing, medicine, and public health, particularly in departments of psychiatry, behavioral sciences, epidemiology, and family and community health, and in newly developing health education programs. It is also relevant in selected courses in departments of psychology, sociology, and social work. The concepts and practical ideas should be particularly useful to nurses, social workers, medical students, physical therapists, occupational therapists, nursing students, and pastoral counselors who work in health settings. They should also be useful in nurse practitioner, physician's assistant, and other types of paramedical training programs. The ways in which patients cope with the personal crisis of illness, hospitalization, and treatment is of central concern to these professional groups.

The book has 11 parts. Part I presents a general perspective on the importance of psychosocial factors and coping processes in health and disease. A conceptual model to help the student understand the crisis of physical illness is presented. Seven basic adaptive tasks and seven basic sets of coping skills are outlined. Part II presents articles dealing with the crisis of illness with special emphasis on stillbirth and birth defects. The articles describe how parents react to an infant with a fatal birth defect, how a mother reacts to the loss of septuplets, and how parents react to a child with Down's Syndrome. Part III deals with the crisis of illness with special reference to cancer. The articles discuss the stresses faced by cancer patients, how women cope with breast cancer, and the role of the family in coping with childhood leukemia.

Part IV deals with the crisis of illness with special reference to cardiovascular disease. The articles describe how patients deal with the period of convalescence following myocardial infarction, how coping processes can assist in the recovery from open-heart surgery, and how the facilitation of adaptive behavior can help patients and their families in rehabilitation from a stroke. Part V deals with the crisis of illness with special reference to severe burns. The material covers the adaptive mechanisms used by severely burned patients and the adjustment problems of the family of the burn patient.

Part VI focuses on the crisis of illness with special reference to chronic conditions in children. The articles discuss the development of adaptive strategies among children dealing with long-term physical illness, and the psychosocial problems involved in handling cystic fibrosis and scoliosis.

Part VII presents material on the crisis of treatment with special reference to unusual hospital environments. The articles discuss the impact of different hospital settings on patients, how patients react to a cancer ward and how these reactions can be changed by staff, and special problems which may arise in the waiting room of a pediatric oncology clinic. Part VIII presents material on the crisis of treatment with special reference to dependence on machines and medical hardware. The articles discuss the response of heart patients to the implantation of an electronic pacemaker, the emotional reactions of patients undergoing maintenance hemodialysis in hospital centers, and the extreme stress which may be associated with chronic hemodialysis. Part IX reviews the crisis of treatment with emphasis on reactions to organ transplants. The material highlights the emotional effects of receiving a transplanted kidney and the adjustments patients make following cardiac transplants.

Part X focuses on the crisis of treatment with special emphasis on the staff. The articles discuss how nurses adapt to working with severely burned children, and the unusual psychological stresses of intensive care unit nursing.

Part XI deals with death and the fear of dying. The articles discuss the disclosure of terminal diagnoses such as cancer, the patient's reaction to the dying process, family responses to the crisis of death, and the personal account of a man slowly dying from a degenerative neuromuscular disease.

I have dedicated this book to Erich Lindemann, whose early descriptions of the ways in which people handle life crises influenced my thinking. He had the unusual gift of clarifying complex concepts so that others could understand them. Erich also faced his own illness, his own increasing pain and incapacitation, and the imminence of his own death better than I thought anyone could. I wish I could have coped with his last crisis as well as he did.

Many other people have influenced me. There is still no better descriptive work on how patients cope with physical illness than that carried out by David Hamburg and his colleagues over 20 years ago. They pointed out that so-called defense mechanisms often had positive adaptive value. These ideas, as well as many ensuing discussions, kindled my curiosity in this field. George Coelho and Bish Lipowski influenced me both by their writings and by our discussions. Kurt Goldstein, Abraham Maslow, and Carl Rogers have influenced me mainly through their writings, which emphasized self-actualization and the notion that people could cope with and transcend major life crises.

I have compiled and organized this book in collaboration with Vivien Tsu, who coped with an overwhelming mass of material, coauthored the overview article and took the major responsibility in preparing the commentaries for each section. Louise Doherty and Susanne Flynn efficiently performed the typing and secretarial tasks involved. The work was supported in part by Grant MH 16026 from the National Institute of Mental Health, Grant AA02863 from the National Institute of Alcohol Abuse and Alcohol, and by Veterans Administration Research Project MRIS 5817-01 to the Social Ecology Laboratory, Department of Psychiatry and Behavioral Sciences, Stanford University, and the Veterans Administration Hospital, Palo Alto.

Bernice, Karen, Kevin, and I know firsthand about the difficulties encountered in handling severe physical illness. We hope that the material presented here can help professional care-givers and patients and their families facilitate effective coping skills and thus enhance the quality of their lives.

R. M.

Palo Alto

Contents

I

Overview and Perspective

The Crisis of Physical Illness: An Overview

RUDOLF H. MOOS and VIVIEN DAVIS TSU

The human capacity to overcome the pain and suffering of severe physical disease is immense. People often continue to function under the most harrowing life circumstances. How can this be? Why don't people simply give up under the stress of severe physical illness? What are the tasks which they must successfully negotiate? What are the coping skills which facilitate effective recovery? How can medical staff enhance the psychological healing process? This book is addressed to these questions.

Consider, for example, the severe problems faced by Eric Lund and Jill Kinmont. In September, 1967, Eric Lund was getting ready to leave for his first year at college. Eric, a soccer star in high school, had been running miles each day to train for the freshman team he hoped to win a place on. His mother noticed some large sores on his legs and insisted he see a doctor immediately; the doctor ordered some blood tests and a bone marrow biopsy. The next day Eric's parents, who had prepared themselves to see their second child off into the adult world, learned instead that he had acute lymphocytic leukemia and probably only six months to two years to live. Eric, who had been told that he had anemia and would have to postpone college, began his first course of chemo-

RUDOLF H. MOOS, M.D. and VIVIEN DAVIS TSU, M.A. • Stanford University Medical Center and Veterans Administration Hospital, Palo Alto, California.

therapy. Two months later when he finally achieved remission, his mother told him the whole truth.

The first remission lasted less than two months. To achieve each subsequent remission, stronger and stronger drugs had to be used with correspondingly more serious side effects like mouth ulcers, vomiting, and bleeding gums. His second remission lasted about a year. That fall he entered college and became cocaptain of the freshman soccer team. More than two years after his illness was diagnosed, and following three months in the hospital during which time all his close friends on the ward died, Eric achieved his fourth remission which lasted almost a year. After working out all summer to rebuild his strength, he was able to return to school and soccer and was even named an All-New England All Star player.

After 3½ years in and out of remission, Eric was put in a sterile air chamber for nearly three months. Despite the stringent precautions he contracted an infection and almost died. After four days of semiconsciousness and raging fever, he fought his way back.

What gave Eric the strength to keep fighting, to pick up the pieces of his life after each interruption, and to live fully whether he was feeling sick or well? How did his parents and younger brother and sister deal with 4½ years of sudden ups and downs, midnight medical emergencies, and the total disruption of family life whenever Eric was hospitalized? After the near-fatal incident Eric lived one more year, a rich and happy year because he was in love with a young woman, a nurse who accepted him and their limited time together. When he knew the arsenal of drugs finally had nothing more for him, he was able to accept the approaching end of the struggle.[10]

In January of 1955 Jill Kinmont was 18 years old; her picture was on the cover of *Sports Illustrated* and she was well on her way to becoming a member of the U.S. Olympic ski team. Years of training and hard work had brought her to this point. In the last major race before the Olympic tryouts she went flying off the side of a mountain and crashed to earth at 40 miles an hour, breaking her neck. Her nearly fatal fall left her permanently paralyzed from the shoulders down.

Six months later, her condition stabilized, she was released from the hospital and entered a rehabilitation center in Los Angeles. She had the use of parts of her arms and wrists, but not her hands. Fitted with a stiff corset (so she could sit up in a wheelchair) and braces on her hands (so she could hold a pen and a special spoon), she began to regain a measure of independence. In order to meet her medical expenses the

Kinmonts had to sell their home in Bishop, a guest ranch the whole family had worked hard to build up. For the first year the family was split up since Jill's mother stayed with her daughter to assist in her care. After six months in the center strengthening and refining her remaining physical abilities and learning self-care skills, Jill was reunited with her family and they moved into a small house together.

Until the accident, competitive skiing had been the focus of all Jill Kinmont's energy; it was the primary source of challenge and pleasure in her life and the basis of the attention, public and private, which she had come to enjoy. Now she had to completely reorient her life, and she hardly knew where to begin. She started with some basic courses at UCLA and later added some volunteer tutoring. Gradually she became convinced that teaching was what she enjoyed most, and that it would be the best way for her to achieve independence and to help others, two goals she cherished. She graduated in 1960, but UCLA's School of Education refused to admit her because of her handicap. Eventually she secured training elsewhere, and in 1964, not quite 10 years after her accident, she began her first regular job teaching remedial reading in an elementary school, her dream finally fulfilled.[14]

In this overview article we present a brief historical introduction focusing on the development of psychosomatic medicine and of crisis theory. We then sketch a conceptual framework of physical disease as a life crisis, and present an outline of the major tasks with which patients must cope and the types of coping skills they use. We conclude by focusing on the central role of medical and paramedical staff in facilitating effective coping by patients, and by their family and friends.

Historical Perspectives

Current approaches to the field of coping with physical illness have been influenced by the evolution of concepts in psychosomatic medicine and by the development of "crisis theory" and its implications for clinical intervention.

Psychosomatic Medicine

During the last half century a number of conceptual approaches have contributed to the development of psychosomatic medicine. The work of Sigmund Freud, Ivan Pavlov, and Walter Cannon contributed significantly to the early development of the field (see Wittkower[16] for a fuller discussion) Much of the initial research in the 1930s and 1940s developed out of a psychodynamic perspective and focused on personality traits or conflicts thought to be characteristic of individuals with particular types of disorders.

Harold Wolff and his colleagues at Cornell took a different tack. They studied the physiological effects of experimental stress situations and evolved a theory that psychosomatic illness is an *adaptive* response to "life stress." This new focus led to attempts to relate aspects of the physical and social environment to the onset and course of diseases such as diabetes mellitus, peptic ulcer, rheumatoid arthritis, and the like. Some investigators focused on the importance of relationships with others, on the psychological effects of divorce and separation, and on the mourning process.[1,7]

Two additional trends have helped to shape this field. First, detailed clinical studies of patients with serious physical illnesses (like brain injuries, severe burns, or poliomyelitis) illustrated the importance of adaptive and coping processes. The other trend, which arose mainly from personality theory and experimental psychology, focused on cognitive appraisal, the perception of threat, and the importance of self-regulation. Lazarus[8] has emphasized that it is not the stress itself that is of paramount importance, but rather the individual's cognitive appraisal of it.

Many of these threads have begun to come together in the last decade, as the multifactorial nature of all illness has become more generally accepted. There has been a striking increase in research on a broad array of psychological and social factors thought to influence not only the etiology and onset of disease, but also the experience, course, and outcome of illness, the response to treatment, the utilization of medical care, including resistance to seeking and cooperating with treatment, and so on. Psychological and social factors are now conceptualized as a class of relevant factors in all phases of all diseases.[9] There is also a more dynamic perspective now which takes into account the importance of feedback mechanisms and of maintaining psychological as well as physiological homeostasis.

Crisis Theory and Research

Crisis theory is concerned with how people can cope with major life crises and transitions. Historically, "crisis theory" has been influenced by four major intellectual developments: evolution and its implications for communal and individual adaptation, fulfillment or growth theories of human motivation, a life-cycle approach to human development, and interest in coping behavior under extreme stresses such as natural disasters.[13] Crisis theory has provided a conceptual framework for preventive psychiatry in general, and for the handling of severe physical illness or injury in particular. The fundamental ideas were developed by Erich Lindemann, who vividly described the process of grief and mourning and the role community caretakers could play in helping bereaved family members cope with the loss of their loved ones. These notions, as well as Erik Erikson's[3] formulation of "developmental crises" at transition points in the life cycle, paved the way for Gerald Caplan's[2] classic formulation of crisis theory.

Similar to people's need for physiological homeostasis is their requirement for a sense of social and psychological equilibrium. People generally have certain characteristic patterns of behavior. When they encounter something which upsets their usual balance, they employ habitual problem-solving mechanisms until the balance is restored. A situation which is so novel or so major that the usual habitual responses are inadequate constitutes a crisis and leads to a state of disorganization often accompanied by anxiety, fear, guilt, or other unpleasant feelings which contribute further to the disorganization.

A person cannot remain in an extreme state of disequilibrium, and a crisis is thus, by definition, self-limited. Within a few days or weeks some resolution, even though temporary, must be found, and some equilibrium reestablished. The new balance achieved may represent a healthy adaptation which promotes personal growth and maturation, or a maladaptive response, which signifies psychological deterioration and decline. A crisis experience may thus be seen as a transitional period, a turning point, which has important implications for an individual's ability to meet future crises.

Severe physical illness almost always represents a serious "upset in a steady state." A person may face separation from family and friends, the loss of key roles in his or her life, permanent changes in appearance or in bodily functions, assaults on self-image and self-esteem, distressing feelings of anxiety, guilt, anger, or helplessness, and an uncertain, unpredictable future. According to crisis theory, the individual is much more receptive to outside influence in a time of disequilibrium. This greater accessibility offers health professionals and others who deal with patients an unusual opportunity to have a strong constructive impact. In addition, the crisis of illness may extend over a relatively long period of time, presenting the patient with a complex set of new issues and circumstances over which he has little control, and leaving him in a state of tentative equilibrium which may be shattered at any moment. This fact increases the leverage of professional care-givers, and underscores the importance of their learning appropriate crisis resolution and psychosocial counseling techniques.

A Conceptual Framework

We have evolved a framework in which serious physical illness or injury is understood as a life crisis. This crisis, through the individual's cognitive appraisal of its significance, sets forth basic adaptive tasks to which various coping skills can be applied. This cognitive appraisal, the perception of the tasks involved, and the selection of relevant coping skills are influenced by three sets of factors: background and personal characteristics, illness-related factors, and features of the physical and sociocultural environment. All these factors together determine the outcome of the crisis. It is important to note that family members and friends, as well as patients, are affected by the crisis, encounter many of the same or closely related adaptive tasks, and use the same types of coping skills. In the next sections we briefly review the basic tasks and skills and the three sets of factors determining outcome.

Major Adaptive Tasks

Although any classification is somewhat arbitrary, we believe that the major adaptive tasks can be divided into seven general categories. Three of these tasks are mainly illness-related, whereas the other four are more general and are relevant to all types of life crises (see Table I).

The first set of tasks involves dealing with the discomfort, incapacitation, and other symptoms of the illness or injury itself. This includes a whole range of distressing symptoms such as pain, extreme weakness, dizziness, incontinence, paralysis, loss of control (in convulsive disorders), the feeling of suffocation (in respiratory ailments), the permanent disfigurement which may occur in disorders such as scoliosis, and so forth.

A second and closely related set of tasks entails the management of

Table I. Major Sets of Adaptive Tasks

Illness-related
1. Dealing with pain and incapacitation
2. Dealing with the hospital environment and special treatment procedures
3. Developing adequate relationships with professional staff

General
4. Preserving a reasonable emotional balance
5. Preserving a satisfactory self-image
6. Preserving relationships with family and friends
7. Preparing for an uncertain future

the stresses of special treatment procedures and of various aspects of the hospital or institutional environment itself. The increasing sophistication of medical technology over the last few decades has created a host of new stressors for patients. Surgical procedures like mastectomy and colostomy, debridement as a treatment for burns, radiotherapy and chemotherapy with their concomitant side effects, the necessity of wearing a cumbersome brace for certain orthopedic disorders, long-term hemodialysis, and organ transplantation—all these represent therapeutic measures which create additional adaptive tasks for patients.

Special technical environments such as the operating and recovery rooms, the intensive care unit, the premature baby nursery, and even the waiting room of an oncology clinic also represent significant new stressors for patients. Separated from family and exposed to unfamiliar routines and procedures, patients (particularly children) find hospitalization itself to be upsetting. We believe that "the crisis of treatment" is an increasingly significant factor in understanding the tasks which must be faced by seriously ill patients (see parts VII, VIII, and IX).

The third set of tasks consists of developing and maintaining adequate relationships with medical and other care-giving staff. From the experience of the patient and his or her family and friends, this can require all the interpersonal skill they can muster. Consider the questions patients may ask themselves: Can I express my anger at the doctor for not coming to see me? How can I ask for additional medication for pain when I need it? How can I deal with the disagreements among different physicians regarding how I should be treated? How can I handle the condescension and pity I sense in the nurses who care for me? How can I tell the physical therapist not to give up on me even though my progress is disappointingly slow? How can I engage my doctor in a meaningful discussion of how I wish to be treated if I am incapacitated and near death? These are problems which plague patients and their families. The frequent turnover and change in personnel, particularly those staff who come into more direct contact with the patient, makes this an unusually complicated set of tasks.

The fourth category of tasks involves preserving a reasonable emotional balance by managing upsetting feelings aroused by the illness. There are many "negative" emotions associated with medical crises, such as the sense of failure and self-blame at giving birth to a deformed child (see part II), the anxiety and apprehension of not knowing the outcome of an illness, the sense of alienation and isolation, and the feelings of inadequacy and resentment in the face of difficult demands. An important aspect of this task is for the patient to maintain some hope, even when its scope is sharply limited by circumstances.

The fifth set of tasks consists of preserving a satisfactory self-image and maintaining a sense of competence and mastery. Changes in physical functioning or appearance, such as permanent weakness or scarring, must be incorporated into a revised self-image. This "identity crisis" can necessitate a change in personal values and life style, as, for example, when permanently disfigured burn victims and their families learn to downplay the importance of physical attractiveness. Patients who must rely on mechanical devices like cardiac pacemakers or hemodialysis to sustain their lives must come to terms with a "half man–half machine" body image.

Defining the limits of independence and readjusting goals and expectations in light of changes brought by the illness are other tasks which belong in this category. The need to depend on others for physical care and emotional support can be very stressful. It is important to find a personally and socially satisfactory balance between accepting help and taking an active and responsible part in determining the direction and activities of one's life. Resuming independent status after a long period of enforced passivity can also be difficult, as, for example, when a successful organ transplant patient is suddenly no longer an invalid (see part IX). This conflict is further complicated for children by the normal developmental drive to gradually increase independence and self-direction, to which illness-imposed dependence and parental protectiveness may represent a serious setback (see part VI).

The sixth set of tasks includes those of preserving relationships with family and friends. A person who becomes ill may feel isolated by his or her new identity as a "patient" or as a "dying person," someone who is different from other people. This sense of alienation, and the physical separation occasioned by hospitalization, often disrupt normal relationships with friends and relatives. Like many of the other sets of tasks, this one applies to relatives and friends as well as to the patient directly. What affects one member within the family system also touches the others, as when the breadwinner is disabled by a stroke or when a child becomes terminally ill. Serious illness may make it extremely difficult to keep communication lines open and to offer comfort and support at the very time when these are most essential.

The seventh set of tasks involves preparing for an uncertain future in which significant losses are threatened. The loss of sight, of speech (for example, after a stroke), of a limb or a breast by surgery, or of life itself, are all losses which must be acknowledged and mourned. Ironically, new medical procedures which raise hope for patients with previously incurable illnesses may make this task more difficult. Patients must prepare for permanent loss of function while maintaining hope that restoration of function may be possible. When death seems likely, patients and family members must engage in anticipatory mourning and initiate the grieving process, while maintaining hope that new treatment procedures may prove beneficial.

Even when the prognosis is certain and death is inevitable, the future that counts is still uncertain. Consider the questions which patients may ask themselves: How long do I have to live? How will I know when death is near? Will I be able to retain bowel and bladder function until the end? Can I die at home in familiar surroundings? Will my death be reasonably painless? Even at the end of life, patients and their families must handle these and many other similar uncertainties.

These seven groups of tasks are generally encountered with every illness, but their relative importance varies widely depending on the nature of the disease, the personality of the individual involved, and the unique set of environmental circumstances. For the person suddenly rendered blind the physical discomfort may be minor, while the difficulty of restoring social relations seems overwhelming. A bone cancer patient, on the other hand, must deal with severe pain. A woman who has had a mastectomy may find that accepting her new self-image is her most significant task. Someone who is physically active, like a professional athlete or a construction worker, will probably have more difficulty adjusting to a wheelchair than a person who has a more sedentary occupation.

These tasks may be as difficult for family members and friends as for patients themselves. Family members must develop adequate relationships with professional care-givers. They must maintain a sense of inner mastery of the divergent emotions aroused in them and attempt to maintain hope. They must try to preserve a satisfactory self-image (helping the patient as much as possible, but not feeling overwhelmed by guilt when they cannot do everything the patient asks). They must handle the task of maintaining family integrity and their relationship with the patient. They, too, must prepare for an uncertain future. The first step for family and friends, as for patients, is to recognize the importance of these tasks, and to understand that they are common tasks which all patients and their families must face.

Major Types of Coping Skills

People respond to severe physical illness in many different ways. We offer here a description of major types of coping skills which are commonly employed to deal with the adaptive tasks discussed above. These skills may be used individually, consecutively, or, more likely, in various combinations. Specific coping techniques are not inherently adaptive or maladaptive. Skills which are appropriate in one situation may not be in another. Skills which may be beneficial, given moderate or temporary use, may be harmful if relied upon exclusively. We do not distinguish between coping skills on the basis of whether they are "mental" or "behavioral" mechanisms. We believe that each of the major types of coping skills can have both mental and behavioral components. We use the word "skill" to underscore the positive aspects of coping, emphasizing coping as an ability which can be taught (as any other skill) and presumably used flexibly as the situation demands.

The first category covers an array of skills based on *denying or minimizing the seriousness* of a crisis. These may be directed at the illness itself, as when a myocardial infarct patient maintains "it was just severe indigestion." Or, after the diagnosis is accepted, they may be directed at the significance of an illness, as, for example, when the parents of a fatally ill child still go from doctor to doctor looking for a cure. Upsetting feelings are often handled by this type of skill. Anger may be suppressed, projected (attributed to someone else rather than oneself), or displaced to a less threatening target (a spouse instead of a doctor) or a more socially acceptable one (a healthy sibling rather than the terminally ill child).

Another skill in this general category is being able to isolate or dissociate one's emotions when dealing with a distressing situation. This occurs, for example, when the parents of a hemophiliac react quickly and calmly in a bleeding episode rather than showing their terror or dismay, or, more commonly, when patients discuss their symptoms with "clinical detachment." These skills have often been described as "defensive mechanisms," because they are self-protective responses to stress. This term, however, does not convey their constructive value; they often rescue the individual from being overwhelmed or provide the time needed to garner other personal coping resources.

The second set of coping skills consists of *seeking relevant information* and, more generally, using intellectual resources effectively. Adequate information can often relieve anxiety caused by uncertainty or misconceptions. Learning about the causes of birth defects can mitigate the sense of guilt or failure felt by the mother of a deformed baby. People who are feeling helpless and useless may find that information-seeking gives them something to do and restores a sense of having some control. For example, parents of leukemic children seek information about the degree of their responsibility for the illness (initially blaming themselves, for example, for not having paid more attention to the early nonspecific manifestations of the disease), about hospital procedures (questioning ward physicians and nurses and scrutinizing newspaper and magazine articles), and about ways of coming to terms with their expected loss.[5]

The third set of coping skills involves *requesting reassurance and emotional support* from concerned family, friends, and medical staff members. Emotional support can be an important source of strength in facing difficult times, but patients and others who keep their feelings "bottled up" or who withdraw from social interaction cut themselves off from help of this type. For this reason, patients are often encouraged to express their feelings, thereby relieving tension and opening themselves up to the comfort and reassurance given by concerned people around them. A related means of seeking support is to join special groups, whether they are national self-help organizations (like Reach for Recovery for mastectomy patients, chapter 6) or smaller ad hoc groups for patients (e.g., stroke patients, see chapter 10), relatives (e.g., spouses of hemiodialysis patients) or staff members (e.g., cancer ward nurses, see chapter 17).

The fourth set of coping skills concerns *learning specific illness-related procedures,* such as feeding and caring for a premature baby, running a home dialysis machine, or giving oneself insulin injections. These accomplishments can provide much-needed confirmation of personal ability and effectiveness at a time when opportunities for independent and meaningful action are scarce. Patients take pride in being able to care for themselves; relatives find relief in being able to offer concrete help.

The fifth set of coping skills entails *setting concrete limited goals,* such as walking again or attending a special event (such as a wedding or graduation). This often gives patients something to look forward to and a realistic chance of achieving something they consider meaningful. The strategy of "progressive desensitization," whereby patients with severe disfiguration gradually "expose" themselves to others and dull their own sensitivity to others' reactions, also falls within this category (see part V). This set of skills includes the ability to break seemingly overwhelming problems into small, potentially manageable bits.

Rehearsing alternative outcomes comprises the sixth set of coping skills. This category includes mental preparation (anticipation and mental rehearsal), and the discussion of various alternative outcomes with family and friends. It is often used in combination with information-seeking, as patients try to prepare themselves to handle expected difficulties by thinking through the steps involved and by acquainting themselves with the demands that might be made on them. This technique is commonly used to allay anxiety, as, for example, when unfamiliar medical procedures are scheduled. Reminding oneself of previous successes in handling difficult problems, in order to ease one's fears and bolster one's confidence, fits into this category. On a broader scale, it also encompasses the anticipatory mourning process in which an expected death or other loss is acknowledged beforehand.

When life's happenings seem capricious and uncontrollable, as with the sudden onset of serious illness, it is often easier to manage if one can *find a general purpose or pattern of meaning* in the course of events. Efforts in this direction constitute our seventh type of coping skill. Belief in a divine purpose or in the general beneficence of a divine spirit may serve as consolation or as encouragement to do one's best to deal with the difficulties one encounters. White and Liddon[15] reported that 5 of 10 cardiac arrest patients they studied experienced a "transcendental redirection" of their lives as a result of their illness and, in that sense, viewed their heart attacks as having been of positive value. Putting an experience into a long-term perspective (with or without religious orientation) often makes individual events more manageable (see chapter 3).

Almost anything a person does can be a coping skill if it serves to deal with an adaptive task, but these seven categories cover the most common types observed in dealing with physical illness. It is important to keep in mind that coping skills are seldom used singly or exclusively. A patient may deny or minimize the seriousness of a crisis while talking to a family member, seek relevant information about prognosis from a physician, request reassurance and emotional support from a friend, and so on. A crisis situation usually presents a variety of tasks and requires a combination or sequence of coping skills. These categories, though arbitrary, provide a useful manner by which the major types of coping skills can be conceptualized.

General Determinants of Outcome

Why does one person respond differently from another to a life crisis like serious illness? What factors influence the overall appraisal of an illness, the perception of specific tasks, the initial choice of coping skills, and subsequent changes in coping strategy? The relevant determinants fall into three categories: background and personal characteristics, illness-related factors, and features of the physical and sociocultural environment.

Background and personal characteristics include age, intelligence, cognitive and emotional development, philosophical or religious beliefs, and previous coping experiences. These factors determine the meaning that the illness carries for an individual (see Figure 1), and affect the psychological and intellectual resources available to meet the crisis. For example, intelligence and the level of cognitive development play a role in determining an individual's ability to seek or use information to counteract uncertainty or a sense of powerlessness. General ego strength and self-esteem also have a significant impact on adaptive ability. An individual who feels insecure or inadequate may rely more heavily on denial or minimization skills than someone with a more positive self-image.

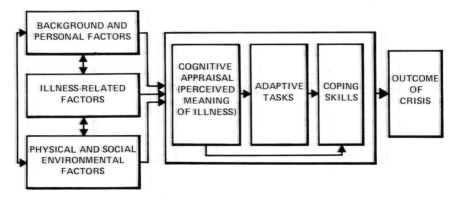

Fig. 1. A conceptual model for understanding the crisis of physical illness.

The timing of an illness in the life cycle is often particularly important. A child invalided by rheumatic heart disease has different concerns from those of an elderly patient incapacitated by heart disease. Some adolescents have a particularly difficult time coping with physical illness, since it imposes an additional stress at a time when the tasks of gaining independence from parents and establishing personal identity and a stable body image already provide difficult challenges (see part VI). Greater maturity and more extensive coping experience may provide the elderly with greater personal resources on which to draw. On the other hand, many elderly patients already have some degree of brain damage and/or severe cognitive disorganization which seriously impairs their coping ability.

Illness-related factors include the type and location of symptoms— whether painful, disfiguring, disabling, or in a body region vested with special importance, like the heart or reproductive organs—and are a major component in defining the exact nature of the tasks patients and others face, and, consequently, their adaptive responses. Different organs and functions may have a psychological significance which has little to do with biological factors related to survival. For example, an injury to the face or amputation of a breast may have greater psychological impact on a person than severe hypertension directly threatening his or her life.

Coping ability may be directly affected by physiological problems like brain damage, hormonal imbalance, or extreme weakness. The rate of onset and the general progression of a disease, including the occurrence of complications, may also affect both the choice of coping strategies and their effectiveness. The parents of a leukemic child in remission may halt the process of anticipatory mourning begun when the diagnosis was first announced, only to have to resume their preparation when the child relapses.

Features of the general physical and social environment can contribute to the stress or can serve as sources of help and support. The physical environment of a hospital, with its unfamiliar sights and sounds and bustle of activity, or of special areas like intensive care units, can further upset patients already trying to deal with a distressing illness (see part VII). The physical milieu of the patient's home may also be important. The esthetic quality of one's surroundings, the amount of personal space available and the usual degree of sensory stimulation may influence the patient's (and his or her relatives') cognitive functioning, mood, and general morale.[11]

The human environment includes the relationships of patients and their families, of staff and patients, the social supports in the wider community (such as friends, clergy, and various social service agencies), and sociocultural norms and expectations. The course of an illness tends to be more stormy and recovery slower than expected when it occurs in the context of serious interpersonal conflict or of recent bereavement. Mutual understanding or empathy on the part of stroke patients and their families is related to the patient's rate of rehabilitation. Patients with intractable duodenal ulcer and other intractable diseases who scored relatively high on a scale of environmental deprivation (including such factors as emotional impoverishment within the family and in other social relations) tended to show poorer outcome of surgery. The ability of family members to help the patient and each other strongly affects the choice of coping strategies and the ultimate outcome.

The Therapeutic Role of Staff

Can anything be done to promote effective coping among patients and others who are involved in the illness experience? Crisis theory maintains that the individuals experiencing a life crisis are more susceptible to external influences at that time than they are during periods of more stable functioning. Outside intervention, even minimal intervention, can play a significant role in facilitating (or hindering) effective adaptive behavior. Therefore, it is especially important that the medical staff and all those who are professionally involved in patient care recognize the opportunity they have to aid the patient and his or her family.

In order to give real assistance, care-givers should be competent in four areas. First, they must know what the usual responses to a given illness situation are, including the sequence of stages in emotional processes like mourning and the inevitability and value of the expression of "negative" emotions like anger or sadness. Understanding the need to express anger may help staff members accept the emotion, especially when it is directed at them.

Staff should understand the time dimension involved, for example, in grieving for a loss (whether of a person, a body part or function, or a cherished ideal). It entails a progression from an initial reaction of numbness or disbelief to a growing awareness of pain, sorrow, and often anger and a preoccupation with the lost object, and gradually to a reorganization in which the loss is accepted and equilibrium is restored. When staff encounter the parents of a defective infant, a patient who is terminally ill, a woman who has just lost a breast, or a disfigured burn victim, for example, they should not mistake numbness for stoicism or label depression or anger as pathological responses. In practical terms, it means that doctors who must announce an impending loss should be prepared to repeat their explanations again when the initial shock has subsided, for very little may be taken in at the first hearing.

Second, staff members should know the major tasks and typical coping strategies, so that they can recognize and respond to the adaptive efforts which their patients make. One of the most important ways in which medical staff can help is to give information: to respond to patients' questions, to clarify misconceptions, to prepare patients or family members by advising them of events or emotions which are likely to occur, and to identify other sources of available assistance like self-help groups and relevant community agencies. Mastectomy patients, for example, should be told that they may have crying spells, trouble sleeping, and numbness in their arms after the surgery. Then, if these occur, they need not fear they are having an emotional breakdown, or, as one woman did, that a nerve was mistakenly cut.[6]

Two other coping skills which can relate directly to staff are individual appeals for emotional support and efforts to maintain or build a sense of personal competence. Care-givers should be aware of the emotional needs of patients and family members and give the reassurances and the understanding that are sought, keeping in mind that frequent repetition of this support may be necessary. Patients often deal with their general physical dependence by asserting their independence and testing their competence in other areas. Family members also rely on this approach to cope with their sense of helplessness, as when parents help with the routine care of their hospitalized child. Staff should treat these not as intrusions in their own spheres but as valuable means of coping with the assault on self-image which illness makes. By offering opportunities for and encouraging independent action and by aiding successful mastery experiences, staff contribute to the maintenance or restoration of a healthy sense of self-esteem.

If those who are vulnerable because of poor use of coping skills can be identified, as Kimball did with a group of open-heart surgery patients (chapter 9), perhaps counseling or some other means of helping them can be obtained (see also Gruen[4]). The relationship of individual coping strategies to compliance with a therapeutic regimen is another area of particular concern for health professionals. Understanding different strategies can also help care-givers deal with problems which arise when patients and family use discrepant and incompatible coping strategies, for instance when a cancer patient is seeking information and emotional support from those around her while her spouse is denying there is anything seriously wrong.

Third, staff need to understand both the background and milieu factors which facilitate or hinder various coping strategies. Particular attention should be directed at the social environment (including friends and relatives, social workers, clergy, and the general community support system) and at the hospital as a stressful environment in itself. Focus on family and friends may enable staff to assist those involved with the patient to be more effective in helping him. Focus on the hospital milieu should help staff to orient and provide information to patients and thereby decrease its negative and confusing impact. This also raises the possibility of changing certain aspects of the hospital environment (both social and physical) to enhance patient care. Staff might use their understanding of this area to make "environmental diagnoses" on which to base individual intervention strategies appropriate to particular patients.[12]

Finally, health care professionals should understand their own reactions to various crises. They need to know that they too face certain tasks, go through certain stages in reaction to patients, and employ certain coping skills (see part X). Full awareness of this process can help staff to deal with the stress inherent in the nature of their work and to keep negative feelings about a particular patient or situation from affecting the quality of care they give (see chapter 17).

Professional care-givers have a special responsibility to help those whose lives have been disrupted by illness. Beyond the realm of physical care, this includes sympathetic understanding of the coping process and recognition of their own role in facilitating that process. Sensitivity to the psychological effects their own routine actions have on patients and their families may lead to alterations of behavior or procedure, with positive consequences for the patients. For example, Golden and Davis's practical suggestions (chapter 4) for the physician who must inform new parents that their child is defective reflect this kind of awareness: the mother should be told with her husband or other close friend present, not alone; the doctor should hold the infant in his or her arms while giving the news (giving a clear "message" that the child is still human and lovable); the clinical findings should be demonstrated directly on the baby; the physician should stress the similarity of the child to normal children; questions should be encouraged and all the information should be reviewed again the next day. It is impossible to enumerate behavioral cues of this type for each illness, but with a general understanding of the coping tasks and skills involved, health professionals should be able to carry out their care-giving, minimizing the negative impact of the illness experience and supporting healthy coping.

References

1. Backus, F. I., & Dudley, D. L. Observations of psychosocial factors and their relationship to organic disease. *International Journal of Psychiatry in Medicine*, 1974, **5**, 499–515.
2. Caplan, G. *Principles of preventive psychiatry*. New York: Basic Books, 1964.
3. Erikson, E. H. *Childhood and society* (2nd ed.). New York: W. W. Norton, 1963.
4. Gruen, W. Effects of brief psychotherapy during the hospitalization period on the recovery process in heart attacks. *Journal of Consulting and Clinical Psychology*, 1975, **43**, 223–232.
5. Hamburg, D., & Adams, J. E. A perspective on coping behavior. *Archives of General Psychiatry*, 1967, **17**, 277–284.
6. Harrell, H. C. To lose a breast. *American Journal of Nursing*. 1972, **72**, 676–677.

7. Insel, P. M., & Moos, R. H. (Eds.). *Health and the social environment.* Lexington, Massachusetts: D. C. Heath, 1974.

8. Lazarus, R. S. Psychological stress and coping in adaptation and illness. *International Journal of Psychiatry in Medicine,* 1974, **5,** 321–333.

9. Lipowski, Z. J. Physical illness, the individual and the coping processes. *Psychiatry in Medicine,* 1970, **1,** 91–102.

10. Lund, D. *Eric.* Philadelphia: J. B. Lippincott, 1974.

11. Moos, R. H. *The human context: Environmental determinants of behavior.* New York: Wiley-Interscience, 1976, Chap. 4. (a)

12. Moos, R. H. Evaluating and changing community settings. *American Journal of Community Psychology,* in press, 1976. (b)

13. Moos, R. H., & Tsu, V. D. Human competence and coping. In R. H. Moos (Ed.), *Human adaptation: Coping with life crises.* Lexington, Massachusetts: D. C. Heath, 1976.

14. Valens, E. G. *The other side of the mountain.* New York: Warner Paperback Library, 1975.

15. White, R., & Liddon, S. Ten survivors of cardiac arrest. *Psychiatry in Medicine,* 1972, **3,** 219–225.

16. Wittkower, E. D. Historical perspective of contemporary psychosomatic medicine. *International Journal of Psychiatry in Medicine,* 1974, **5,** 309–319.

II

The Crisis of Illness:
Stillbirth and Birth Defects

The birth of a child is usually a momentous and happy occasion. Within a short time after delivery, the hopes and expectations built up by the parents during months of preparation are finally confronted by reality. For the parents who lose their child through miscarriage, stillbirth, or premature birth, or for those whose child is born with a serious defect, the experience can suddenly become an unexpected nightmare. The hospital setting in which these events usually occur encourages attention to the physical problems, but a full return to health requires emotional readjustment as well as medical treatment.

There are four major areas with which these unfortunate parents may have serious problems. The most immediate issue is the loss of the beautiful baby of their fantasies. The parents often experience a sense of failure and guilt due to their lack of success in producing a healthy infant. They may also feel anger at whomever or whatever they perceive as having caused their loss. In addition to the loss of the idealized child the couple may face the death of the real child. As long as the survival of the child is uncertain, parents must live with a high level of anxiety. Third, if the baby dies within a few days of birth, the normal grieving process is complicated by the feeling of the wasted physical and emotional preparations made during pregnancy—the futility of the preceding nine months.[1,6] Finally, if the baby lives, the couple must deal with the special procedures and hospital care often required by an ill or handicapped child. Parents commonly feel inadequate in meeting the child's critical needs and resent the many demands made on them.

At this time of emotional crisis parents may use a variety of coping skills. The most immediate protective reaction is a denial of the seriousness of the situation and a temporary rejection of or withdrawal from the baby (see Mori,[4] Rozansky & Linde[5]). Other skills include seeking information about the cause of the disease and about the care and prognosis of the child, redefining parental expectations and goals taking into account the child's physical or mental handicaps, and building a sense of parental competence on each small success (despite major difficulties and setbacks).

One of the most important elements in achieving a healthy readjustment is the supportive interaction of relatives and friends.[2] The person who can reach out for, or at least accept, the concern and reassurances offered by others is likely to handle the situation better.[3,7] Successful adaptation to the difficulties at hand is significant, not only for the future care and development of the child, but for the preparation and skills gained by the parents which may aid them in dealing with later stressful events.

In the first article Pat Jackson describes a young couple who lost two children because of birth defects. Their first child, born with a serious cardiac defect, lived five months. For these inexperienced, first-time parents one of the most troubling aspects of the baby's condition was the special care she required. Anxiety and feelings of inadequacy coupled with frequent separations for medical attention made it difficult to develop a comfortable and satisfying relationship with the baby. Ann was able to get some relief for her feelings of guilt and inadequacy by placing blame on the medical staff, criticizing them freely. As she learned how to care for the baby more effectively, she derived some satisfaction from her successes (for example in feeding the baby) and from the belief that her daughter needed her personal attention. The father found some comfort in learning all he could about his daughter's medical condition.

When the baby finally died Mark and Ann went through the usual grieving phases— first shock and disbelief, then painful awareness of the loss and finally acceptance of the new reality. In time they were able to deal with their anger and ambivalence (sorrow *and* relief) about their daughter's death. When their second child was born with a different defect and died two days later, they had to go through this stressful mourning process again. With reassurance and support from family, friends, and concerned health professionals, and the strengths gained in their previous experience, it was hoped this young couple could again cope with this crisis and achieve a reasonable adjustment.

In the second article George Burnell discusses the reaction of a woman to the premature birth and immediate death of her septuplets. Unlike those parents of babies who survive with congenital defects, who require special care, and whose life span is uncertain, this woman's loss was immediate and complete. After three years of unsuccessful attempts to become pregnant and then the abrupt loss of all her babies, the patient's feelings of inadequacy and failure as a mother and a woman were nearly overwhelming. She used her time alone to weep and then to try to put the loss into perspective. The availability of professional counseling and the supportive concern shown by her husband helped her work through her grief. Within a few weeks she resumed her previous work as a teacher, an activity in which she could rebuild her sense of competence and well-being. Six months later the couple adopted a baby girl and then decided to attempt another pregnancy. With frequent reassurances from her obstetrician and support from her husband, the patient was able to manage her considerable apprehensions and, a year and a half after the septuplets' death, delivered a healthy baby boy.

Health professionals often play a crucial role in the physical care of a child with a congenital defect, but the importance of their intervention in the emotional crisis which results from such a birth is not always well understood. In the third article Deborah Golden and Jessica Davis discuss the impact of professional intervention on parents of children with Down's Syndrome. This condition carries a particular stigma as it affects both physical appearance and intellectual capacity. Its known genetic basis contributes to the parents' sense of responsibility in producing an imperfect child. Doctors can minimize this stigma and guilt by stressing the similarity to normal infants, especially the need all babies have for parental nurturing. Care-givers' actions (for example, holding the baby) and explanations of the cause of the defect and the probable course of development (i.e., a delay rather than a standstill in achieving usual milestones) may also reassure parents.

When long-term arrangements are considered, it is vital that decisions be based on the needs of the specific child and parents involved. Doctors and social workers should discuss the value of home care and institutional placement fully, as well as intermediate alternatives like foster care or small group homes. Golden and Davis suggest that home care is feasible in most cases (when constant medical attention is not needed), but recognize that in some families it would create unacceptable stress (as, for example, when career-oriented parents feel unable to devote the extra attention and effort a severely handicapped child requires). Bolstered by professional intervention in the form of detailed information and a clear offer of continuing support and advice most parents can redefine their expectations of the child, make plans based on a realistic appraisal of the situation, and resolve their ambivalent feelings of resentment, guilt, and inadequacy.

References

1. Cain, A. C., Erickson, M. E., Fast, I., & Vaughan, R. A. Children's disturbed reactions to their mother's miscarriage. *Psychosomatic Medicine,* 1964, **26,** 58–66.
2. Caplan, G. Patterns of parental response to the crisis of premature birth. *Psychiatry,* 1960, **23,** 365–374.
3. Johnson, J. M. Stillbirth: A personal experience. *American Journal of Nursing,* 1972, **72,** 1595–1596.
4. Mori, W. My child has Down's syndrome. *American Journal of Nursing,* 1973, **73,** 1386–1387.
5. Rozansky, G. I., & Linde, L. M. Psychiatric study of parents of children with cyanotic congenital heart disease. *Pediatrics,* 1971, **48,** 450–451.
6. Stanko, B. Crisis intervention after the birth of a defective child. *Canadian Nurse,* 1973, **69**(7), 27–28.
7. Stone, N. D., & Parnicky, J. J. Factors in child placement: Parental response to congenital defect. *Social Work,* 1966, **11,** 35–43.

Chronic Grief

PAT LUDDER JACKSON

I first met Ann and Mark about two weeks after their daughter Heidi was born. They had brought her to the medical center (where I worked as a graduate student) from the hospital where she had been born. At birth she was slightly cyanotic and at four days of age was found to have cardiac abnormality.

Ann and Mark were 18 and 21 years old respectively. Both were high school graduates and Mark was currently enlisted in the U.S. Navy. They had been married approximately 11 months before Heidi was born. Ann had had a vaginal infection in the first trimester of pregnancy and edema and excessive weight gain during the last trimester. During labor she became preeclamptic and was treated with magnesium sulfate.

Parenthood, especially for the first time, is a crisis situation for most couples, even when their child is born healthy.[1] When a defective child is born, this crisis is magnified. The fears an expectant mother has of giving birth to a deformed child have come true. Solnit and Stark hypothesize that, when this damaged child arrives in place of the wished-for, fantasized child, the mother reacts as if the fantasized child had suddenly died and grieves and mourns its loss.[2] They define grief as follows:

> . . . the characteristic response to the loss of a valued object, be it a loved person, a cherished possession, a job, status, home, country, an ideal, a part of the body,

PAT LUDDER JACKSON, B.S., M.S. ● Hospital for Sick Children, London, England.

Reprinted from *American Journal of Nursing,* 1974, **74,** 1289–1291. Copyright by the American Journal of Nursing Co. Reproduced by permission.

etc. Uncomplicated grief runs a consistent course, modified mainly by the abruptness of the loss, the nature of the preparation for the event, and the significance for the survivor of the lost object.[3]

The fantasized, desired child was much valued by Ann and Mark, and the loss of this child, which occurred when the defective child was born, was severe because of its abruptness.

Solnit and Stark believe that to resolve the loss of the fantasized child the parents go through the mourning stages of shock and disbelief, developing awareness, and finally the last stage of grief in which "intense reexperiencing of the memories and expectations gradually reduces the hypercathexis of the wish for the idealized child."[4] In comparing the mourning of parents for a dead child with parental reactions to the birth of a defective child, the main difference is that, since the defective child requires continual care, parents cannot complete the final phase of mourning.

Parents do indeed grieve when a defective child is born or from the time the defect is first diagnosed. Olshansky says:

> The permanent, day-by-day dependence of the defective child, the interminable frustrations resulting from the child's relative changelessness, the unaesthetic quality of mental defectiveness, the deep symbolism buried in the process of giving birth to a defective child, all these join together to produce the parent's chronic sorrow.[5]

Mark and Ann were excited about having had the baby but also anxious, fearful, and dubious about their ability to care for her, in light of her serious cardiac defect. The baby's extended hospitalization hindered their relating to her. During this separation, the parents' anxiety and feelings of inadequacy and failure tended to grow. "What if we do something that hurts her," Mark asked, "or are too rough with her so that she gets too tired?" Ann didn't say anything, but was obviously anxious about her ability to mother her child. She was hesitant about holding Heidi and continually sought reassurance from the nurses that she was doing things correctly, such as folding the diapers or positioning the baby.

Often the parents' anxiety is heightened when their baby is finally ready for discharge, particularly when, as with Ann and Mark, they are not familiar with the infant's routine. Shortly after Heidi was taken home, Ann expressed concern because the baby at one month old "did not smile much and made funny faces, sometimes letting her eyes roll back into her head." Ann believed this was probably normal, but it scared her.

About three days after Heidi came home, she started to vomit and regurgitate some formula after feeding. The first time this happened was after Ann had first prepared the formula herself. Previously, Heidi had been taking formula sent home from the hospital. Ann expressed feelings of guilt, failure, and rejection. Even after repeated assurances that the vomiting was probably coincidental or Heidi's normal initial reaction to a slightly different formula, Ann continued to feel like a failure.

For the first two months, Heidi had few symptoms of her cardiac condition, but then she developed signs of congestive heart failure that grew steadily worse. Whereas feeding usually had been a pleasing, rewarding experience for both mother and child, it now became a time of great stress due to the baby's increasing cyanosis, constant wet cough, and frequent vomiting. Because of her cardiac condition, she was extremely susceptible to respiratory tract infections, which intensified her symptoms. As a result, and because further diagnostic studies had to be done, she was hospitalized repeatedly. Even though the progression of symptoms was inevitable, her parents took each setback as a sign of personal failure and of their inadequacy in caring for Heidi.

Because parents experience chronic sorrow, however, they are not necessarily immobilized or prohibited from carrying on their daily activities and receiving some satisfaction and joy from their child. Unlike acute grief, which is intense and limited in time, chronic grief is prolonged and recurrent. But it follows the same stages as acute grief, except that it is unresolved.[5]

Although Ann and Mark appeared to have accepted their child's heart condition from the beginning, they either did not realize its gravity or were denying its seriousness and the potentially fatal aspects of her anomalies. When I asked Mark after my first home visit how his daughter was doing, he happily replied, "Fine. I think she's going to be all right." They spoke of putting money away each month so that when Heidi grew up she would have enough money saved for a car or for school. But they also often spoke of the child's probable need for open heart surgery at a later date. Once Ann even said that she was glad the baby was a girl because she would be more content to do quiet things like cooking and sewing when she grew up, whereas a boy would want to play football or baseball and he wouldn't be able to because of his heart.

As Heidi's condition deteriorated, it was more difficult for her parents to deny the probable outcome. Where initially they had hoped corrective surgery would completely repair her defect, they now hoped that pulmonary banding would relieve the worsening symptoms so that Heidi could live until open heart surgery could be performed. But after the doctors told them that the tests indicated that banding would not help Heidi, and that her anomalies were more extensive and complicated than originally thought, Ann and Mark realized the condition would probably be fatal.

In the second stage of grief, developing awareness, the common feelings are of guilt, anger, and failure. Ann wanted to know if she had done something during her pregnancy to cause the defect. She wondered if perhaps the medication she had taken for the vaginal infection in the first trimester or the extra weight she gained and the preeclampsia in the third trimester had affected her baby? She needed to discuss her pregnancy over and over again and to be continually reassured that she had done nothing that could have caused her daughter's defect. Later, Mark expressed feelings of guilt and inadequacy when it became necessary for Heidi to be rehospitalized. They both needed praise and repeated assurance that they were caring for their child more than adequately, and that the child's condition deteriorated because of the natural increase in strain on her heart, and not because of something they did or did not do.

Ann was able to displace many feelings of guilt, inadequacy, and failure onto the medical personnel in charge of Heidi. Whenever she believed her child's care was faulty or inadequate, she leaped at the opportunity to berate the physicians and nurses and express her dislike of them. She believed that each time Heidi was hospitalized she became sicker than when she had been at home under her care.

She had learned how to care for Heidi and knew how to alleviate much of her distress. She could spend an hour feeding her and be successful, but the nurses were unable to spend this much time. This gave Ann a feeling of being important and needed by her child which helped diminish her sense of failure.

Mark sought information about the child's condition and treatment as a means of alleviating his feelings of guilt and failure. He did not do this to excess, which can be harmful, according to S. B. Friedman.[6] By learning more about his child's condition and the treatment given and discussed, he seemed better able to accept the situation realistically and aid in Heidi's care.

In the third stage of grief—restitution—support and consolation are given the grieving person by the family and community. The person's grief is shared and thereby lessened. Instead of the funeral ritual, which usually helps a bereft person acknowledge his loss and accept it, parents experiencing chronic grief have individual rituals involved in the care of their child to help them to not deny the situation and to acknowledge the presence of the defect. For instance, Ann and Mark made biweekly visits to the pediatric cardiologist to have Heidi's condition evaluated, fed her a special low salt formula, and gave her a daily dose of digoxin.

Because of the continued presence of the grief-producing object, parents of a defective child cannot move on to the final stage of grief—resolution—until after the death of the child. When Heidi died, her parents went through the first three stages of grief again. Even though the death had been anticipated, it came as a shock. However, the first phase of shock and disbelief did not last long because of the anticipatory grief that had preceded. As Mark said, "Her death came as a surprise, but not as much as if she had been hit by a car or choked to death."

These parents moved quickly into the stage of developing awareness. They cried openly and expressed their sorrow. They found it difficult to discuss Heidi's death or even say the words "she died." Instead, they used words like "she didn't make it" or "she is no longer with us" to tell people of Heidi's death.

Mark vented his emotions by being angry to others. For instance, he was extremely angry at his superior officer, who almost denied him a pass to come to the hospital because of his daughter's rapidly deteriorating condition. He also expressed anger at his parents, who disagreed about the funeral arrangements.

Both parents expressed guilt and ambivalence about Heidi's death. Mark felt guilty about possibly having contributed to the child's final cold by not bundling her up sufficiently after a sweat test. Though they were both sorry Heidi had died, they were also relieved that her suffering was over. Ann said, "It's really better this way. She would have been sick all her life and we didn't want that. Now she won't suffer any more. She's probably much happier in heaven. She won't have to go through all the suffering of life."

The parents also felt relieved of their burden. They had been through a stressful five months. Following is an excerpt from their conversation the day Heidi died:

Ann: Things should go better now. Heidi was the main problem. After her, every little thing became a big problem.

Mark: Yes, we've been fighting over little things. Now, maybe we can start anew.

Ann: Before, we didn't know what would happen to Heidi or how we could get money to pay for her care. All sorts of questions.

Mark: It sounds sort of bad, but now we can start enjoying ourselves again and doing things we haven't been able to do for a long time.

By the day after Heidi's death, Ann and Mark seemed to have overcome their bewilderment and confusion, which are characteristic of the initial grief reaction.

Because of Ann's and Mark's chronic grief it was easier for them to resolve the loss of their child and resume their daily activities in a happy productive manner. For about two weeks they stayed pretty much by themselves, reliving their experiences with her, resting after the stress of the funeral, and making plans for the future. Soon they were able to speak of Heidi realistically, neither idealizing nor rejecting her. They frequently looked through their picture album and had favorite pictures of Heidi enlarged.

Both Ann and Mark expressed fear of having another defective child. Although physicians and nurses may have tried to reassure them that Heidi's defect was an accident of nature and not likely to happen again, Ann and Mark still knew only the one experience and feared it would be repeated. They were somewhat reassured by the physician's interpretation of the autopsy report, which was that there was only a slight chance that Heidi's condition would be repeated, although it had resulted from the parents' genes. The physician stressed that the child's condition was not caused by anything the parents could have prevented. This information seemed to relieve some of their guilt feelings.

Approximately six months after Heidi's death, Ann and Mark moved, but we continued to correspond. They were eager to have another child and were thrilled when Ann became pregnant again about one year later. I encouraged her to obtain complete and thorough medical care because I was concerned about her developing toxemia again. I did not tell her that everything was going to be all right this time and that she would have her "perfect" baby because I knew my reassurances would never erase the memory of Heidi and the fear that her next child would be defective.

Mark called me shortly after their child was born. They had had a boy who died two days after birth. All Mark could tell me was that the child's heart was normal but his head was "large and soft."

Needless to say, Ann and Mark were terribly upset and had to go through the grief process again. I felt quite helpless trying to give them support and reassurance from so far away. I could only hope that there was another health professional with them who understood what they must be going through and would take the time to give them the help they most surely needed.

Parents in similar situations need a great deal of help, especially during the initial phases of shock and disbelief and developing awareness. Because of their feelings of guilt and failure, they need continual reassurance that they were not responsible for what happened They need to express their feelings of guilt over and over again and receive assurance that these feelings are acceptable and normal.

Feelings of failure and inadequacy can be relieved greatly by including parents in the care of their child and letting them know they are an important part of the health team. When they are able to help and feel a sense of need, their thinking may turn from despair, blame, or guilt to better problem solving.

The professional health worker should help the parents gain some satisfaction from their child. The positive aspect of his development should be stressed and the parents praised for even the smallest accomplishment. This should help parents focus on their accomplishments instead of their perceived failures.

Rapoport summarizes much of the professional health workers' interventions well. She classifies the necessary interventions as follows:

1. Keeping an explicit focus on the crisis by helping with cognitive mastery; doubt, guilt, and self-blame; grief and mourning; and anticipatory worry.
2. Offering basic information and education regarding the child's development and care.
3. Creating a bridge between the family and other personnel and community resources.[7]

Successful intervention may mean the difference between a mentally healthy solution to the family's grief, and a mentally unhealthy solution that can plague family members for the rest of their lives.

References

1. Le Masters, E. E. Parenthood as crisis. *Marriage and Family Living* **19**:352–355, Nov. 1957.
2. Solnit, A., & Stark, M. Mourning and the birth of a defective child. *Psychoanalytic Study of the Child* **16**:523–537, 1963.
3. Engel, G. L. Is grief a disease? A challenge for medical research. *Psychosomatic Medicine* **23**:18–22, Jan.–Feb. 1961.
4. Solnit, A., & Stark, M. Mourning and the birth of a defective child. *Psychoanalytic Study of the Child,* **16,** 526, 1963.
5. Olshansky, S. Chronic sorrow: A response to having a mentally defective child. *Social Casework* **43**:191, 1962.
6. Friedman, S. B., and others. Behavioral observations on parents anticipating the death of a child. *Pediatrics* **32**:614, Oct. 1963.
7. Rapoport, L. Working with families in crisis: An exploration in preventive intervention. *Social Work* **7**(3):48–56, 1962.

3

Maternal Reaction to the Loss of Multiple Births

GEORGE M. BURNELL

Throughout history the experience of multiple births has been associated with emotional and social stress for most mothers.[1] This is particularly true because of the element of surprise, the concern over prematurity, and the anxiety over the potential loss of babies shortly after delivery.[2] In this communication I report the emotional adjustment by parents who experienced a rare event: the birth and loss of a set of septuplets.

There have been only five confirmed sets of septuplets since 1900, and according to Hellin's rule, only one such delivery occurs at a mathematical frequency of $1:80^3$ or one such delivery in every 26,214,400,000 births.[1] But, because of the increasing use of gonadotropins, superovulation occurs in a substantial percentage of cases and therefore the problem of multiple births is becoming more common.[4,5]

A summary of the literature on the clinical use of menotropins (Pergonal) revealed that out of a total of 1,286 patients multiple births occurred in 20% of the pregnancies, and of these, three-fourths were twins and one-fourth (or 5% of all pregnancies on the drug) involved three or more concepti.[6]

GEORGE M. BURNELL, M.D., • Department of Psychiatry, Kaiser Permanente Medical Center, Santa Clara, California.

Reprinted from *Archives of General Psychiatry,* 1974, **30** (Feb.), 183–184. Copyright 1974, American Medical Association.

The psychological sequelae of having multiple births should be known to physicians since it could bring about an emotional crisis and serious psychiatric complications in the mother or even both parents.

Report of a Case

Predelivery Period

A 26-year-old primigravida, high school teacher, was admitted, in labor, to the obstetrical service of the Kaiser Foundation Hospital in Santa Clara, March 1972. She was in her 26th week of pregnancy and had been on complete bedrest for almost her entire pregnancy. She had received some human menopausal gonadotropin (Pergonal) in the course of an infertility diagnostic work-up after trying to become pregnant for three years. The husband, a 27-year-old engineer, was most cooperative and desirous of having a family. Both the patient and her husband had been told about the possibility of having twins or even triplets since this is known to occur with the administration of gonadotropins. However, this eventuality was acceptable to both of them.

The patient was admitted three days before her birthday. Being in her sixth month, she became concerned and anxious about the prematurity and possible complications. She was tense and apprehensive, but remained in good contact with reality and maintained good communication with her husband, her obstetrician, friends, and the hospital staff. During the initial period of hospitalization many friends called, showed concern, and gave support.

When she went into labor she was told that she would have a set of triplets. All necessary measures were taken for multiple premature births and several pediatricians and other specialists were standing by. The delivery took place March 17, 1972. The first and second infants were vertex presentations, the third was delivered by breech extraction, the fourth was a vertex presentation and anencephalic, the fifth was a breech extraction, the sixth was anencephalic, and the seventh a breech. There was no cervical or vaginal laceration and the uterus clamped down immediately.

The patient had been slightly drowsy, and when she became alert her husband told her the news of having given birth to a set of septuplets. He also added that the chances of their survival were quite precarious. There had been four boys and three girls, two of which were stillbirths.

Because of her desire for privacy and wish to be alone, every attempt was made by her obstetrician and the medical and nursing staff to shield her from the press and television news media. The obstetrician agreed to appear on television and at press conferences, but asked newsmen to respect the mother's and father's privacy.

Aside from the two stillbirths, the remaining five infants died within 12 hours despite special facilities and treatment availability for complications associated with prematurity. The infants' average weight was 681 gm.

A psychiatric consultation was offered to the patient at this point to see if she could be helped to cope with the multiple stresses of this experience. She was most cooperative and receptive to the interview. She was an attractive, light-haired, articulate, intelligent, and spontaneous young woman who displayed appropriate affect, well-organized thought process and content, and good contact with reality. Upon talking about the experience of losing the babies, which she referred to as "the experience," she became tearful and added, "I've been trying to put together a lot of things in a short time."

She looked upon this event as another experience to learn from, and as a basis for further growth for her and her husband. She indicated that she was concerned about his reaction to this loss but later discovered that he had been warm and supportive and seemed to share the same feelings she had about "the experience." She stated that she was not religious and seemed content to accept life or death as an integral process of nature. At another level she felt she had let her husband and parents "down" by this experience and expressed feelings of inadequacy as a mother. She was not much of a housekeeper and cook, but had succeeded as a straight *A* student and as a good teacher. She admitted doubts about functioning in the mother role.

Her past history revealed that she was the oldest of three siblings, and both siblings were in good health. She grew up in a close-knit family and thought she had a happy childhood and a good relationship with her parents. Her father was a successful engineer and so was her husband. She herself had special interest, ability, and talent in science and mathematics. She had met her husband in college. They were happily married for five years and had both worked full time for four years. She saw herself as a happy, active, and healthy person and had a good relationship with her husband.

Postdelivery Period and One-Year Follow-Up

For two to three days following the delivery the patient asked to have "as much privacy as possible." She remained in a single room and desired only a few visitors. Later, she volunteered that she needed the time "to cry without interruption." In subsequent visits, she talked readily about the loss, which she perceived as a single loss rather than a multiple one. She stated that she wanted a "rest" for a few months, but that she would try again to become pregnant this year. She felt a determination about being a mother and wished to prove it to herself and to her husband. After a few weeks off, the patient became active again with her work as a teacher, and with her favorite sport—tennis. In September the couple adopted a 3-month-old girl and she consented to have another course of menotropins.

Eight months following the loss of the septuplets the patient became pregnant. She reported that both she and her husband were quite happy. One year following the loss of the septuplets she added that she had not dwelled on the "experience," had not had any "bad feelings," and had not experienced any further grief. However, she expressed fears about the current pregnancy that occurred again following the administration of human menopausal gonadotropin. Her fears related to the anticipation of potential prematurity, birth defects, or of another loss. She was prepared to consider an abortion if there were any indications of potential complications.

The patient continued to express anxiety and apprehension throughout the pregnancy. She feared the possibility of multiple concepti, and the occurrence of abnormalities during the pregnancy, delivery, or birth. Between the fourth and fifth month she was reassured of having one baby. At the seventh month, x-ray film revealed a well-formed head. Subsequently the delivery took place under local anesthesia on Aug. 29, 1973, and a baby boy, weighing 4,338 gm, was born. The infant's Apgar score was 9.

The patient and her husband had an intense emotional release with joy, tears, and total relief.

There were no subsequent complications at the six-weeks follow-up. The patient was advised not to go on birth control pills because of possible complications.

It should be emphasized that the close, frank, and open communication between the doctor, the patient, and her husband contributed greatly to allaying fantasies and fears generated during this traumatic experience. The psychiatric consultant reinforced the need for continuous feedback and encouraged the patient and her husband to participate in all decisions suggested by the obstetrician.

Comment

Admittedly the experience of unusual multiple births is a stressful event because of the following considerations: (1) There is an element of unknown and unexpected occurrence. (2) The event is rare, and attracts immediate attention and publicity. (3) The prematurity raises anxiety about possible complications and loss of life. There may be grief about a partial or total loss. (4) The event may bring on personal feelings of inadequacy, ambivalence, or guilt in certain predisposed individuals. (5) The reactions of the spouse, grandparents, and friends can be supportive or further stress-producing.

In the case reported here the mother made a satisfactory physical and psychological recovery and adjustment. Contributing to her favorable postpartum course were the following factors: (1) The patient was given the privacy needed for her to go through the expected grief and the need to have some time alone. (2) She was offered the opportunity to talk about her grief, her feelings of inadequacy, and her future goals with a psychiatrist.[3] (3) She was shielded from the pressures for publicity in the press and television. (4) Her spouse remained supportive, protective, and hopeful of the future. (5) She received much support from her obstetrician, in whom she had complete trust. (6) The nursing staff was protective and very responsive to all of her needs.

In addition to these important factors one can assume that this patient's happy childhood, successful personal growth, good self-image, and happy marital relationship all contributed to the appropriate grief reaction. Actually, this reaction was relatively short (less than two weeks). In her mind the patient conceptualized the loss as a single experience rather than a multiple loss. One could speculate that this mechanism was a form of denial and rationalization in the service of the ego. Her subsequent return to a full range of activities, her decision to adopt a child, and her ability to get pregnant again within months further helped erase the traumatic event and reverse the doubts about her motherhood she had acquired from the years of sterility and the experience of loss.

Because of the increasing likelihood of future multiple pregnancies due to ovarian hyperstimulation among women taking gonadotropins, physicians should become more aware of the psychological and social factors operating in these cases. Psychiatric consultation should provide additional insights into the specific factors and needs of special importance to the mother faced with such an unusual and stressful experience.[3]

The psychiatric intervention has several functions: (1) It is to prevent unresolved guilt or grief; (2) it is to facilitate the grief reaction by giving the patient an opportunity to review the meaning of the loss in her own life-experience; (3) it is to make appropriate recommendations for psychosocial supports in her environment and to provide support and guidance to the father and other relatives if necessary.

Because of the complexity and multiplicity of physical, psychological, and social factors, it is concluded that a team approach, combining obstetrical, pediatric, and psychiatric specialties, is the best approach for patients experiencing the crisis of multiple births and the occurrence of loss.

(In view of the inevitable publicity in this case, the medical and administrative staff of the hospital should be congratulated for keeping the patient's privacy and handling the situation with much care and consideration for the family.)

Nonproprietary Name and Trademarks of Drug

Menotropins—*Pergonal, Humegon, Pregova.*

References

1. Mayer, C. F. Sextuplets and higher multiparous births: A critical review of history and legend from Aristoteles to the 20th century. *Acta Genetica Medicae et Gemellologiae (Roma)* **1**:242–276, 1952.
2. Kaplan, D. M., & Mason, E. A. Maternal reactions to premature birth viewed as an acute emotional disorder. In H. J. Parad (Ed.), *Crisis intervention.* New York: Family Service Association of America, 1965. Pp. 118–128.
3. Caplan, G. *Concepts of mental health and consultation.* Washington, D.C.: Department of Health, Education and Welfare, Children's Bureau, 1959.
4. Gemzell, C., & Roos, P. Pregnancies following treatment with human gonadotropins, with special reference to multiple births. *American Journal of Obstetrics and Gynecology* **94**:490–496, 1966.

5. Turksoy, N. R. et al. Birth of sextuplets following human gonadotropin administration in Chiari-Frommel syndrome. *Obstetrics and Gynecology* **30:**692–698, 1967.

6. Thompson, C., & Hansen, L. Pergonal (menotropins): A summary of clinical experience in the induction of ovulation and pregnancy. *Fertility and Sterility* **21:**844–853, 1970.

4

Counseling Parents after the Birth of an Infant with Down's Syndrome

DEBORAH A. GOLDEN and JESSICA G. DAVIS

Approximately one in every 600 babies born in this country is diagnosed as having Down's Syndrome. The condition has lifelong implications for physical appearance, intellectual achievement, and general functioning. It is usually suspected at the time of delivery or shortly thereafter. The clinical diagnosis must be confirmed by chromosome studies for the child with this syndrome has extra genetic material, usually in the form of an entire extra chromosome.

The physical characteristics that a doctor generally finds in a baby thought to have Down's Syndrome may include upward-slanting eyes, simple ears, somewhat protuberant tongue, short stubby fingers, and, sometimes, an unusual crease in the palm of his hand. Although babies with mongolism seem to have more heart defects, as well as more colds and respiratory infections than normal infants, the use of antibiotics and

DEBORAH A. GOLDEN, M.S.W. • Assistant Director, Social Work Consultant, Child Development Center, Genetics Program, North Shore University Hospital, Manhasset, New York. JESSICA G. DAVIS, M.D. • Director, Child Development Center, North Shore University Hospital, Cornell University College of Medicine, Manhasset, New York.

Reprinted from *Children Today*, 1974, 3 (March–April).

the development of modern heart surgery have increased the life expectancy of these children.[1]

The intellectual functioning of the children varies but a majority will be moderately retarded and trainable. A small proportion of individuals with this condition function in the range of mild retardation, while others are severely retarded.

The birth of an infant with Down's Syndrome—mongolism—represents a major crisis for physicians and parents alike. We believe that it is crucial at this time that doctors and other involved professionals view each child as a human being and each family as unique. We also believe that frightened, hysterical, and grieving parents should not be offered stereotyped solutions or be pressed for lifetime decisions.

At a time when they have not yet begun to come to terms with the diagnosis, or to understand what the child-rearing alternatives are or might mean to them in the future, parents should not be urged, as they so often are, to place their child in an institution. Rather, we believe that they should be given initial and ongoing medical support and be helped to reach community resources that can aid them. With this kind of help, many families can care for young children with Down's Syndrome at home and those who subsequently decide to place their children in residential care will have done so in a more thoughtful and rational frame of mind.

This article is based upon our clinical experience at the Genetic Counseling Program of the Rose F. Kennedy Center for Research in Mental Retardation and Human Development, Albert Einstein College of Medicine, and on a series of 100 structured interviews held with families of children with Down's Syndrome. The interviews were conducted with parents and sometimes other relatives who had come to the Center for genetic counseling and to discuss other concerns about the children. They took place after we knew the families and had asked them to "think back about your experiences" and then discuss them with us and other doctors, nurses, social workers, and counselors at the Center. Since our purpose was to study and evaluate the informing process, we talked about how and when they were told of their children's defect. We also learned what information and advice had been given to them regarding the care of their children and the effect this advice had had on their lives then—and now.

Professional Response to the Birth

The discovery of an affected infant is disturbing to the obstetrician, the pediatrician, and the nurse. Any one of them may be immediately confronted with decisions as to when and what to tell the parents about their new baby.

Most doctors tend to give the diagnostic information as soon as possible after the time of delivery. This approach would seem to be a good one, rooted as it is in the recognition that parents have a right to know about their infant. Moreover, delays in relaying the information can lead to misunderstandings and, since information is disseminated and distorted quickly in hospitals, the likelihood that the parents will learn about their child from some unexpected and inappropriate source increases as each day passes. If a couple learns about their infant's condition from another person, the family's relationship with their doctor and with any others they might consult may be jeopardized.

Informing the family early of the diagnosis of Down's Syndrome, however, does have one major pitfall that causes several difficulties: the family does not yet know their infant as an individual. In addition, they may know nothing about children with this medical problem or have only scanty and often incorrect information about it. Therefore, their view of the child—of what he is like now and how he will be in the future—will be very much determined by the doctor's statements regarding cause, manifestations of the condition, and his prognosis. Since he may be viewed as an omnipotent figure whose recommendations the family frequently feels compelled to follow, the doctor's opinions and advice are often crucial.

In their initial discussions of Down's Syndrome with parents, physicians often give specific advice regarding planning for the baby's immediate and eventual care, in addition to their explanation of the infant's condition. The experiences of the patients known to our facility confirm findings that the recommendations of many physicians constitute an "unqualified dictum for institutionalization."[2] Such a suggestion on the doctor's part, regardless of the family's eventual decision about placement, can have profound, long-lasting implications for the life of both the child and his family.[3,4]

Why do physicians in such large numbers continue to press automatically for immediate institutionalization of newborns with Down's

Syndrome? First, perhaps because some doctors perceive the baby's condition to be a hopeless one. They may know little about this disorder or how children with it develop. The physicians initially consulted by parents now active in our clinic often indicated that the child essentially would be a vegetable and reach few, if any, milestones. They implied it would not be worth the family's effort to bring up the baby. Children with Down's Syndrome were frequently portrayed as presenting overwhelming management problems and parents were told their presence would be destructive to other members of the family unit. Unaware of the guilt, denial, and struggle present even in parents who appear to have completely rejected the child, physicians may also tend to focus on the child's possible eventual need for special care and on arranging for this before everyone becomes involved with and attached to him or her.[2]

Placement may also be advised because the physician is transmitting his own negative feelings. Recommendation of institutionalization may become a way of obliterating a situation he considers unbearable.[4]

Parents' Reactions

Whatever their race, religion, or socioeconomic background, families are devastated to learn their new baby has Down's Syndrome. Frightened by the implications of this disorder with respect to the child's appearance, intelligence, and capacity for independent function, their joy in the new baby is compromised. When placement is mentioned at this juncture, there are several characteristic responses.

Some families seize on the idea, welcoming the apparent opportunity it offers to escape the problem. They then proceed to place their child. However, many such families often find that their problems only begin once the infant is institutionalized. Since they never knew their child, they may now wonder whether he would have done better had he been kept at home. They find their sorrow at having produced a retarded child is still present, as is the attachment to the infant which began long before birth.[4] The Allen family, with whom we spoke, clearly illustrates the difficulties which can arise from premature placement.

Polly was born when the Allens were in their mid-30s. They were told immediately that Polly was "Mongoloid," a condition which meant, they understood the doctor to have said, that she would not develop at all and should be "put away." The Allens responded to the physician's "order" by arranging for immediate institutionalization, despite the great financial burden it would impose. The baby developed poorly. However, despite the seeming confirmation of the doctor's dire predictions, the Allens kept wondering if their child would do better at home. Finally, when she was five years old, they decided to take Polly home, even though she could not stand, feed or toilet herself, and had no language development. Within six months, Polly was walking, feeding herself, and beginning to comprehend what was said to her. She was then accepted into a day school program for severely retarded children.

While the Allens know that residential placement will probably be necessary eventually, they feel Polly will now function better in such a setting. Moreover, they have benefited from having Polly at home to love and nurture. The Allens feel betrayed by the doctor who urged placement initially and they wonder how their child might have developed had she been with them from the start.

For various reasons, many families reject the recommendation for placement. Nevertheless, the fact that such a plan was proposed often has a substantial and continuing deleterious effect on their relationship with the child and the professionals who deal with him. Parents may view the child as unworthy and useless or at least believe that others perceive him this way. Such an attitude may inhibit them from giving the child needed attention, stimulation, and discipline. Other parents may be very surprised when their baby achieves certain milestones and then feel that they have been misled by those who were supposed to know better, a feeling that is often translated into a generalized hostility toward physicians and other professionals.[4] Thus their necessary future relationships with doctors and others often become uncomfortable, unproductive, or cease to exist. The Brandon family story illustrates such a sequence of events.

The Brandons are a young couple whose first child was diagnosed immediately after birth as having Down's Syndrome. Immediate institutionalization of the baby was recommended because, they were told, Robert had no future and would bring them only unhappiness. Although distraught, the Brandons instinctively felt that their son should be with them. They took him home and located a new pediatrician to oversee his routine care.

Robert achieved virtually normal milestones. By age two he was walking, toilet-trained, and saying a few words. As the Brandons realized the capacities of their youngster, they became increasingly angry with the physician who had recommended placement. Later they transferred their negative feelings about their first doctor to all physicians, believing that they could not risk discussing Robert with anyone. By chance, when Robert was four, the Brandons learned about the local Association for Retarded Children and then sought services through that agency.

Gradually these parents began to feel comfortable enough to trust professionals by consulting with them in relation to Robert and their decision to have another child, a decision they had postponed until then.

Robert is now a sociable, verbal 7-year-old who is learning to read. The Brandons are still very angry with the doctor who pressed them to institutionalize him, and they are frightened by the thought that they might have heeded his advice.

The Carrs are another family that remains disturbed by an early recommendation for placement of their child, even though the parents rejected the advice.

The Carrs were told that their third child had Down's Syndrome soon after their daughter was born. Both the attending obstetrician and the pediatrician advised that they place the child and the Carrs were on the verge of acceding to this pressure when they sought another opinion. At this point, the way in which the Carrs talked about their infant and handled her showed the consulting doctor that placement was really the last thing the family desired. Once they were encouraged to keep their baby at home, the Carrs were enormously relieved and they assumed their parental roles confidently. Their daughter is now an alert, active toddler whose developmental milestones are only slightly delayed.

The Carrs are delighted with their youngest child, as are her 10- and 12-year-old siblings. However, they still become distressed when they consider that they might have followed their first doctors' advice and placed the child in an institution.

Discussing Down's Syndrome with Parents

How can the physician, who usually has primary responsibility for communicating with the family, and other professionals enable parents to deal with the crisis that occurs when a baby is born with Down's Syndrome?

First, all involved have to recognize and understand their own feelings about the affected infant. The professional must strive for an objective approach to each separate family situation. The parents need support and assistance so that they can get to the point of planning rationally for their child. The eventual solution, such as placement, may not be appropriate at this time. Rather, the major goal then is to help the family deal with the acute grief and chronic sorrow that invariably accompany a diagnosis of Down's Syndrome. This obligation cannot be discharged in one or two discussions with the family.[3,4] If the doctor tries to deal with what has happened, the family will usually try to cope also. It helps, whenever possible, if the doctor (obstetrician, pediatrician, or general practitioner) knows and is trusted by the family.

Any information about Down's Syndrome should be discussed in the presence of both parents. The physician may first wish to discuss his impressions with the child's father before they go in together to talk with the mother.[5] If the father is not available, arrangements should be made for a relative or close friend to be present when the doctor initially conveys the diagnosis. The vulnerable new mother should not be alone during this time, as she so often is.

The physician can begin his talk with the family by voicing his concerns and suspicions about the baby. If possible, he should be holding the infant in a respectful and caring way during the discussion. His willingness to hold the infant so will help convey to the family that the baby is human and capable of being accepted. The doctor may wish to demonstrate some of the clinical findings directly in order to support his belief that the baby probably has Down's Syndrome. He should talk about confirmatory studies that need to be made. In addition, he must mention the possible presence of any other medical problems, such as congenital heart disease, and explain what can be done about them. He should indicate that such a child can be born into any family, regardless of their circumstances, and that genetic counseling is available for parents like them.[6]

In speaking about the baby, the doctor should point out that the young infant with Down's Syndrome has the same needs as most babies and that it is anticipated that he will respond to those who care for him and show development over time. The doctor should explain that the baby is not expected to remain in a vegetative state, although his or her achievement of normal psychomotor milestones will probably be delayed. The parents should also know that there is absolutely no way to predict any baby's exact course of development at the time of birth and that this fact also applies to those with Down's Syndrome.[1,3,6] Parents should also be reassured about the baby's physical appearance; in particular, that the infant will not be a "freak" or a "monster."

After the doctor completes his explanation, he should be prepared for and encourage questions. It is important that he demonstrate his willingness and capacity to accept the upsetting behavior parents may exhibit. When he finally leaves the couple to talk alone, he should promise to come again the next day to continue the discussion. This second visit is essential because many parents are unable to communicate effectively so soon after hearing the diagnosis.

No attempt should be made at this time to keep the baby from the mother unless specifically requested.

Much of the initial information should be reviewed when the doctor returns to talk with the family. The parents are certain to have more questions, including some regarding the long-term prognosis for their infant. The family must be told that the child with Down's Syndrome will almost certainly be slow or retarded. Simultaneously, the parents need to hear that there is no cure for this disorder and that their child will not outgrow his difficulties. Again, however, it must be stressed that at birth there is no way of measuring a child's ultimate capabilities. These are dependent both upon endowment, which in this condition sets known upper limits on the individual's development, and on the child's environment. Nevertheless, although there is a wide range of possible functioning, a child with this condition will need special education and supervision throughout his or her life.[6]

Upon learning about the lifetime implications of Down's Syndrome, families usually fall into one of two groups. Some parents will begin to accept their fate and commence the necessary mourning process; at the same time, they will begin to mobilize themselves to care for the baby. These parents need to know that their doctor and other appropriate professionals, such as a public health nurse or social worker, will be there to help them through the very difficult period of adjusting to having a Down's Syndrome baby and telling other family members about his condition, as well as dealing with any medical or management problems the baby presents.

The Duncan family was introduced to their baby's condition in the manner described and the way they were informed seems to have had a great deal to do with the quick progress they were able to make in adjusting to the infant's problems.

Mark was the Duncan's first child. Mr. Duncan was told first about the baby's difficulty and he then told his wife in the doctor's presence. The physician gave them a positive but realistic view concerning their son's probable development during his first few years of life and later. In discussions with the Duncans, the doctor indicated his belief that Mark could be raised at home and that all concerned would profit from his presence there. The Duncans left the hospital with good feelings about their baby, correctly anticipating his slow but steady development. Moreover, they felt a strong bond with the pediatrician who respected the child and their feelings for him.

Other groups of parents, as they begin to come to terms with the fact their child is irrevocably retarded, will ask about placement. In response to their questions, they should be told that this is one alternative and that it has specific implications for both the infant and his parents. Unless a child needs continual medical attention, the doctor may tell them, "Most mongoloid infants can be cared for at home in the interest of both the child and the family—and many such children in the past have been inappropriately placed."[2,3,7,8,9]

Since the overall needs of a child with Down's Syndrome do not differ greatly from those of other children during infancy, there is no reason why a young mongoloid child should make undue demands on its parents or other family members. The parents can be told they can always place their child later on if they can't manage but that they and their child will probably never be able to regain what is lost if the infant is in an institutional setting during his early years. Parents, as well as their children, lose a great deal when they are unable to nurture their child.

It is also vital for physicians and families to understand that public institutions in the United States may not accept infants and that private facilities which often have long waiting lists can be very expensive. Doctors often suggest institutionalization as an alternative to home care without having any knowledge of the availability, quality, or cost of such care. Doctors may also fail to mention other options that may be open, such as foster care or small group nursing home placement for children. Once again, when families subsequently discover that their doctor offered them unrealistic and unacceptable solutions in this area, their confidence in him and in physicians generally can be seriously undermined.[4]

A major issue often raised by parents and professionals alike concerns fears that unless a child is placed in an institution immediately, the family will become so attached to him or her that it will never be ready to place the child even when such a step becomes imperative. However, families can be told that they were involved with the baby long before his birth and that once they have tried to raise him, they will be able to make whatever plans are necessary for their child with considerably fewer and less destructive feelings of guilt than if they had never made any effort at all. Perhaps most significantly, parents and professionals should plan for a child on the basis of their knowledge of each child and his particular needs and not on the basis of a stereotyped image of children with Down's Syndrome. Such awareness is not possible at the time of the child's birth. For many families who realize this, such an approach will result in a decision to take their baby home, even though they realize that institutionalization may become necessary later.

The Arthur family, for example, first considered placement of their daughter Barbara immediately after she was born. After discussing the alternatives, however, they decided to take her home and soon became very attached to her.

Barbara developed exceptionally poorly, and at 18 months she was functioning at the level of a 3-month-old. She required such constant attention that an older son was neglected. Consequently, when a social worker suggested that Barbara's name be placed on a waiting list of the state institution, the Arthurs agreed. However, they stated that whatever happened in the future, they were glad that they had taken their daughter home and tried to help her.

We recognize that some families, to whom the idea of knowingly raising a retarded child is intolerable, will have to place the child immediately. However, such a plan should be the result of discussion and the decision should be made after all other possibilities have been fully explored.

If the parents do choose institutionalization, they will require support during the process of arranging for the baby's care and afterwards. The feelings and conflicts aroused by the birth of a defective child and its placement are not resolved simply when the institution doors close behind the baby. The following case eloquently pinpoints these issues.

When his second child was born with Down's Syndrome, Mr. Frank, a very immature man, perceived the condition of the baby as an assault on his masculinity. Mrs. Frank was even more upset. She had a severely physically handicapped sister who, she felt, had destroyed her childhood and she could not contemplate living again with another abnormal person. As a result, the Franks' infant went directly into placement from the hospital.

After several months Mrs. Frank became extremely anxious and phobic. Preoccupied with the fear that she would do something to hurt her normal son, she required long-term psychotherapy to help her function.

Summary and Conclusions

Down's Syndrome infants and young children can be in a home environment. Except under unusual circumstances there is no compelling reason for these youngsters to be placed elsewhere. When such a plan is suggested, it should reflect specific needs of the child or parents and not the negative feelings professionals may hold about retarded children generally or those with Down's Syndrome in particular. We believe it is possible to take such a strong position because the majority of families, no matter how unhappy, upset or angry they are initially, can be helped to deal with their situation.[3] With adequate professional attention, they come to realize that their Down's Syndrome babies are human beings whose needs are comparable to those of other babies. Families can then recognize that their child's special problems will be revealed only gradually and can be dealt with as they occur.

Parents also need to be aware of the fact that they are not alone. There are physicians, other health professionals, and parent groups, such as local associations for retarded children, who are available to help them in managing their child. Parents should be encouraged to work through private organizations and their elected government representatives for the improvement and extension of programs for the retarded.

If families are to be helped to keep their "special" children with them and institutionalization for all but the most severely retarded is truly to be eliminated, there must exist a thriving network of community services to provide programs and counseling to children and their families from, literally, the cradle to the grave.

References

1. *Facts about Mongolism for women over 35.* National Institute of Child Health and Human Development. NIH (DHEW Pub. No. (NIH) 74–536), 1974.
2. Giannini, M. J., & Goodman, L. Counseling families during the crisis reaction to Mongolism. *American Journal of Mental Deficiency,* March 1963.
3. Breg, W. R. Family counseling in Down's Syndrome. *Annals of the New York Academy of Sciences,* 1970.
4. Zwerling, I. Initial counseling of parents with mentally retarded children. *Pediatrics.* April 1954.
5. National Association for Mental Health Working Party. The birth of an abnormal child: Telling the parents. *Lancet,* November 1971.
6. *Antenatal diagnosis and Down's Syndrome.* National Institute of Child Health and Human Development. NIH (DHEW Pub. No. (NIH) 74-538), 1974.
7. Stedman, D., & Eichorn, D. A comparison of the growth and development of institutionalized and home reared Mongoloids during infancy and early childhood. *American Journal of Mental Deficiency,* November 1964.
8. Shipe, D., & Shotwell, A. Effect of out-of-home care on Mongoloid children: A continuation study. *American Journal of Mental Deficiency,* March 1965.
9. Centerwall, S., & Centerwall, W. A study of children with Mongolism reared home compared to those reared away from the home. *Pediatrics,* April 1960.

III

The Crisis of Illness: Cancer

Cancer, the lay term given to a multitude of different malignant growth processes, is a particularly frightening illness because its cause is unknown, its treatment can involve great discomfort or even disfigurement, and its cure is uncertain. In addition to the physical symptoms of the disease the patient must deal with severe emotional stress, including the threat of recurrence and ultimately death. In this section we focus on the general problems encountered by cancer patients and on specific tasks associated with particular types or stages of the disease.

In the first article John Hinton explores the reactions of people who have developed cancer, their problems in accepting the diagnosis and their altered status, and their attempts to resolve these problems. The cancer patient must deal with the discomfort of various physical symptoms, with treatment procedures such as radiotherapy or surgery which are painful or disfiguring, with the loss of personal dignity which becoming a patient often entails, and with the prospect of an early death. The increase in dependency (for example, the loss of the work role, the financial burden on the family, and the necessity of relying on other people for meeting personal physical care needs) is very disturbing to many people. The sense of total dependence on the doctor is often accompanied by a fear of displeasing him, a fear which makes many patients become passive, uncomplaining, and overly cooperative.[1] Another major source of distress is the growing sense of alienation and isolation. Friends and family often have great difficulty relating warmly and openly with the person diagnosed as having cancer. Individual

defenses on both sides can become a barrier to meaningful communication, adding further to the isolation caused by hospitalization and the
interruption of normal home life.

Hinton identifies several of the coping skills which people use to
deal with these stresses. One of the most common protective devices is
for the person to deny that there is any real cause for distress, for
example, ignoring symptoms or explaining them as the result of some
other, less threatening, disease. Alternatively, setting limited goals
provides the person with some hope and an opportunity for at least
small successes at a time when the ultimate goal of survival or return to
normalcy is clearly impossible. Many people are disturbed by the question "Why me?"; they may blame their own past wrongdoings, their
heredity, the doctor, or the hospital staff, and thus find a target for their
pent-up anger. When improvement no longer seems likely, those who
can achieve some acceptance of their situation (based on religious
beliefs, for example) find some relief from the frustration and terror of
their illness.

Other coping strategies have been described in the professional
literature and in personal accounts by cancer patients. Fear of the
unknown is a major component in the general anxiety patients
experience. One of the most basic ways in which people allay this fear is
to seek out information about their problem situations and about what
to expect. Klagsbrun[5] describes a librarian who, upon learning that she
had cervical cancer, went through recent medical journals reading about
her illness, survival statistics, and preferred treatment procedures.
Anticipation of the probable future course of the disease and mental
rehearsal for it is another way of dealing with anxiety. After learning of
his tongue cancer John Bennett[2] spent some time imagining what lay
ahead of him, examining it, becoming accustomed to it, and reassuring
himself that he would be able to manage it. Some people are reassured
by reminding themselves of past difficulties with which they have coped
successfully. Others may displace their anxiety onto someone else, worrying about the other person's problems rather than their own.[7]

The issue of dependence can be handled in several ways. The
librarian described by Klagsbrun,[5] by reading up on her illness and
treatments and discussing them thoroughly with her doctor, was striving
to maintain a sense of control of her own destiny. Many turn to family
and close friends for comfort, admitting their need at a critical time for
support and assistance (see, for example, Bennett & Sagov[2]). A few may

resolve the conflicting independence–dependence drives by giving in to the latter and relying heavily on others for physical care and extensive emotional nurturing.

Our second article is Lester David's account of one woman's personal experience with breast cancer, a disease which strikes tens of thousands of women annually. Marvella Bayh's reactions to this crisis provide a good example of the interplay of previously established ways of handling problems and current external circumstances in determining immediate coping responses. She deals with anxiety by keeping active (attending a large party the night before her biopsy), by seeking detailed information about what to expect, and by using this to prepare herself mentally. External circumstances in this case were compatible with her characteristic methods of coping, as her doctor carefully explained all procedures and her husband was reassuring and supportive.

The importance of such outside help in bolstering a patient's emotional resources is seen clearly in the case of Helen Harrell.[4] She was depressed and anxious after her mastectomy because no one had told her to expect crying spells, trouble sleeping, or continuing numbness in her arm, nor had she been given any information on breast prostheses. Her fears about recurrence and death almost overwhelmed her. It was not until she became active in Reach for Recovery (a program organized by women who have had breast surgery to help other mastectomy patients) that she received the information, support, and sense of usefulness necessary to overcome her paralyzing fears. Mrs. Bayh was visited by a Reach for Recovery volunteer who brought practical information and encouragement, and served as an example of the good adjustment she could hope to achieve. The breast cancer patient faces three major psychological tasks: Accept the loss of the breast, build a satisfactory postmastectomy self-image, and deal with the uncertainty of possible recurrence.[6] Health professionals and others concerned with the patient's well-being can help by acknowledging her feelings of anxiety and depression, by giving her information about her illness and what to expect, and by helping her family understand her feelings and their own.

In the third article David Kaplan, Aaron Smith, Rose Grobstein, and Stanley Fischman discuss family interaction and coping with childhood leukemia. They point out that with each phase of the illness— whether diagnosis, remission, exacerbation, or the terminal state—the patient and the family face a different set of psychological tasks. They give examples of adaptive measures which some parents use, including the open acknowledgment of feelings of sadness and loss and general anticipatory grieving. Seeking information about the illness and its treatment and finding a deeper meaning in the experience also serve an adaptive purpose.[3] Persistent denial either of the leukemia or of its terminal prognosis, hyperactivity or embarking on major life changes which can serve as a distraction from the central issue, and open hostility to health workers (blaming them for the child's condition) represent less successful attempts to deal with these tasks, in that they create serious additional problems. Discrepant parental coping strategies can also create adaptive problems. The authors maintain that it is important for those trying to help the child with leukemia to understand the adaptive strategies employed by the child's family, how they affect the parent–child relationship, and their impact on treatment efforts.

Cancer in its different manifestations and stages presents the individual with a variety of challenges requiring a whole repertoire of coping skills. Hinton has made the additional observation that a person has several psychological needs at any given time and may manifest different needs with different people, for example, presenting a facade of hopefulness with one person while confiding his or her despair to someone else. It is important for the individuals who are struggling with cancer, and for those trying to help them, to understand the adaptive process and the situational and psychological requirements which affect it.

References

1. Abrams, R. D. *Not alone with cancer.* Springfield, Illinois: Charles C Thomas, 1974.
2. Bennett, J. B., & Sagov, S. E. An experience of cancer. *Harper's,* November, 1973, **247,** 94, 97–98, 100, 102.
3. Friedman, S. B., Chodoff, P., Mason, J. W., & Hamburg, D. A. Behavioral observations on parents anticipating the death of a child. *Pediatrics,* 1963, **32,** 610–625.
4. Harrell, H. C. To lose a breast. *American Journal of Nursing,* 1972, **72,** 676–677.
5. Klagsbrun, S. C. Communications in the treatment of cancer. *American Journal of Nursing,* 1971, **71,** 944–948.
6. Klein, R. A crisis to grow on. *Cancer,* 1971, **28,** 1660–1665.
7. Peck, A. Emotional reactions to having cancer. *American Journal of Roentgenology, Radium Therapy and Nuclear Medicine,* 1972, **114,** 591–599.

5

Bearing Cancer

JOHN HINTON

It is an honor to give this lecture in remembrance of Dr. David Kissen. His disciplined investigations into the relationships between psychological factors and diseases such as lung cancer provided information of great value and gave insights into the complex field of psychosomatic processes. The second Kissen Memorial Lecture was devoted to reviewing many of the problems involved in the psychosomatic aspects of neoplasia. After considering the relevant factors in the premorbid personality and life experience of those with malignant disorders, Professor Crisp discussed the influence of psychological factors on the onset and course of the disease.[8] In this lecture another aspect is considered—the reactions of people who have developed cancer. Hence the title, *Bearing Cancer*. There are a variety of meanings and nuances in the word *bearing* which are relevant to cancer. The dictionary definitions include the following: to produce, to bring forth, to carry about upon one, to support a strain, to sustain successfully, to sustain something painful or trying, to stand a test, to tolerate, to hold aloft, to put up with, to endure.

To appreciate the kaleidoscopic patterns of people's adjustments to bearing cancer demands an understanding of so many things at once. It compares with attempts to understand the flight of a bird, where innumerable factors interact, such as aerodynamic principles, differences

JOHN HINTON • Professor of Psychiatry, Middlesex Hospital Medical School, London, England.

Reprinted from *British Journal of Medical Psychology,* 1973, **46,** 105–113, by permission of Cambridge University Press.

between species, evolution, ethology, instinct, migration, types of flight, weather, or the values of the spectator. This may illustrate our problems in understanding the behavior of people who bear cancer. There are so many factors of personality, illness, courage, quality of available care, relatives, passage of time, attitudes of those nearby, etc., which interact one upon the other in an ever-changing dynamic equilibrium. Although it may be convenient to consider some aspects in isolation, sooner or later regard must be given to the whole complex. In this discussion attention will be given, firstly, to the reactions in the early stages of recognizing cancer; secondly, to the stresses borne by those with cancer; and, lastly, to the ways people endure and cope with this disease.

Initial Reactions to Bearing a Cancer

In a paper published in 1951 Shands et al.[24] discuss the disruptive effect of the idea "I have cancer." The individual must needs make an abrupt reorientation toward the future and life expectancy, together with other changes in attitudes toward the more immediate world. The patients described by this group characteristically felt stunned and dazed, just as if they "had received a heavy blow on the head." Initiative was paralysed for a while and they could feel unreal or numb. Presumably, such a reaction follows the sudden open recognition of having cancer. Abrupt realization does occur quite frequently, but often other factors may intervene. The onset of the disease and its recognition may be insidious or psychological coping mechanisms may come into play even as the evidence of cancer emerges.

The clinical onset of a neoplastic lesion does not necessarily announce the diagnosis. It may give rise to only minor nonspecific alterations of health or symptoms more characteristic of other diseases and cause the individual to be justifiably ignorant for some while of the fact that he has a cancer. Later continued changes in health, or the advice to have further investigations, may be accompanied by growing suspicions—is this something serious?—have I got cancer? In this context, there comes the important question of the time interval before a patient approaches a doctor after developing symptoms of cancer. Is delay usually due to ignorance which could be largely overcome by disseminating more information or is there much more to it than that?

Investigations have confirmed the obvious. Delay in seeking

medical advice for cancer is not due solely to ignorance. There is commonly a considerable period of time between the development of symptoms and attending a doctor. Rowe-Jones and Aylett[21] reported that the average time before a patient sought advice for symptoms due to cancer of the colon or rectum was 7–10 months. Several studies have been carried out in patients with breast tumors. Few adult women in our culture could not have been informed in some way that lumps developing in the breast are to be regarded seriously because they could be due to cancer. Yet in the U.S.A. Pack and Gallo[20] found that 57% of patients delayed more than 3 months before consulting a physician. Using the same 3 months criterion, Henderson et al.[15] in Canada reported that 64% delayed, Aitken-Swan and Paterson[5] in Manchester reported 62% delayed, Henderson[14] in Scotland found 70% delayed, although in our inquiry in the surgical wards of the Middlesex Hospital only 23% waited more than 3 months.[7]

Many women in the group we studied responded to finding a lump in the breast in what appears to be the logical way, attending their doctor within a week or two. Asked why they came promptly, the answers were along the lines that early diagnosis and treatment were advisable; several patients used the word *cancer*. Those who delayed spoke of fear or of domestic reasons for putting it off or said they had felt there was no cause for concern. This resembled the reasons given for delay in the other studies quoted: "I didn't think it was serious," "there was no pain," "I couldn't spare the time." Most investigations report fears of hospital, of doctors, of operations, of what they would be told, and in some studies expense has been a deterrent.

As is apparent, the given reasons for delay in reporting breast tumors often include rationalizations, part of the important but enigmatic problem of hidden feelings and knowledge to be discussed later. Admitted anxiety appears to hasten patients to the doctor more than it delays them. In our investigation we found that the group of patients who said that they were not worried or no more than slightly worried on discovering the breast tumor delayed more than the majority, who were frankly anxious. Many admitted fear of operation but this anxiety was not more common in those who delayed. Aitken-Swan and Paterson[5] reported that people who "knew" they might have cancer were slower to consult a doctor. This contrasts with the finding of Harms et al.,[13] who reported that patients admitting that they thought they had breast cancer came more promptly.

This last apparent contradiction had been partially resolved in the studies of Goldsen et al.[10,11] She took into account other aspects of the subjects' attitudes and experience. Certain people had shown in the past a general tardiness in consulting their doctors, a trend not confined to the present cancer symptoms. People with a lower level of education or occupation delayed more. Perhaps most important was the finding that suspicion of having cancer did not of itself hasten or delay medical consultation. But suspicion of having cancer in a person who had previously shown a noticeably worrying attitude to cancer, or had indicated a belief that there was no cure, did produce delay. This explains in part the varied effect of self-diagnosis in people with cancer. It should also be noted that Aitken-Swan and Paterson[5] deliberately put inverted commas about patients "knowing" they might have cancer, because some of their subjects were both hiding and revealing their "knowledge."

The Burden of Cancer

What are the stresses people with cancer have to bear? Unfortunately, it could be a long list. There are the immediate physical symptoms caused by the lesion. There are other indirect somatic changes due to perhaps anemia, involvement of the central nervous system, altered endocrine function, and so on. The symptoms may be intrinsically distressing, such as pain or nausea, or be disturbing because of the implications of damaged function, for example, incontinence or paralysis. For the patient the future may now appear a source of foreboding rather than hope, anticipating discomfort, mutilation, or death. Other changes may bring stress, altered physical appearance, a loss of social status, separation from the family, and all the implications of being a patient rather than just a person.

To obtain some idea of the relative frequency of severe stresses experienced by people who found their situation hard to bear, I have looked back over the records of a hundred patients in hospital with neoplastic conditions who were referred for a psychiatric opinion and advice. Many of them with little or no prompting spoke of their particular problems. The troubles to be mentioned here appeared to play a significant part in causing distress, as judged by the fact that they were volunteered as particularly trying circumstances by 5% or more of this group. *Pain* was a significant source of stress. In some cases it was directly due to the neoplasm and needed further treatment to bring it under better control. In other cases it appeared to be partly or largely a manifestation of psychological disturbance. As usual, the subject of pain crosses all our attempted classifications, and here it could be not only a stress but a manifestation of strain.

Disfigurement could threaten pride or cause extreme embarrassment. For women general wasting, mastectomy, hair loss following radiotherapy, or facial palsy could be hard to bear. Men could be equally and understandably ashamed if their strength had seemed to them to have wasted to skin and bone or if, for example, nasopharyngeal cancer had made ugly their face and distorted the voice. Deep *concern over the future* was voiced by some but even more often it was implied. One or two people were very troubled by continued deterioration and the possibility of dying. Another elderly person was more fearful of treatment than the disease itself.

The other three common sources of stress among these 100 people affected social status and relationships. The *loss of work role* could bring distress. A successful and ambitious young policeman with Hodgkin's disease who was discharged from the force and a conscientious nursing sister who did not know what to do now she could not look after her ward were examples of this group. *Dependency* and fear of being a burden on others was another aspect of social and psychological disruption. This could arise when function was specifically limited as, for instance, with hemiplegia. The dependency could come in a more general form as in the case of a young graduate who had less and less independent life out of hospital and came to question the value of being given repeated transfusions in order to maintain an existence he viewed as progressively unrewarding. The sense of *alienation* was another theme. Patients sensed that many did not care about them as individuals any longer and some people positively wanted no more to do with them. Special circumstances could contribute to this feeling of being a nuisance; for example, people who had had laryngectomies might find the frustrations of failed communication could enhance their sense of isolation.

These are examples of the stresses; what strains are experienced by the people concerned? There may be the shock of sudden recognition of having cancer. The common reaction of anxiety may be expressed in terms of the problems of the present or of the future. But other emotions arise. A monograph by Achté and Vauhkonen[3] describes the psychological symptoms found on psychiatric interview in a group of 100 cancer patients attending hospital clinics at Helsinki. From their list of overlapping symptoms the following have been selected: tenseness, 65%; fear of death, 58%; depression, 58%; aggressiveness, 39%; affect lability, 30%; paranoid trends, 25%; reduced interest in life, 15%; and hypomania, 12%.

These were symptoms discovered in a group unselected from the psychiatric point of view except to exclude the elderly. The picture is not so very different from the formal psychiatric diagnoses given to the previously mentioned 100 cancer patients seen in psychiatric consultation, except that the referred group included 15 patients with organic confusional states. Depression was noted in 49% of the psychiatric group, more common in this series than anxiety states, which were diagnosed in 30%. Although aggressiveness was not included as a diagnosis in the 100 patients I saw, it was a noteworthy feature in several. Excluding the organic psychosis group, paranoid symptoms were marked in 3 depressed patients and hypomania was diagnosed in 2 cases.

This brief outline of the stresses and strains occurring when malignant disease develops leads on to consideration of the ways in which the burden is borne.

Coping with Cancer

Although cancer imposes particular stresses, individuals have their own susceptibilities and they have preestablished tendencies to cope in their own special patterns. In this context Lipowski[18] has defined coping as all "cognitive and motor activities which a sick person employs to preserve his bodily and psychic integrity, to recover reversibly impaired function and compensate to the limit for any irreversible impairment." He goes on to distinguish an individual's coping style, which is the enduring disposition to use certain techniques, from the coping strategy actually employed by the sick person dealing with an illness. This approach to the problem of coping does, of course, include the use of psychological defense mechanisms, to which other workers such as Shands et al.[24] have given pride of place.

Lipowski has included an emphasis on cognitive coping styles whereby an individual may either minimize the available information or he may focus with vigilance upon perceived dangers and attempt to reduce uncertainty. With these cognitive elements go the responses of behavior which tended to take active, passive, or avoiding styles. These styles and their attendant strategies do, of course, overlap with familiar concepts of suppression, denial, dissociation, regression, sublimation, and so forth.

At this point it is appropriate to give recognition to the fact that personality attributes which have been investigated for their bearing upon the etiology of cancer may well influence, or may even be influenced by, the development of cancer. This is an intricate tangle to unravel. The psychosomatic inquiries into the etiology of cancer may be said to contain two broad approaches. One approach, typified by the work carried out at the Rochester Medical Center by Greene[12] and Schmale and Iker,[23] explores the effect of loss and separation resulting in the person giving up and running out of psychological resources. If this reaction to circumstances attends the bearing forth of cancer, then such attitudes are likely to influence the subsequent response to the manifest disease. Conversely, patients troubled by cancer could give a biased account of the antecedent situation.

The second psychosomatic approach, where so much was done by David Kissen, is into the field of the personality of those developing cancer. Bahnson and Bahnson[6] have explored the repressive ego defences of subjects with neoplastic disease. Dr. Kissen and his co-workers[17] have produced a great deal of evidence to indicate that patients with lung cancer have a "poor emotional outlet." Once again there is likely to be an interplay between the preceding state and the reactions to the subsequent lung disease. In David Kissen's controlled studies it appeared that the cancer patients did not know the diagnosis at the time of making the assessments. Huggan[16] has discussed and tried to explore some of the interplay of factors. He found that people receiving radiotherapy for cancer were apt to answer more direct questions about anxiety in a negative fashion, although other indirect inquiries denoted that anxiety was there. These patients also distorted other answers in a negative way. It is not clear whether this was a generalized development of a denying tendency in those who had developed cancer or whether it was just a continuation of the previous personality trends of the lung cancer patients described by David Kissen.

Whatever the approach to the repressive or minimizing mechanisms of people with cancer, it is clear that these patients often appear unaware of some of the threats that face them. It is also to be noted that the vast majority of their friends, relatives, nurses, and doctors will collude with this tendency. When Aitken-Swan and Easson[4] in Manchester ensured that 231 patients with curable cancer were clearly informed of the diagnosis, although two-thirds were glad to have been told, 19% denied that they had been told. The repressing forces are powerful.

Nevertheless, surveys of groups of people with cancer have shown that many are well aware of the diagnosis although others appear ignorant or deny the possibility. In the 100 patients investigated by Achté and Vauhkonen[3] 68 appeared to know and 31 did not. The 31 who did not realize included 7 who had been told the diagnosis by the doctor, 2 of them at the patient's own request. All physicians and surgeons with experience in this field will have seen blatant examples of the denial mechanism at work. Patients with large fungating growths may blandly deny that it is a source of concern. Moses and Cividali[19] explored a little further to see what factors could influence the awareness of 30 people with cancer. They graded their patients along a continuum of awareness. They found no correlation between the level of awareness and age, sex, marital state, or ethnic origin (this work was done in Israel). There was, however, a significant association of greater awareness with higher education. It is of interest that studies in North America and in London have also found that those with a longer period of education tend to consult their doctors earlier if they develop cancer.

It is often said, with truth, of people with cancer that many know but do not speak of it. In a recent study, not yet published, of 60 people with progressive malignant disease reaching the terminal stage, I asked them if they thought much about their illness—using approximately those words. Eight percent said it was on their mind for "most of the time" and 37% were often thinking of their condition; in some cases the symptoms were a frequent reminder. Hence it was clear that many admitted to being only too well aware of the situation. One in five spontaneously used the word *cancer,* although others employed euphemisms. There were remarks like "With cancer you always wonder." Twenty-eight percent said they sometimes thought about their condition and the remaining 27% said they either forgot about it or tried to. Some remarks of theirs may reveal the problem they had: "I try to forget," "I've got to forget about it," "I live from day to day," "No point in dwelling on it," "I don't think about it, I've got cancer," "I won't let myself, I'd go crazy if I did.'' It would appear that the majority of people have considerable uneasy awareness of having cancer, although varying degrees of repression or suppression may be employed.

Apart from some ignoring the burden, this same group of people with cancer illustrated coping styles of which they were often conscious. In about a third the pattern was to maintain hope, often setting a limited goal toward independence, such as wanting to walk again, to cope at home, to return to work or to drive a car. Others were well aware of the lack of progress and spoke in terms of acceptance of despondency. Uncertainty was rife; it could be troublesome, although for some it was a preferable alternative to finality. ''How's it going to end?'' ''Should I talk to the wife?'' ''*If* I get out of hospital,'' ''How much do they really know?''

Some workers in this field have examined how patients with cancer prefer rationalization to the unknown. Abrams and Finesinger[2] noted the marked tendency to explain the cause or the responsibility for the disease developing. A half of their 60 patients blamed their own past actions, be it a fall or a sin. Nearly all the remaining half attributed it to someone else, either as contagion or due to what the other persons had done to the patient. Twenty of Moses and Cividali's[19] 30 cancer patients blamed others, whether it be heredity, rejection, poor medical care, etc., while 8 blamed themselves. This last trend demonstrates the fragility of such boundaries as guilt and self-blame if used in this situation to separate troubled patients from those with a classic picture of depression.

Planned investigations into the way people cope with cancer have tended to focus more on people with progressive malignant disease than those who get better. There is the evidence that most of those with curable cancer have appreciated being told openly about their condition.[4,9] Not all feel this way, and many still believe all cancer is incurable in spite of evidence to the contrary. Sometimes psychiatric advice is sought to help people whose cancer is probably cured but who remain devoid of hope. When previous pessimism and memories of others with fatal cancer combine with current depression, the therapeutic problems are not easily resolved. Even when the prognosis is excellent cancer introduces a serious uncertainty about the future. Despite favorable circumstances, the struggle to regain confidence can be a hard one. There is much anecdotal evidence from people who are in good health years after their cancer treatment that it took them a long time before they could again take life for granted. The apprehension before follow-up appointments, the relief when the doctor gave another clean bill of health, the significance attributed to the doctor's demeanor or the time interval before the next appointment are familiar reactions. Others appear to have coped well by using repressive mechanisms. It is likely that more consistent studies of people's feelings and behavior in this situation would have practical and theoretical value.

Clinically, doctors are more likely to be made aware of the processes involved when the disease progresses and the stresses bear down so heavily that the behavior of patients in treatment becomes disturbed. Earlier in this paper the emotional changes and psychiatric diagnoses of troubled patients were mentioned. Many came to notice because their behavior had crossed conventional limits. Social withdrawal could be overlooked, but aggressive, demanding, excessively complaining behavior could both reveal and pass on to others the turmoil the patient felt. The manner in which some individuals made their complaints of pain, etc., could show these elements. Suicidal attempts carried similar messages of appeal, anger, and despair in this situation as they do for those with other sources of distress. Although some of the studies of people committing suicide have not found an increased incidence of cancer among them, others, including Sainsbury's[22] classic study, found this disease to play a significant role.

The adaptation—or maladaptation—of one or two of the cancer patients referred was to refuse treatment and, consistently enough, they could also refuse to see a psychiatrist. The refusal of help can indicate the degree of emotional upset and despair. Illogical refusal to cooperate in treatment also highlights the intricacies of the enforced dependency of individuals when they become patients. The doctor–patient relationship has been discussed widely. Its significance in people with cancer merits discussion in its own right. Here brief consideration can be given to only one or two elements. There is a background of a potentially fatal disease being involved. The reactions of both parties may appear illogical for, among other reasons, the logic of mortality may be unacceptable to either or both. The doctor–patient relationship in this context is another example of all the problems of interpersonal involvement. It is not solely the patient who has a burden to bear when cancer comes.

Some of the interpersonal problems are illustrated by the issues of communication. This aspect of personal relationships is significant throughout the course of the disease. Henderson's[14] study indicated that a poor relationship between a person and his doctor contributed to delay in reporting the symptoms. When cancer is recognized, doctors in the country have considerable reluctance to reveal the diagnosis to the patient. Instead, contrary to the usual practice of regarding the patient as the best entitled to information, a responsible relative may well be informed. It is reminiscent of discussing the child's illness with the parent.

In some places, as in a report from Minnesota,[9] doctors have been more prepared to be informative and a clear majority of patients, whether they have had curable or progressing cancer, said they felt this was the correct policy. In Scandinavian countries the trend is also for physicians to tell their patients of cancer; but not all patients appreciate being told, and a few are distressed. Achté and Vauhkonen,[3] for example, showed that some of the patients repress what the doctor has said, and whether the studies on telling the patients were carried out in Minnesota or Manchester not 100% wanted to know. Some individuals cope best with burdens by ignoring their existence.

It is not only doctors who are reluctant to communicate with cancer patients; relatives and friends often believe it is wrong for the patient to be told. They will join vigorously the collusion to deny anything but hope. During some recent interviews with 45 terminal cancer patients, when we discussed their attitude to being ill, well over half volunteered that their disease could prove fatal. The wives or husbands of these patients had been told of the diagnosis and prognosis yet apparently only 10 of these pairs had discussed it openly between themselves at any time. This appeared to be a failure in communication over progressing cancer. Overtly it was, and there were occasions when there seemed to be room for improvement. But nearly all of these married couples also said that they were closer to each other now, rather than the opposite. They were bearing the situation together in many, if not all, respects.

Communication between people is not limited to one obvious message in the used words. It depends not only on what is said, but on how and when information is conveyed and how it is received. Many patients are aware that they have cancer, even fatal cancer, although no one has told them. Some have been told and do not know. When cancer patients discuss the conversations they have had with medical staff, it is clear that often more than one message has been communicated, including items which were not meant to be transmitted. Moses and Cividali's[19] patients confirmed what many, but not all, doctors recognize. Categorical denials by a physician about cancer often do not shake the convictions of patients who know otherwise, but only serve to establish the nature of the current relationship between doctor and patient. The physician's nonverbal behavior often conveys unmistakably to the cancer patient both the diagnosis and how the doctor is preparing to cope with the situation.

No simple rules apply. The patient's relationship with others, including his level of communication, may alter during the progress of the illness.[1] It is not uncommon for a patient's first attitude of free communication and faith in the physician to evolve into a more guarded approach if the disease advances. The need to depend on the doctor may be stronger, but also that bond may be criticized or tested by the patient's behavior. Moreover, in my experience, such ill people may seek to meet different needs through different people—perhaps demanding optimistic reassurance from one source and yet welcoming a realistic, if somber, exchange of words with another.

If the situation is nearly unbearable, anger, rejection, withdrawal, importunity, jealousy, or an excessive surrendering of independence may well become manifest. Each of these coping strategies merits much discussion in its own right. Acceptance often follows, even though its presence may only be shown by comparative silence. Occasionally, the cancer is borne in the sense of bearing aloft. The diagnosis is proclaimed and assurance may come from having all questions answered, all plans known, and reasons given. More often the experience is borne with quieter courage, aided by the discreet support from those close to the person who has developed this disease. There is often an extraordinary quality of care given by those whose professional life involves the treatment of people with cancer. It is also apparent that individuals with malignant disease gain a great deal from the example and the support given by other people around them who also have cancer and bear it well.

There is much more to be discovered and applied in this whole field of people's reactions to having cancer. If we can use clinical skill and precise methods of investigation in the way that Dr. David Kissen combined so well, this subject will make worthwhile advances.

References

1.   Abrams, R. D. (1966). The patient with cancer: His changing pattern of communication. *New England Journal of Medicine* **274,** 317–322.

2. Abrams, R. D., & Finesinger, J. E. (1951). Unpublished observations quoted by Shands et al. (1951).

3. Achté, K., & Vauhkonen, M. (1970). Cancer and psyche. *Monographs from the Psychiatric Clinic of the Helsinki University Central Hospital no. 1*, pp. 3–44.

4. Aitken-Swan, J., & Easson, E. C. (1959). Reactions of cancer patients on being told their diagnosis. *British Medical Journal* **1**, 779–783.

5. Aitken-Swan, J., & Paterson, R. (1955). The cancer patient: Delay in seeking advice. *British Medical Journal* **1**, 623–627.

6. Bahnson, M. B., & Bahnson, C. B. (1969). Ego defences in cancer patients. *Annals of the New York Academy of Sciences* **164**, 546–557.

7. Cameron, A., & Hinton, J. M. (1968). Delay in seeking treatment for mammary tumours. *Cancer (Philadelphia)* **21**, 1121–1126.

8. Crisp, A. H. (1970). Some psychosomatic aspects of neoplasia. *British Journal of Medical Psychology* **43**, 313–331.

9. Gilbertsen, V. A., & Wangensteen, O. W. (1962). Should the doctor tell the patient that the disease is cancer? *American Cancer Society Symposium* (1961), pp. 80–85.

10. Goldsen, R. K. (1963). Patient delay in seeking cancer diagnosis: Behavioural aspects. *Journal of Chronic Diseases* **16**, 427–436.

11. Goldsen, R. K., Gerhardt, P. R., & Handy, V. H. (1956). Some factors related to patient delay in seeking diagnosis for cancer symptoms. *Cancer (Philadelphia)* **9**, 1–7.

12. Greene, W. A. (1966). The psychosocial setting of the development of leukaemia and lymphoma. *Annals of the New York Academy of Sciences* **125**, 794–801.

13. Harms, C. R., Plaut, J. R., & Oughterson, A. W. (1943). Delay in the treatment of cancer. *Journal of the American Medical Association* **121**, 335–358.

14. Henderson, J. G. (1966). Denial and repression as factors in the delay of patients with cancer presenting themselves to the physician. *Annals of the New York Academy of Sciences* **125**, 856–864.

15. Henderson, J. G., Wittkower, E. D., & Lougheed, M. N. (1958). A psychiatric investigation of the delay factor in patient to doctor presentation in cancer. *Journal of Psychosomatic Research* **3**, 27–41.

16. Huggan, R. E. (1968). Neuroticism, distortion and objective manifestations of anxiety in males with malignant disease. *British Journal of Social and Clinical Psychology* **7**, 280–285.

17. Kissen, D. M., Brown, R. I. F., & Kissen, M. (1969). A further report on personality and psychosocial factors in lung cancer. *Annals of the New York Academy of Sciences* **164**, 535–544.

18. Lipowski, Z. J. (1970). Physical illness, the individual and the coping processes. *Psychiatry in Medicine* **1**, 91–102.

19. Moses, R., & Cividali, M. (1966). Differential levels of awareness of illness: Their relation to some salient features in cancer patients. *Annals of the New York Academy of Sciences* **125**, 984–994.

20. Pack, G. T., & Gallo, J. S. (1938). The culpability for delay in the treatment of cancer. *American Journal of Cancer* **33**, 443–462.

21. Rowe-Jones, D. C., & Aylett, S. O. (1965). Delay in treatment of carcinoma of colon and rectum. *Lancet* **2**, 973–976.

22.   Sainsbury, P. (1955). *Suicide in London*. London: Chapman & Hall.
23.   Schmale, A. & Iker, H. (1966). The psychological setting of uterine cervical cancer. *Annals of the New York Academy of Sciences* **125**, 807–813.
24.   Shands, H. C., Finesinger, J. E., Cobb, S. & Abrams, R. D. (1951). Psychological mechanisms in patients with cancer. *Cancer* (*Philadelphia*) **4**, 1159–1170.

6

A Brave Family Faces Up to Breast Cancer

LESTER DAVID

On a gray morning in early October of 1971, Birch Bayh, junior senator from Indiana, faced a hushed group of reporters, photographers, and
television cameramen in the Caucus Room of the Senate Office Building. In this chamber, where many historic decisions have been made,
the 43-year-old Bayh announced he was ending his unofficial candidacy
for the presidency of the United States.

His reason was simple and compelling.

A totally unexpected blow had struck his family. His wife, Marvella, to whom he had been married 19 years, had just undergone major
surgery for cancer of the breast.

"I must put first things first," he said, his voice faltering only
slightly. "During this time I want to be at her side. My wife and her
well-being and rapid recovery are more important to me than seeking
the presidency."

Two miles away, Marvella slept fitfully in her hospital bed. Later
that day with the senator, she watched a television news broadcast of
the announcement and reached out to grip his hand.

The Bayhs are unusual people, but the medical crisis that
confronted them, with its physical and emotional traumas, is all too
common. This is their story, untold until now.

It is the story of a remarkable young woman and how she coped

Reprinted in abridged form from *Today's Health,* June 1972, **50**, 16, 18–21. Published by the
American Medical Association.

with the crisis that entered her life, and of a husband whose support
was essential to meet the potentially devastating impact of her illness.
But more than anything else, it is a story that offers hope to other
families who may face the same cruel dilemma.

Breast malignancy, when unchecked, is the No. 1 cancer killer of
women. This year alone, the American Cancer Society estimates,
72,000 women will be stricken and 32,000 will die in the United States.
This year alone, 8,500 women in New York State, 6,500 in California,
and 5,000 in Pennsylvania will hear the same diagnosis. Dr. Arthur I.
Holleb, A.C.S. senior vice-president for medical affairs and research,
predicts that "we can anticipate more new cases in the next ten years
than the entire population of the city of Boston."

Small wonder the A.C.S. past president, Dr. H. Marvin Pollard,
recently called it "the foremost cancer."

Addressing the Second National Conference on Breast Cancer in
Los Angeles last year, he said: "It is the most feared of cancers, the
most frequently self-discovered, the most controversially treated. . . . In
the area of psychological effects, it is also foremost. One cannot compute
its ranking in heartache and suffering."

Marvella Bayh is just one of many thousands who were alert
enough to have a malignancy diagnosed in the early stages, when the
chances for cure are immeasurably improved. *If the cancer has not
spread beyond the breast, some 85% of patients who undergo treatment
show no evidence of the disease at the end of five years.*

The Bayhs live in a 10-room Georgian house on a quiet hilly street
on the edges of Georgetown, about three miles northwest of the Capitol.

Soon Marvella, seated on a couch in the living room, is telling her
story. She talks easily, smiling frequently, with no hint of doom or
tragedy in her voice. And because she tells it so simply, the impact of
her ordeal is all the more powerful.

I'm a greater believer in preventive medicine," she is saying.
"Throughout her life, my mother was in very poor health, and I saw
how much easier it was to correct something if it's caught in the beginning. Believe me, I'm not a fanatic. I don't run to the doctor for every
little thing! But I don't ignore symptoms that can lead to something
serious, like a bad cold that can lead to a strep throat, or worse.

"And so, in February of last year, I just began to be aware of my
right breast. It had always been somewhat larger than the other, but the
doctors had told me it's quite normal for breasts to be of unequal size.

I'd always gone regularly to my gynecologist for a checkup, but that month, when I began to have these fleeting sensations, maybe two or three a day, I called for a special appointment."

In his office on Connecticut Avenue, Dr. Stafford W. Hawken detected nothing by palpation, a manual examination of the breast tissue, but, to make sure, he ordered a mammogram. This is a special x-ray of the soft tissues which can detect tumors, even tiny ones the size of a pencil eraser, too small to feel. The results were negative and, since the sensations had disappeared, Marvella forgot about them.

But six months later they returned. This time they were constant, though still not painful. "They didn't bother me," she said, "I was simply aware of that part of my body." Once again she saw Dr. Hawken, who ordered new mammograms. But once again the x-rays showed no evidence of a tumor or an abnormality.

"Not only that," Marvella said, "there was no lump, nothing at all that you could feel." Once again the x-rays were negative, and physical examination disclosed no dominant tumor, but this time Dr. Hawken noticed a slight skin change below the nipple, a lack of mobility in the area that aroused his suspicions. He suggested a biopsy. Surgical removal of a small portion of tissue for microscopic examination in the laboratory—a biopsy—is the only way of diagnosing a tumor with total accuracy.

Four days after Dr. Hawken suggested a biopsy, Marvella received a call from the Columbia Hospital for Women on L Street, not far from Georgetown, saying that she could be admitted the following day. That night, Marvella Bayh did an extraordinary thing: she sang and danced, gaily and exuberantly, at a Democratic women's organization fund-raising at the Sheraton Park Hotel! Only she and her husband knew that at one o'clock the next day she would enter the hospital for her crucial biopsy.

At eleven o'clock the next morning, Marvella was wheeled to the operating room in the east wing, Bayh walking beside her to the double-door entrance to the surgical suite. He returned to sit in her room and wait.

Usually when breast cancer is suspected, the patient remains on the operating table while the tissue fragment is examined. Then, if the pathologist reports a malignancy, the doctors proceed with major surgery. But two days before, Marvella had asked Dr. Hawken, who is senior consultant at Columbia, to perform only the biopsy.

"I can face almost anything," she said, "as long as I *know*. It's the uncertainty I find hard. I've got to know, when I go under, what you are going to do. This way," she explained, "I can prepare myself for what could happen."

Dr. Hawken removed a piece of granular tissue of the breast right beneath where he had seen the changes in the skin. Later, in the recovery room adjoining the operating suite, Marvella began to emerge from the light anesthetic and called for Dr. Hawken. In a moment, he appeared, Birch Bayh at his side.

Still only half awake, Marvella formed the words, "Is it or isn't it?" She now realizes that she could have seen the answer in the faces of the doctor and her husband as they stood at her bedside.

"Bad news, bad news," Dr. Hawken said. "Malignant."

Dr. Hawken had always reminded Marvella of the old-fashioned family doctors in the rural area in Oklahoma where she grew up. He had a no-nonsense air about him which never hid the fact that he truly cared.

"He just told it like it is," Marvella recalls. "He had always told me exactly what he believed. At the same time, I knew how deeply he felt."

Senator Bayh leaned over the bed. He took his wife in his arms and wept. For husbands, too, the ordeal can be agonizing, and it was especially so for Birch Bayh, whose mother had died of cancer when he was 12.

The surgery took about two hours. Once more, Birch Bayh had walked alongside the stretcher to the operating suite, returning to wait in Marvella's room. Dr. Hawken, assisted by Dr. James Scully, removed her right breast, a portion of the chest muscle, and the lymph glands in the armpit. He did not perform a classic radical mastectomy, which includes, in addition to the breast, removal of all the pectoral muscles and axillary lymph nodes. In "extended radical mastectomy," the internal mammary node chain under the breast bone is also excised.

In the recovery room, emerging once again from the haze of the anesthetic, she saw Dr. Hawken and Birch at her bedside. Simply, in his matter-of-fact tones, Dr. Hawken told her, "Everything's fine."

The senator leaned over her and kissed her. "That wonderful doctor has saved your life," he said.

It was all over.

Marvella was surprised to discover that there was no pain and little discomfort. "It astonished me because the breast is such a sensitive, easily injured part of the body and you would think that any surgery connected with it would be extremely painful. I had absolutely none. Any discomfort I had resulted from the removal of the lymph glands under the arm."

Five days after the operation, she had a visitor, someone with a message of incalculable value to Marvella and all other women who have undergone the experience of breast removal.

By this time she had been in the hospital for a week. "My hair had lost its set and needed washing," she recalls, "and I was feeling dowdy. In walked this woman looking like a million dollars in a slit midi skirt, boots, and a jersey blouse and her hair all fixed up. 'I'm from Reach for Recovery,' she told me, 'and I want to talk to you!'"

It was Marvella's first introduction to a remarkable organization of breast surgery patients who conduct a rehabilitation program designed to help women who have had mastectomies meet their psychological, physical, and cosmetic needs. Reach for Recovery was founded in 1953 by Mrs. Terese Lasser, herself a patient, with funds made available by her husband, J. K. Lasser. Since 1969, it has been part of the service and rehabilitation division of the American Cancer Society and Mrs. Lasser is its national consultant. The organization's fame and work have spread far beyond this country, to South Africa, India, Japan, New Zealand, and Israel. In the United States alone, there are more than 2,000 volunteers who made 8,000 visits to patients last year.

With the approval of the attending physician, an organization volunteer visits a patient while she is recovering from her mastectomy in the hospital and discusses all the problems that lie ahead, including suggestions for bra comfort and clothing adjustment, particularly bathing suits. All medical questions are referred to the patient's physician.

Marvella found it hard to believe her visitor had had breast surgery. "I just stared at this woman who looked like a model," she said, "and I thought to myself: If she can do it, I can too!" The woman talked to her for more than an hour and left a 38-page yellow booklet filled with facts. There were chapters on exercises, clothing, fashions, and "do's and don'ts":

Do act as you always did with your family and friends. They will feel more at ease, and so will you.

Do go back to your normal way of life as soon as possible, whether it be home or career. You'll feel much better for it.

Do resume such sports as golf and tennis (or find new ones) and drive your car just as soon as your doctor gives the green light.

Don't overdo in any way. Getting overly tired will only retard your recovery, and it won't help your disposition.

Don't have blood pressure taken or injections given in arm on side of surgery, or garden without gloves—thorns and cuts may cause an infection.

Don't neglect your appearance.

Don't allow yourself to become discouraged. Keep busy so there won't be time for brooding. Don't create hurdles which will be hard to overcome when you return home.

In large black type toward the end was this message: REMEMBER THAT YOU ARE THE SAME PERSON TODAY THAT YOU WERE BEFORE SURGERY—IN EVERY WAY!

Reach for Recovery also publishes a small folder called "A Letter To Husbands" which tackles squarely one of a mastectomy patient's most profound fears: that her husband will no longer find her attractive. In a society as bosom-conscious as America, it is a real enough worry.

"Uppermost in the mind of every married woman," the folder says, "are the nagging thoughts: Will my husband react with revulsion to my body? Will it create a barrier between us? Will our sexual relations be affected? Will he pity or be ashamed of me?"

For Marvella, the question was settled once and for all in a conversation that lasted only a few seconds.

The night before the surgery she said to her husband: "Just think. I'm 38 years old and I'm going to have to go through the rest of my life with only one breast."

A smile twitching at the corners of his mouth, Bayh replied: "Don't let that upset you, dear. I'm five years older than you are and I've gone through life this far without any." Then, seriously, "Do you think I married you for your breasts? I married you for what you are."

Marvella declares: "I think the hottest place in hell should be reserved for men who might make a wife feel she is any less of a woman, because it's not true at all!"

As Mrs. Lasser puts it: "A woman has retained her ability to love, her femininity and her intellect. She can do everything and be everything she was—but only with your (a husband's) encouragement."

Six months after her surgery, Marvella resumed her normal life, taking care to rest every afternoon for at least an hour. She has curtailed some of her traveling and speaking, but by no means all. Last April, she accompanied her husband to the Cameroons in Africa to attend sessions of the International Parliamentary Union, which meets biannually in various parts of the world to promote understanding and cooperation between legislative bodies around the world.

"I'm giving myself time to recover," she says, "I'm doing almost everything I ever did before, but in moderation. If I rest in the afternoon, I find I can go out in the evening to a meeting, a lecture, a party, even dancing. I accept some speaking engagements, go places, help run the house and raise my son, help Birch all I can."

She paused a moment. "You know," she continued, "things really haven't changed a greal deal."

There, in that simple statement, lies the most important thing the Bayhs have discovered from their experience. For when breast cancer is caught and treated in time, things don't really change very much—not for a woman, not for her husband, not for a family, not for anyone.

7

Family Mediation of Stress

DAVID M. KAPLAN, AARON SMITH, ROSE GROBSTEIN, and STANLEY E. FISCHMAN

Serious and prolonged illness such as childhood leukemia is a common source of stress that poses major problems of adjustment, not only for the patient but also for family members. It is important to emphasize family as well as individual reactions in coping with stress since the family has a unique responsibility for mediating the reactions of its members.

When individuals belong to families, they do not resolve their own problems of stress independently, nor are they immune to effects of stress that may be concentrated in another member of the family. Vincent states that the family is uniquely organized to carry out its stress-mediating responsibility and is in a strategic position to do so.[1] No other social institution has demonstrated a comparable capability for mediation that affects as many people in the community.

Because the family has a commitment to protect its members under a wide range of stressful conditions and over long periods of time, physicians, social workers, and other professionals working with a severely ill child must extend their concern beyond the child, as least to members

DAVID M. KAPLAN, Ph.D. ● Director, Division of Clinical Social Work, Stanford University Medical Center, Stanford, California. AARON SMITH, M.D.H., M.S.W., ROSE GROB-STEIN, B.A., and STANLEY FISCHMAN, M.D. ● Departments of Pediatrics and of Community and Preventive Medicine, Division of Clinical Social Work, Stanford University School of Medicine, Stanford, California.

Reprinted from *Social Work*, 1973, **18** (July), 60–69. By permission of the National Association of Social Workers.

of the immediate family and perhaps to other close relatives. They must offer parents and other family members, as appropriate, help when they need it to handle and resolve specific problems of stress. If stress is great enough and sufficiently prolonged, the role of a family as a buffer for its members can be permanently impaired or even destroyed. To prevent this, more must be learned about effective individual and family coping—and more help given to improve this coping.

A better understanding of the process of coping with severe stress would have substantial clinical and preventive value. Adaptive coping by the family and its individual members—that is, mastery of the sociopsychological problems associated with stress—offers the greatest protection for family members confronted by stressful situations and the best assurance that the family will continue as a viable unit, able to meet the changing needs of its members after they have gotten over the stress.

This article describes the effect of serious illness on the family, delineates the family's critical role in resolving problems related to stress, and provides data needed for organizing preventive and clinical programs that will protect the family's stress-mediating function and mitigate the impact of stress on individual family members. The article is based on the authors' clinical review of more than 50 families with a child diagnosed and treated for leukemia at the Stanford University Department of Pediatrics. Each family was studied from the date the parents were informed of the diagnosis until two months after the child died.

Identifying Early Reactions

The aim of the study was to identify adaptive and maladaptive coping responses by the family as early as possible after diagnosis—within three weeks or four at most. It was hoped that developing a method of early case-finding would make intervention feasible during this crucial period and reduce the incidence of families who failed to cope adequately.

Early identification was attempted because studies of the concept of crisis suggest that both individual and family reactions to such threats as prolonged illness are fashioned from one to four weeks after the diagnosis is confirmed.[2] Both adaptive and maladaptive coping responses become evident then. These responses tend to persist and to be reinforced throughout the course of the illness, which may run for years. Rapoport indicates that coping patterns are not as fixed and unyielding during these first weeks as they become in time.[3] Therefore, the ideal time to discover that families are coping inadequately is during this early phase.

Families with a leukemic child constitute a high-risk group. The severe stress precipitated by the diagnosis of the illness generates many problems in addition to those involved in caring for the leukemic child. Both clinical and research observations indicate that a disturbingly large number of families who face this situation fail to cope successfully with the problem it poses.[4] Binger et al. reported that following this diagnosis, at least one member in more than half the families in a 1969 study required psychiatric treatment.[5] Bozeman et al. noted that in families with a leukemic child, school difficulties with the healthy children, divorce, and illness occurred frequently.[6] In the study on which this article is based, 87% of the families in the sample failed to cope adequately with the consequences of childhood leukemia, and this failure created a variety of individual and interpersonal problems that were superimposed on the stresses posed by the illness itself. The success or failure of the family's coping behavior was assessed on the criterion that Friedman and his associates outlined: "Coping mechanisms observed in parents should be viewed in terms of how such behavior contributes or interferes with meeting the needs of the ill child and other family members."[7]

In addition to demonstrable risks associated with a fatal illness such as childhood leukemia, many critical problems of management that involve the family confront medical and social work personnel. Research has not yet provided data helpful for resolving these problems. The following are among the common unsolved questions of management:

1. What should the parents, the leukemic child, healthy siblings, and members of the extended family be told about leukemia—that is, about its course, treatment, and prognosis?

2. Who should give each family member the information deemed appropriate?

3. What advice should be given to parents who consider major family changes after they hear about the child's diagnosis—for example, having another child soon, separating from each other, remarrying, or moving to a new community?

4.   What should be done to help parents who seriously disagree about the handling of fatal illness in the family?

5.   What help can be offered to single-parent families faced with long-term illness?

6.   During the period in which the parents are preoccupied with the leukemic child and tend to neglect the healthy siblings, how can the needs of these other children be protected?

7.   What should be done to help parents who avoid visiting the leukemic child during hospitalization—and to help the child?

8.   How can morbid preoccupation over the lost child be avoided?

Coping Tasks

The tasks of coping with stress occur in order and relate to the characteristic, sequential phases of the illness—that is, diagnosis, remission, exacerbation, and terminal state. These phase-related tasks must be resolved in proper sequence within the time limits set by the duration of the successive phases of the illness. Failure to resolve them in this manner is likely to jeopardize the total coping process of the entire family and the outcome of the stressful situation faced.[8]

Successfully resolving any crisis depends largely on each individual's ability to experience with minimum delay the immediately painful consequences of a stress-producing event and to comprehend and anticipate, even though dimly, the later consequences—that is, the pain, sorrow, and sacrifice that the trauma will cause. Comprehension in this context means learning to accept one's new life circumstances, however painful, and then acting in accordance with the new conditions that follow the original crisis-precipitating event. The family, primarily through its adult members, can either facilitate or obstruct individual efforts to master a situation of stress.

The development of preventive or clinical programs that are capable of reversing maladaptive coping responses to any illness is contingent on having detailed knowledge of the process of adaptation specific to each illness, including relevant coping tasks and methods of task accomplishment. Because coping tasks vary significantly from one illness to another, it is first necessary to identify the problems posed by each illness.

The birth of a premature infant, for example, requires the family to anticipate the infant's possible loss. If it survives, the family must face the possibility of its being defective. Even when the prognosis is favorable, the parents must prepare themselves to care for an infant who has special early needs that yield in time to normal patterns. Many families with premature babies manage these tasks well, but a large minority do not. This minority continues to think of and treat the premature baby as though it were permanently damaged, even after its development follows normal patterns.[9]

The family with a leukemic child is also suddenly confronted with major alterations in its circumstances that threaten cherished hopes and values for all its members and involve drastic alterations in their lifestyle. Each family member must comprehend these new circumstances and adapt to them by making suitable role changes, despite an understandable reluctance to face painful losses. While coping problems are unique for each illness, crises do fall into common groupings. Principles relevant for coping with leukemia apply with some modification to problems of family coping with other severe and fatal illnesses in children and adults.

Family Coping

For any serious illness, coping demands and responses are not static, but change as the medical treatment of the illness changes. At any point in time, families confronted by childhood leukemia will have dissimilar experiences that reflect differences in the course of the illness as well as variations in medical treatment. Physicians and hospitals also have important differences in their philosophy of "managing" families who have a fatally ill member.

From the authors' observations, it is clear that certain methods of medical management facilitate family coping, while others hinder families struggling to master the consequences of leukemia in a child. For example, some physicians are vague and obscure when communicating with families concerning the diagnosis and prognosis. Others realistically describe the illness and its prognosis, but are eager to sustain hope by emphasizing possible breakthroughs in research. Still another group describes the illness realistically, but tries to focus the family's hopes on lengthy remissions during which the child may live comfortably and actively at home. The authors' experiences indicate that describing leukemia and its prognosis honestly and holding out hope of good remissions is the most helpful approach in dealing with patients and their families.

The marked differences in the medical management of families must be delineated before a demonstration program aimed at enhancing family coping with childhood leukemia can be established. However, it is possible and important at this point—without analyzing how this significant variable affects the coping process—to describe the essential factors in adaptive and maladaptive family coping with this fatal illness.

The typical experience with childhood leukemia today begins when a community physician who suspects a child of having leukemia refers that child to a medical center to confirm the diagnosis. The center usually makes this diagnostic evaluation with the child admitted as an inpatient. The family and the child (if old enough to understand the situation) await the news of the diagnosis with considerable apprehension; the parents may have received forewarning that serious illness is possible. However, the symptomatic behavior of the leukemic child prior to diagnosis rarely prepares the family adequately for the bad news to come, since the symptoms are rarely severe or frightening to the layman and may have been evident only for a short time.

Adaptive Coping

Although what physicians tell parents about the diagnosis varies considerably, it is important for both parents to understand the essential nature of the illness as early as possible, preferably before the hospital that makes the initial diagnosis discharges the child.

According to the authors' observations, in families that achieve adaptive coping, parents understand that leukemia is a serious, ultimately fatal illness involving remissions and exacerbations but moving progressively toward a terminal state. These parents often reach this understanding within a few days after the diagnosis is confirmed. They do not spend an inordinate amount of time blaming themselves or others for the illness; instead, they accept the fact that the etiology of leukemia does not seem to be related to genetic characteristics or certain patterns of child care.

These parents do not arrive at this realistic understanding of the illness and what it holds for the future without considerable anguish. As a prelude to making the necessary changes in living that the child requires, they must accept the fact that they have a chronically and seriously ill child instead of a normal one. The realization that a child until recently considered healthy is seriously ill in itself provides reason for family mourning. Furthermore, the recognition that there is neither a cure nor a good prospect of long-term survival (over five years) adds to the shock and grief these parents experience initially as they anticipate the eventual loss of their child.

Early comprehension of the consequences of a stress-producing event does not mean having detailed knowledge of what the future holds. The parents cannot know at the outset how long the child will live or what symptoms he will experience at each stage of the illness— but they should understand that since leukemia is a chronic and fatal disease, the diagnosis constitutes bad news and will involve painful losses and sacrifices for the family. The course of the illness varies with the type of leukemia; some forms have a rapid development and are short-lived, while other types continue for many years with proper treatment. The average life expectancy after diagnosis is from two to three years.

It is important for both parents to inform the family about the true nature of the illness. At the outset it is sufficient to tell all family members that the child suffers from a serious illness which will require regular and continuous medical care. Medical care is aimed at bringing the child home from the hospital.

Communicating the nature of the illness within the family leads to a period of grief that involves many if not all members. The diagnosis ushers in a phase of shared family mourning and mutual consolation that includes the leukemic child.

Those in the fields of health and social services have long known that mourning is a healthy, natural response to the news of impending loss. They realize what patients and family survivors must experience to accept fatal illness and death.[10] In the instance of childhood leukemia, each family member should have the opportunity to experience grief for current anticipated losses. This should include the leukemic child, who gathers from his hospital experience and the behavior of staff and family that he is seriously ill.

The family as a group offers its members the potential of mutual support and access to its collective coping experience. When a healthy child becomes seriously ill, all members of the family need to find comfort and solace in each other in their grief. With such support they can face losses and make the sacrifices required by severe trauma.

Mourning may extend over a long period and be an intermittent process in which family members participate. Many losses are associated with a child's serious illness—such as goals that must be postponed indefinitely or relinquished forever. Some families are able to face the inevitable outcome realistically and talk about it frankly.

> John D was the eldest of seven children, an active 12-year-old boy involved in many activities. The family was close, and Mr. D's job provided them with a reasonably good financial situation. The parents were understandably shocked when told that John had leukemia. Their initial reactions were typical of those of other parents, but they expressed their shock and grief openly and together. They understood that leukemia is a fatal illness for which there is no cure, respected and trusted the physicians, and made no attempt to seek corroborative or contradictory diagnoses from other physicians. The parents did not try to hide their feelings from each other but found strength and encouragement in grieving together.
>
> From the start, Mr. and Mrs. D knew they must talk to their son about the diagnosis. They told him he had a serious illness that most children did not survive and encouraged him to trust the physicians, who would do everything within their power to keep him as well as possible as long as they could. John and his parents were able to cry together over the implications of the illness. Mr. and Mrs. D also talked with John's 10-year-old sister about the situation, since the two children were especially close.
>
> The parents clearly wanted to be as honest as possible with John. The limited time remaining was doubly precious and was not to be wasted playing games or jeopardizing relationships. The pain of accepting their child's impending death would be even more unbearable if he turned away from them and no longer trusted them. They had never lied to him and were sure their frankness allowed them to trust, respect, and love each other.
>
> At times the family had to express feelings of sadness by crying and mourning and no one tried to inhibit this. Mr. and Mrs. D allowed John time to himself but he was always free to go back to one or both of them with questions that were bothering him. He was a remarkable child whom everyone enjoyed. He was a bright, sensitive boy who wrote a science paper on leukemia for which he received an *A*.

The D family's open discussion of survival with the child at an early stage attests to their unusual strength as a family. Not all families need to be as frank at the outset. Some may prefer merely to indicate to the child the seriousness of the diagnosis.

Maladaptive Coping

Of the families studied, 87% failed to resolved successfully even the initial tasks of coping—that is, the tasks associated with confirmation of the diagnosis. Parents' reactions vary but fall into certain recognizable classes. Their most common reaction is to deny the reality of the diagnosis in as many ways as possible. Such parents avoid those who refer to the illness as leukemia. They themselves use euphemisms (for example, virus, anemia, blood disease) in speaking of the child's illness. They may even be fearful that the child will hear the news from someone outside the family.

> Mr. and Mrs. R refused to allow anyone to tell their 8-year-old daughter what her illness was or what implications it had. When the child asked her father what was wrong, he told her not to worry—there was nothing seriously wrong—she had the gout, just as he did. One evening he called his neighbors for a meeting at which he asked them not to tell their own children that his daughter had leukemia for fear they would reveal the secret.

Reality-denying parents seek convincing reasons for their actions.

> Mr. and Mrs. H said their 15-year-old son was not emotionally strong enough to be told about his diagnosis. When the child asked his parents what was wrong, they told him he had a long-term virus but would be O.K. After the child died several months later, his best friend informed the parents that their son knew he had leukemia but cound not tell them he knew.

Parents who strongly reject facts cling to the possibility of a mistaken diagnosis and often seek other medical opinions to confirm their suspicions. Interestingly enough, parents who deny the existence of leukemia, who fight on many fronts to block out both thoughts and feelings associated with this illness, rarely deny their children the medical treatment offered for leukemia.

> Mrs. T, 24 years old, was devastated when told her 4-month-old son had leukemia. Her mother encouraged her not to accept one physician's opinion but to see others, hoping that the diagnosis was wrong. As a result, the family was almost overwhelmed by financial problems, with bills from seven physicians and two university medical centers.

In some cases these parents deny the obvious symptoms of the illness and the effects of treatment.

> The face of the once slender and attractive 4-year-old son of Mr. R became puffy and round soon after steroid treatment began. The physical change in the child

was obvious to everyone except his father. When his wife reminded him of these changes, he became angry and refused to talk to her for several days.

Often these parents take elaborate precautions to keep the child unaware of the diagnosis.

Mr. and Mrs. B insisted that their 12-year-old son be protected from knowing the nature of his illness or how serious it was. They mounted a 24-hour watch over his hospital bed, never leaving the child alone. One parent or family member was always present. The child asked his parents to explain why they never left him as other parents did.

Fear of Disaster

Such extreme precautions seem to stem from fear that the child's knowing about the illness will lead to disaster—for example, mental breakdown or suicide. Parents use this fear to justify concealing the diagnosis, but it often reflects their own inability to face the facts. One parent's open expression of fear or depression is perceived as confirming the other's worst fears and may lead to the other's repression of grief. One parent's emotion is frequently seen as "weakness," requiring the partner to inhibit expression of feeling because "someone has to be strong." The strong spouse who suppresses his own fears and grief is the one to be concerned about, not only for his sake but for the rest of the family, whose coping he jeopardizes.

Mr. and Mrs. D, although quite close, seemed to have disparate ways of handling their grief. Mr. D was an open, sensitive person who cried whenever his son had a serious exacerbation of the illness. Mrs. D was secretive about her feelings, stating that both of them could not afford to break down because there were six other children to consider.

Some parents talk about postponing grief until the illness has reached advanced stages. These parents may have severe reactions in the later phases.

Mrs. W, the mother of six children, resisted everyone's efforts to get her to express her feelings about the illness of her 4-year-old boy. Even when tears would have been appropriate, she refused to express any emotion. She rationalized the importance of remaining strong because she had to think of the other children. Because no one would promise her it would be better if she cried, Mrs. W insisted on waiting until later to cry and mourn. When her child's condition worsened, she was completely unprepared for the change. She became frantic and hysterical and required sedation. Even when her child called for her to be with him, she was so overwhelmed that she proved ineffective.

"Flights into activity" may accompany inability to grieve. Parents may try to escape from grief by becoming involved in new activities that keep them from thinking about the illness or the future—such as starting a new pregnancy, making other changes in family composition, or moving to a new home. Unfortunately, such activities increase the family's burdens and divert resources urgently needed to contend with the illness and its demands.

Hostile Reactions

Parents who refuse to accept the diagnosis occasionally display overt and massive hostility to members of the health center staff. If this lasts long, it usually evokes a counterhostility among the staff toward the family. The leukemic child is generally the chief victim of such family–staff warfare.

> Mr. and Mrs. A seldom left their child during his hospitalization. They refused to allow anyone to talk with them about his illness. Mrs. A would run away if anyone mentioned the word "leukemia." Both parents expressed great hostility toward everyone. Mr. A would curse the nurses; he refused to share pertinent information concerning his son's prior illnesses and infections with the physicians. As a result, the staff questioned his sanity.

Some families accept the diagnosis, but refuse to believe that leukemia is incurable or fatal even when the course of the illness confirms both facts. Shopping for a cure, resorting to faith healing, and placing the child on a special diet in the belief that food restriction will cure or arrest the illness are not uncommon practices among these families.

> Mr. H, a dairy farmer, refused to believe there was no cure for leukemia. He was sure the disease was transmitted to his 14-year-old son by the farm animals and therefore refused to allow the boy to eat milk products, restricting him to vegetables and grains. Mr. H also believed that iron-rich foods such as liver would enrich his son's blood. His theory involved overcoming his son's "bad blood" with "good blood."

In a few families the parents can accept the diagnosis and also can anticipate the additional care the illness will require of them. However, they fail to cope by refusing from the start to take on the actual care of the leukemic child because it is "too much for them to handle." These parents claim that they cannot help the child and should not be expected to care for him. This early abdication of parental responsibility is not to be confused with the later abdication that occurs in families only after the parents have taken care of the leukemic child for months or years.

> Mr. and Mrs. K could admit to themselves and others that their 3-year-old son had leukemia, but they could not cope with or adjust to the illness. They refused to visit the child when he was hospitalized, explaining that it was too hard on him when they left. Mrs. K claimed she was too ill to drive from their home to the hospital. Furthermore, since they couldn't take care of him when he was really sick, they didn't see why they should bother to visit him. They also refused to allow their 17-year-old son to visit the ill boy, stating that his school work would suffer and he would not be able to graduate with his class. The leukemic child was literally abandoned by his family and no appeal from the staff changed their attitude. The child became withdrawn and frightened during each hospitalization.

Discrepant Coping

However capable one parent may be in facing and resolving the issues, the family's success in coping with childhood leukemia is in jeopardy if the parents take opposing positions at an early stage of the coping process. The family's ability to manage the illness depends on successful coping by both parents in the tasks that follow diagnosis. When the parents have different emotional reactions to leukemia and when they disagree on how to define the illness, whom to discuss it with, and what to tell others about it—then the essential ingredients for failure in individual and family coping are present.

> From the time the diagnosis was confirmed, Mr. and Mrs. D had difficulty communicating with each other. Mrs. D wanted to talk with her husband about their child's illness. He insisted that nothing could be accomplished by talking or crying over the situation. He offered no support to his wife, who constantly needed and expected him to comfort her. This gap in communication and mutual support continued for over two years. Mrs. D's anger toward her husband finally became quite apparent. She was on one occasion able to receive comfort from her father, with whom she did not usually feel close, but never from her husband.

Discrepant parental reactions to the coping tasks that follow diagnosis may be responsible for (1) producing garbled and dishonest communication about the illness or preventing communication about it, (2) prohibiting and interrupting individual and collective grieving within the family, and (3) weakening family relationships precisely when they most need to be strengthened. Relationships between parents are undermined by dissatisfaction with the amount of support one gives to the other. Dishonest communication about the illness creates distrust and undermines relationships between parents and children. When parents fail to accomplish coping tasks that follow diagnosis, the net result is to compromise the family's ability to address itself to the next coping tasks, that is, preparing for and making the adaptations necessary in the siege phase of serious illness. Successful early resolution of the tasks following diagnosis is considered a most critical coping assignment because achieving further coping tasks depends on the effectiveness of this initial effort.

In the family system of reciprocal relationships, in which one function is to provide mutual assistance to members under stress members expect others in the family to help them meet their needs—whether these needs are for emotional support or assistance with family functions and labors. When one family member fails to respond to what another considers legitimate expectations under stress, the inevitable resentment and dissatisfaction that follow decrease the effectiveness of the joint effort essential for successful family coping. The parents' failure to cope successfully with the initial tasks after diagnosis largely precludes sound coping by the rest of the family.

A family must have the closest possible cooperative relations to attain the discipline it requires for living through the siege imposed by a child's serious illness. Such close relations are based on trust, honesty, and mutual support and are virtually impossible to maintain if the family fails to handle the initial coping tasks adequately.

One purpose of the authors' study was to provide the groundwork for effectively assisting at an early stage those families who experienced difficulty in coping with severe illness—specifically, childhood leukemia. Preliminary attempts have been made to correct maladaptive family responses to the diagnosis of leukemia. The following case summary is an example of early efforts to develop appropriate techniques of intervention:

> The reaction of Mr. and Mrs. S to the diagnosis of leukemia was typical of many parents. The mother recognized the seriousness of the illness and felt frightened and depressed. When she cried and sought consolation from her husband, he became angry. "What in hell are you crying about?" he asked. He refused to believe or accept the diagnosis. Mrs. S became angry with his failure to support her and they fought frequently.
>
> Peter, their 13-year-old leukemic boy, resisted treatment procedures during his first hospitalization and an early rehospitalization, loudly proclaiming that

the medication did not help and he knew he was "going to die." His parents had steadfastly refused to talk to Peter about the seriousness of his illness. When the project worker insisted, they finally consented to let the physician discuss Peter's illness with him because staff had continuing difficulty in managing him. The physician told the boy, while his mother was present, that he had a serious illness requiring continuous hospital and clinic care. Peter became upset and cried, but soon was less agitated. Just before his mother left the ward, he asked her to lean over so he could whisper to her. He threw his arms around her and they both sobbed bitterly. Then Peter said, "I'm all right now. You can go home." His mother, after a day or two, expressed pleasure that she and Peter were close once again. She was relieved that she no longer had to evade his questions or lie to him about his illness. He told her he now understood why she and his father were worried about him and why she cried. She had thought she had successfully concealed her worry and tears from him.

This case illustrates one method of reopening the clarifying communication in families whose members refuse to talk honestly with one another about leukemia. It is also clear that since coping is a family problem, coping tasks cannot be successfully resolved if key family figures are not included. In this instance, the reopening of family communication did not involve the father and an adolescent sister. After the boy died, the sister refused to go near his room. The family had to sell the house and move to a new home. These omissions limited the success of this interventive effort.

Guidelines

Certain guidelines for clinical management can be outlined at this point on the basis of the limited research data available. The following principles were derived from the authors' study findings, plus consultation with a physician who had broad clinical experience.*

1. The successful management of the seriously ill child and his family is based on a trusting relationship with the physician treating the child. The psychiatrist is not a practical alternate for the physician, although he may serve as a consultant. Social workers, nurses, technicians, and other health and social service personnel who may be available can help deal with these problems, but they cannot take over for the physician.

* The authors discussed clinical management of the leukemic child and his family with Dr. Dane Prugh, Department of Pediatrics, University of Colorado Medical Center.

2. Perhaps the most important function the physician or social worker can fulfill is to share the anguish, the grief, and the fears of these families without "turning them off." Listening without offering false hope is essential. Giving them long, intellectual descriptions of disease processes and chemotherapy alone is of small value.

3. The parents' denial of the significance of the illness is natural at the outset; however, persistent denial lasting for weeks and months should be probed gently but persistently. Sources of denial such as guilt may be mentioned to them as natural feelings. That the physician and the social worker can face the bad news with them offers the parents the hope that they can somehow survive the child's death.

4. Since families often must endure years of siege with a leukemic child, it is important to help them conserve their energies and resources for the long haul. Physicians and social workers should anticipate and discourage common family reactions that lead to such flights into activity as early pregnancy, divorce, remarriage, and changing jobs or residence. The most useful advice to families contemplating these activities is "Don't just do something, stand there." Each additional major change adds stress to an already overloaded circuit.

Appointments with the parents after the child's death are extremely valuable in assessing whether the family is managing adequately or needs additional help. All members of the family should be considered at that time since all are vulnerable as a result of the leukemic experience. Unresolved problems of grief are not uncommon long after the death of the child. The physician or social worker can help resolve problems of grief by indicating that such reactions are normal and that mourning often takes months to complete.

References

1. Vincent, C. E. Mental health and the family. *Journal of Marriage and the Family* (February) 1967, 22–28.
2. Caplan, G. *Principles of preventive psychiatry.* New York: Basic Books, 1964. Pp. 39–54.
3. Rapoport, L. The concept of prevention in social work. *Social Work,* 6 (January) 1961, 3–12.
4. Bozeman M. F. et al. Psychological impact of cancer and its treatment, III: The adaptation of mothers to the threatened loss of their children through leukemia, Part I. *Cancer* 8 (January-February) 1955, 1–20; and Maurice B. Hamovitch,

The parent and the fatally ill child. Duarte, California: City of Hope Medical Center, 1964.

5. Binger, C. M. et al. Childhood leukemia: Emotional impact on patient and family. *New England Journal of Medicine* (February 20) 1969, 414–417.

6. Bozeman, M. F. et al. Psychological impact of cancer and its treatment, III. The adaptation of mothers to the threatened loss of their children through leukemia, Part I. *Cancer* **8** (January–February) 1955, 12.

7. Friedman, S. B. et al., Behavioral observations on parents anticipating the death of a child. In Robert I. Noland (Ed.), *Counseling parents of the ill and the handicapped.* Springfield, Illinois: Charles C. Thomas, 1971. P. 453.

8. Kaplan, D. M. Observations on crisis theory and practice. *Social Casework,* **49** (March) 1968, 151–155.

9. Glasser, P., & Glasser, L. (Eds.). *Families in crisis.* New York: Harper & Row, 1969. Pp. 273–290.

10. Lindemann, E. Symptomatology and management of acute grief. *American Journal of Psychiatry,* **101** (September) 1944, 1–11.

IV

The Crisis of Illness: Cardiovascular Disease

Traditionally the functioning of the heart has been equated with life itself. Because of this special association a serious disruption of cardiovascular functions can pose a significant threat emotionally as well as physically. The reciprocal impact of the emotional state on the cardiovascular system adds yet another dimension to complicate the problem. The sudden onset of a heart attack or stroke, or the decision to undergo major open-heart surgery, can create a psychological crisis for the patient and for his or her family as well.

In the initial period after a myocardial infarction (MI) or heart attack has occurred, the primary reaction is one of intense anxiety. Coronary patients commonly deal with this anxiety through various forms of denial. Some people use denial in a maladaptive way when they first experience frightening symptoms like chest pains or breathlessness. Either they try to ignore the symptoms or they attribute them to some ailment less threatening than a heart attack, such as indigestion. In this way they are able to control their anxiety, but at a cost of delay in receiving medical attention in a situation where delay can be fatal.

During the acute period while the MI patient faces the threat of sudden death, he must remain totally passive. The severe physical restriction, necessitated by monitoring and body maintenance equipment, compounds the sense of helplessness and frustration. Because of the influence of emotions like anxiety and frustration on cardiac functioning, some doctors maintain that in the early stages of hospitalization denial is an effective protective device. In the high-tension atmosphere of an intensive care or coronary care unit (for more on these special environments see part VII) the patient who ignores or denies the diagnosis of myocardial infarct, who shuts out the risk of sudden death, or who minimizes his discomfort or his fear, may get through the crisis period more easily.[4] Intervention by those caring for MI patients can include measures to alleviate anxiety (such as giving information on what to expect and clarifying misconceptions), to provide orientation in the CCU, and to reinforce the patient's sense of competence by letting him participate in his own care.[3]

Once the patient has survived the acute period, he must anticipate a convalescence lasting several weeks to several months. In the first article Howard Wishnie, Thomas Hackett, and Ned Cassem discuss the stresses encountered in post-MI convalescence and the importance of adequate preparation and support. The shift from the security of hospital care to home convalescence in itself causes some patients to be anxious. In addition, those who were active and in relative good health just prior to the attack are often surprised and dismayed to discover how weak they are when they try to move about at home. General (often vague) instructions by the doctor about permissible exercise, diet, and so forth, are a source of frustration and conflict for the convalescent and his family. Family members, especially spouses, tend to be overly protective and restrictive in interpreting these instructions, hovering over and attempting to control patients who feel increasingly humiliated and resentful. The authors suggest several ways by which staff can alleviate these stresses and facilitate the coping process during convalescence, e.g., providing careful explanations of the likelihood of feeling weak and uncertain to prepare the patient and relieve his anxiety, and formulating an explicit program of mental and physical activity. Medical care-givers must also give practical advice on methods by which well-intentioned patients could alter initial risk factors like obesity, smoking or drinking (e.g., mutual support groups, behavior modification programs).

The development of open-heart surgical techniques has brought some hope of significant relief to people with debilitating heart disease or structural defects. Those who elect this life-saving surgery must also face some risk of dying, either during the operation or shortly thereafter. The period immediately after open-heart surgery is often critical, and the emotional state of the patient (as with MI) can be a significant factor in the recovery process. The second article discusses a study in which Chase Kimball divided people undergoing open-heart surgery into four adaptive types on the basis of preoperative interviews. He found that patients showing considerable anxiety or depression preoperatively had a greater risk of dying during the surgery and a greater morbidity after surgery than others who had been able to manage their anxiety and maintain a hopeful future orientation. Other studies of general surgery patients have also found significant relationships between preoperative anxiety levels and postoperative physical and emotional outcome.[1,5] These findings demonstrate the possibility and the importance of strategic professional intervention, particularly among those who are identified as coping poorly with the crisis at hand.

The emotional state and psychological resources of the individuals have also been related to the common phenomenon of postoperative delirium among cardiac patients. Lazarus and Hagens[6] suggest there are three sets of contributing factors: the preoperative psychological state of the patient, the CCU or ICU environment (such as the monotony and the interruption of sleep), and the surgical procedure (for example, the time on the heart–lung machine). Preoperative efforts to provide reassurance and support, and postoperative nursing procedures designed to reorient the patient to time and place, have been shown to decrease the incidence and duration of this delirium.

While a cerebrovascular accident, or stroke, does not have the same symbolic significance as illnesses affecting the heart directly, it is similar to a heart attack in the suddenness of its onset, in its life-threatening seriousness, in the restricted physical activity of the acute period, in the long convalescence, and in the threat of recurrence. Unlike heart attacks, though, the effects of a stroke—weakness, paralysis, speech difficulties—can be quite noticeable. For C. Scott Moss,[7] aphasia (speech and thought disturbance) was the primary residual effect of his stroke, but it necessitated significant adjustments in his personal life and his professional life as a psychologist. Espmark[2] has described several common coping strategies used by stroke patients, such as suppression (a conscious effort to keep busy and distracted from the central problems), rationalization (making up more tolerable explanations for situations which seem unacceptable), avoidance (refusing to acknowledge any need for medical care), and projection (attribution of disturbing feelings to someone else). People sometimes deal with their temporary loss of independence by regression (giving in to their desire to be taken care of), or, at the other extreme, by a pseudoindependence and hostility toward their caretakers.

For a successful adjustment the stroke victim must mourn his losses, deal with his fears, and rebuild his life taking into account the changes in his circumstances. In the third article Judith D'Afflitti and Wayne Weitz describe their experiences with discussion groups organized for stroke patients and their families. They divide the grieving process into three stages. The initial reaction is shock ("How could this happen so fast?"), which is commonly handled by denying the sudden stress or the possibility of serious consequences (for example, "It can't be real" or "Soon I'll be good as new."). In the second stage, as the extent of damage becomes clearer and the patient becomes more aware of all the ramifications of the stroke, feelings of grief and anger tend to surface. Family members must also deal with their feelings of resentment toward the one who is ill and their guilt over these feelings.

The third phase is a time of restitution and resolution. Patients reminisce about former good times and begin to define and accept the limits their stroke disabilities will place on future activities. Oredai and Waite[8] have also reported the use of reminiscence by stroke patients and the citing of famous people who overcame similar handicaps. Group members offer one another support throughout the different stages, sharing feelings and practical information. Gradually patients gain self-assurance and begin to reintegrate an acceptable self-image.

References

1. Cohen, F., & Lazarus, R. S. Active coping processes, coping dispositions, and recovery from surgery. *Psychosomatic Medicine*, 1973, **35**, 375–389.
2. Espmark, S. Stroke before 50: A follow-up study of vocational and psychological adjustment. *Scandanavian Journal of Rehabilitation Medicine* 1973, **2**(Suppl.): 1–107.
3. Foster, S., & Andreoli, K. G. Behavior following acute myocardial infarction. *American Journal of Nursing*. 1970, **70**, 2344–2348.
4. Gentry, W. D., Foster, S., & Haney, T. Denial as a determinant of anxiety and perceived health status in the coronary care unit. *Psychosomatic Medicine*, 1972, **34**, 39–44.
5. Janis, I. L. *Psychological stress*. New York: Wiley, 1958.
6. Lazarus, H. R., & Hagens, J. H. Prevention of psychosis following open-heart surgery. *American Journal of Psychiatry*, 1968, **124**, 1190–1195.

7. Moss, C. S. *Recovery with aphasia: The aftermath of my stroke.* Urbana, Illinois: University of Illinois Press, 1972.

8. Oredai, D. M., & Waite, N. S. Group psychotherapy with stroke patients during the immediate recovery phase. *American Journal of Orthopsychiatry,* 1974, **44,** 386–395.

8

Psychological Hazards of Convalescence Following Myocardial Infarction

HOWARD A. WISHNIE, THOMAS P. HACKETT, and NED H. CASSEM

Three decades ago physicians commonly imposed a six-month convalescence upon patients recovering from myocardial infarction (MI). Since that time recommendations have undergone a liberal transformation. Not only has "early mobilization" become the aim for patients with an uncomplicated hospital course,[1] but those discharged are now expected to return to normal activities and employment much earlier than ever before. Indeed, for asymptomatic patients with uncomplicated coronary disease, Friedberg permits resumption of occupation after six weeks of convalescence.[2] Despite these liberal trends, there is a growing body of evidence to show that at least half the patients permitted to return to work are reluctant to do so and remain inactive for a prolonged period.[3-10] If capable of work, why should a patient procrastinate? A number of authors have indicated psychosocial factors such as

HOWARD A. WISHNIE, M.D. • Assistant Professor of Psychiatry, Harvard Medical School, Cambridge, Massachusetts. This investigation was supported by Public Health Service contract PHS-43-67-1443 from the National Institutes of Health.

Reprinted from *Journal of the American Medical Association,* 1971, **215,** (8), 1292–1296. Copyright 1971, the American Medical Association.

fear of recurrent infarction, anxiety, and depression.[5-8,11,12] In a more recent comprehensive review, Miller and Brewer[11] classify factors which influence progress in rehabilitation and cite psychological problems as heavy contributors to delayed convalescence.

The most complete and detailed account of the psychological hazards of cardiac rehabilitation is that of Alan Wynn.[6] He found that unwarranted emotional distress and invalidism were present in half of the 400 patients he studied. In most of the patients who remained unemployed for more than six months, the major reason was psychosocial and might have been averted with proper management. Furthermore, nearly half of the 107 patients who remained unemployable were disabled by psychiatric problems which Wynn also regarded as preventable.

The present report is an extension of an earlier study on the psychological hazards of the Coronary Care Unit (CCU).[13] We followed our original patients after their discharge from the hospital in an effort to identify and investigate sources of emotional distress in convalescence. Our observations corroborate Wynn's findings and emphasize remediable shortcomings in patient management during cardiac rehabilitation. Based upon our data suggestions are offered for improving the psychological difficulties of this period.

Methods and Materials

All patients initially had been seen by one of the investigators in the CCU. From the original population of 50 patients, 24 were available for followup. Of the remainder, 11 had died, 4 had left the area, 1 had a change of diagnosis, and 10 were unable or unwilling to cooperate.

In the 24 cases under consideration there were 18 males with a median age of 59.9 years and 6 females with a median age of 58.4 years. All were lower-middle-class in background. Sixteen were interviewed at home and 18 were seen with the families present. The interviews averaged 1 hour and 15 minutes and took place between three and nine months after discharge; they were tape-recorded with the patient's permission.

Findings

Physical and Mental Status

Although each of the 24 patients was eager to go home, 11 felt totally unprepared for the physical limitations they experienced, 9 recalled wishing they were back in the hospital during their first week at home. The most common complaint was weakness. Twenty were distressed by it, 14 to a degree they had not anticipated. Ten interpreted weakness as a harbinger of cardiac decline. A typical example is that of a 39-year-old teacher who did very well following his MI until he returned home. In his words: "I felt great in the hospital. No matter what anyone told me I pictured myself breaking records getting back to work. The first week home I could hardly walk the length of the house without feeling exhausted. I felt like a cooked goose, like I was done for. It took another two weeks before I started to feel better."

Twenty-one patients rated themselves as anxious or depressed or both during the first month at home. Their families concurred and, in 10 instances, added "unstable" to the description. This usually meant irritable and quick to take offense. In nine patients his mood alteration persisted for several months. Through a combination of anxiety and anger one patient ground through a new set of dentures. Another developed a foot-and-finger-tapping habit that continued for months after his successful return to work. By and large these convalescent personality traits were exacerbations of premorbid tendencies and did not arise from the illness itself. As one spouse phrased it, "He was always selfish, even before his heart attack. We used to call him a bear. Now we call him a brute."

Activities

Twenty-three patients spontaneously complained of feeling frustrated at being inactive during the first months at home. Six engaged in mild physical exercise (walking), which was planned by the physician in only two cases. The other 17 spent their time puttering about the house or watching TV. Only 3 were able to turn to hobbies for relaxation. All felt the lack of structure in their lives when unable to work and claimed they had been altogether unprepared for the sense of foundering which resulted.

Sleep

Sleep was characterized as disturbed if the patient had trouble fall-ing asleep or awoke regularly for reasons other than pain or bathroom needs. Fifteen patients had disturbed sleep which lasted weeks to several months after discharge. Eleven patients stated spontaneously that they thought about their hearts before going to sleep. Six had persistent insomnia and seven admitted they feared the possibility of death during sleep. One woman regularly reported anginal pain upon getting into bed and waiting for sleep to come. Nocturnal preoccupation with heart function accompanied by some degree of insomnia persisted for months after MI in all 11 cases.

Habits

Of the 14 patients who resolved to stop smoking, 9 failed to keep their resolutions. Seven out of 9 patients who determined to lose weight failed to do so, and 5 out of 6 patients who vowed to stop drinking alcohol failed in the attempt.

Return to Work

Thirteen of the 24 patients successfully returned to work either part or full time. Of these, 5 disclosed the fear of sustaining another MI because of work stress; 3 others experienced increasing bouts of angina, dyspnea or both during the two weeks preceding the return. These symptoms abated once the patient was established in his job.

Eleven patients did not return to work. Of these, five used their heart attacks as reason to retire. Two went back for one day, but both became so frightened they chose to retire prematurely at considerable financial sacrifice. Another was stricken with a second MI during con-valescence and still another with a cardiovascular accident. The tenth, a housewife, took up domestic duties, but on a diminished scale. The eleventh patient was so incapacitated by anxiety she would not consider returning to work.

Correlating the seriousness of the patient's illness with whether or not he returned to work revealed a less positive relationship than one would expect. Of those patients under retirement age (65 years), the most seriously ill, as determined by the Peel score, were working part time. Those who were employed full time had Peel scores averaging only four points lower than part time workers.

Family Conflicts

Eighteen of the 24 patients had families with whom they resided. Nine of the 24 had a major alteration in living plans as the result of their heart attack. Four were forced to sell their homes. Three had to live elsewhere during convalescence. Two others had to make drastic relocations within their homes.

A steady, eroding conflict over the implications of the illness was noted in all 18 families. In 11 there was marked controversy over the specific meaning of the physician's instructions. Vague terms, such as *use in moderation, a few times a day,* and *use your own discretion,* were seized upon by family and patient and interpreted in an entirely personal way. Arguments resulted, the manifest content of which centered about the patient's activity, diet, and "nervousness."

All of the 18 families interviewed demonstrated significant anxiety about the patient's recuperation and their role in promoting or retarding the process. In 13 families the anxiety was exaggerated and disproportionate to the patient's current degree of disability. These families attempted to shield the patient from all unpleasant information and physical exercise. The patients resented this attitude and spoke of it as humiliating.

The wives in particular tended to overprotect their husbands in an aggressive way. They felt guilty at having been somehow instrumental in the genesis of the heart attack and were frustrated at being unable to express grievances and anger lest such action bring on another MI. Their solicitousness often took on a punitive quality which was thought to represent an indirect expression of suppressed anger. It had a deleterious effect on marriage as demonstrated by the following example. A patient was describing a medication and started to get up to fetch a pill box within five feet of his chair. His wife, who was seated far across the room leapt to her feet, exclaiming, "Wait now, let me get it for your dear. You know the doctor doesn't want you to get up more than you have to." He was months into convalescence and was doing well. His response was to bolt angrily from his chair and thrust the box of pills at the investigator while gazing sullenly at his wife.

These conflicts between patient and family occurred even when the marriage and premorbid home life had been quite stable. Although long-standing marital problems tended to worsen after MI, particularly when they involved dependency/independency issues, those described in this presentation are predominantly interpersonal friction. They largely hinge on misunderstanding the nature of coronary disease and on misinterpreting the physician's orders.

Doctor–Patient Relationship

Physician's Orders. Eight of the 24 meticulously adhered to their physician's instructions. This exaggerated compliance correlated positively with the presence of overt anxiety and depression. The families of all 8 described the postinfarction behavior of each as overly cautious and strongly motivated by fear. Two patients consistently disregarded physician's orders while the remaining 14 tended to comply with instruction although with some indiscretions.

Follow-up Care. Patients were slow to complain about symptoms during office visits. Seven failed to report troublesome insomnia; five deliberately denied nervousness and irritability and three consciously withheld information about overexerting and overeating. Two patients neglected to mention increases in anginal pain. The excuse given, in all of the above instances, was that the doctor failed to ask the specific question.

Medication. Eighteen of the 24 patients were judged by the investigator to require a tranquilizer or antidepressant. This opinion was based upon the following factors: (1) patient's undisguised complaint of fear, apprehension, anxiety, or depression; (2) bodily agitation such as pacing, sweating, finger tapping, and hand or foot tremor during interview; (3) insomnia and inability to relax during the day; and (4) despondency and emotional lability as related by family. Eleven of the 18, while acknowledging the need for medication, refused to ask their physicians for it or to take sedatives already in their possession because they feared "getting hooked on pills." The remaining 7, while admitting fear or depression or both, did not want to discuss it with either the investigator or their physicians because emotions were equated with weakness and lack of virility.

Comment

Klein's finding that anxiety mounts and catecholamine excretion increases markedly on the day of transfer from the CCU underlines the significance of transitions in the treatment of MI.[14] If the passage from an intensive care setting to a convalescent unit occasions such psychological alarm, then certainly the change from hospital to home can be expected to posit stress of equal or greater magnitude. Patients seldom foresee the problems that convalescence will present and whatever reservations they have about leaving the protective custody of the hospital become dwarfed at the anticipated joy of homecoming. The physician himself is apt to underestimate the importance of losing the security intensive care provides; furthermore, he may not fully appreciate the hardship of adhering to a cardiac regimen and the rigors of rehabilitation.

Our findings indicate that most patients in early convalescence suffer from anxiety, depression, a feeling of physical weakness, insomnia, and ennui. Moreover, few of them succeed in altering habits that might adversely influence their coronary disease. Nearly half failed to return to work. Those who succeeded did so despite apprehension about another heart attack or increased angina or dyspnea or both. These results agree with those of investigators already cited.[3,7,8,11,12] The high incidence of intrafamily conflict and quarreling has not been specifically noted before although Adsett and Bruhn[13] called attention to the fact that the wives of patients with coronary disease suffered marked inhibition in the expression of hostility. The tendency of the postcoronary patient to minimize symptoms and deny emotional troubles during follow-up visits with his physician has not, to our knowledge, been reported before.

Since the population under study is small and predominantly lower middle class and was followed in the outpatient clinic by house officers, one might argue that it is not a representative model for coronary convalescence across the country. Even though each patient was followed by the physician who had treated him in the hospital, the doctor–patient relation was probably not as close as would be the case if the patient had had a family physician. In the latter instance the patient might be better informed at the time of discharge and the family would almost certainly be included in the planning. Also a private physician would probably pay more attention to the patient's emotional well-being. As a consequence, convalescence might not be as uncertain and trying as we have described. However, since a recent study of ours comparing white-collar with blue-collar responses in a CCU has demonstrated surprisingly little difference in the emotional reaction patterns of these two groups to the early stages of coronary illness, we are by no means sure that convalescence will prove an exception.

Despite the small number of patients in this series and a disproportionate representation of blue-collar families, the fact remains that our
findings agree with those of other investigators working with different
populations. As information on cardiac convalescence accumulates there
will undoubtedly be differences between the responses of one group
against another. However, the principal message of this communication
is simply to underscore the fact that a large number of patients with
coronary disease undergo more psychological distress during rehabilitation than is warranted.

On the basis of the data presented, a few suggestions for management can be offered. First, prepare the patient for feeling weak, fearful,
and uncertain when he returns home. By anticipating the homecoming
response in this way and explaining that it does not reflect a more
serious impairment of the heart, the physician can save his patient
unnecessary anguish. Telephone contact at regular intervals during each
convalescence is often reassuring. A call to the patient's home to answer
those questions that could not have been asked before discharge was
found to be of great help with our patients. A program of mental and
physical activity should be set up with the patient and his wife in which
the exact amount of exercise and work requiring mental concentration is
spelled out. Avoid vague terms which place the responsibility for deciding what is correct on the patient or spouse. Wives should be cautioned
against totally suppressing appropriate annoyance or anger as these
responses may emerge in the guise of zealous overprotection, among
others, and cause more disruption than in the original form.

A regimen of hypnotic drugs should be ordered for the first month
just as though a sleep disturbance existed. Minor tranquilizers should
also be given routinely during this period. In order to insure the control
of anxiety the physician should sanction the use of tranquilizers by
emphasizing the importance of being calm and by awarding these agents
the same status as cardiac drugs. Finally, it is good for the physician to
remind himself that the successful adaptation to coronary disease often
requires that the habits of a lifetime be altered. The pleasures of bed,
board, and bar must yield to the alien and often unwanted edicts of
restraint and moderation. Few of us are able to change our life-styles
without becoming angry, sad, and bad-tempered. There are ways of
reducing the sting of deprivation through substitute gratifications, the
use of comparable alternatives, and psychoactive drugs. We would
probably enjoy more success in the pruning of bad habits as well as in

the redirecting of misguided, deleterious behavior if more use were made of these methods.

The problems of return to work and family conflict require far more investigation. We mention them because they add emphasis to the important insight of Sir James Spence: "If clinical research is to be used to get the full picture of disease, it must equip itself to carry observations beyond the hospital."[16] The CCU itself has probably exhausted most of its possibilities for mortality reduction in acute MI. With this realization a great deal of attention has been given to the prehospital phase.[17,18] However, it is becoming increasingly clear that no program for the reduction of morbidity and mortality in patients with coronary heart disease will be complete until the difficulties of the posthospital phase are attacked as well.

Before these problems can be solved, mass attitudes may have to be changed toward the recuperative potential, employability, and reliability of postinfarction patients. Other resources have already been effectively used in the form of rehabilitation centers.[3,6,7,10] and group therapy for patients alone or with their wives.[15] All these means are growing in importance. Yet it is our belief that the most basic help must come from the personal physician who will anticipate these problems prior to discharge, discuss them thoroughly with the patient, and remain accessible and supportive throughout the rehabilitation period.

References

1. Early mobilization after myocardial infarction, editorial. *Lancet* **1**:821, 1969.
2. Friedberg, C. K. *Diseases of the heart.* Philadelphia: W. B. Saunders, 1966. Pp 922.
3. Gobel, A. J., Adey, G. M., & Bullen, J. F. Rehabilitation of the cardiac patient. *Medical Journal of Australia* **2**:975–979, 1963.
4. Wincott, E. A., & Caird, F. I. Return to work after myocardial infarction. *British Medical Journal* **2**:1302–1304, 1966.
5. Weinblatt, E. et al. Return to work and work status following first myocardial infarction. *American Journal of Public Health* **56**:169–185, 1966.
6. Wynn, A. Unwarranted emotional distress in men with ischaemic heart disease (IHD). *Medical Journal of Australia* **2**:847–851, 1967.
7. Kellerman, J.J., Levy, M. et al. Rehabilitation of coronary patients. *Journal of Chronic Diseases* **20**:815–821, 1967.
8. Groden, B. M. Return to work after myocardial infarction. *Scottish Medical Journal* **12**:297–301, 1967.

9. Klein, R. F., Dean, A., & Willson, I. M. et al. The physician and postmyocardial infarction invalidism. *JAMA* **194:**143–148, 1965.
10. Aldes, J. H., Stein, S. P., & Grabin, S. A program to effect vocational restoration of "unemployable" cardiac cases. *Diseases of the Chest* **54:**518–522, 1958.
11. Miller, G. M., & Brewer, J. Factors influencing the rehabilitation of the patient with ischaemic heart disease. *Medical Journal of Australia* **1:**410–416, 1969.
12. Birock, G. Social and psychological problems in patients with chronic cardiac illness. *American Heart Journal* **58:**414–417, 1959.
13. Hackett, T. P., Cassem, N. H., & Wishnie, H. A. The coronary care unit: An appraisal of its psychological hazards. *New England Journal of Medicine* **279:**1365–1370, 1968.
14. Klein, R. F. et al. Transfer from a coronary care unit: Some adverse responses. *Archives of Internal Medicine* **122:**104–108, 1968.
15. Adsett, C. A., & Bruhn, J. G. Short term group psychotherapy for postmyocardial infarction patients and their wives. *Canadian Medical Association Journal* **99:**577–584, 1968.
16. Julian, D. G. *Acute myocardial infarction.* Baltimore: Williams & Wilkins Co, 1968.
17. Bethesda conference report: Early care for the acute coronary suspect. *American Journal of Cardiology* **23:**603–618, 1969.
18. Goldstein, S., & Moss, A. J., (Ed). Symposium on the pre-hospital phase of acute myocardial infarction: Part I. *American Journal of Cardiology* **24:**609–688, 1969.

9

Psychological Responses to the Experience of Open-Heart Surgery

CHASE PATTERSON KIMBALL

Since heart surgery was first performed in the early 1950s, the incidence of postoperative emotional reactions and long-term readjustment problems has been noted to be greater and perhaps different in kind from responses to other types of surgery. This phenomenon has been the subject of several reviews,[19] and many authors have focused their attention on one aspect or another of the surgical experience in an attempt to delineate factors involved in these responses.

Untoward responses to surgery, not directly related to the technology of the procedure, have long been noted to occur with greater frequency following specific operations. Lindemann[22] and Hollender[14] have described high incidences of "rage" and depressive reactions in patients undergoing hysterectomies. Weisman and Hackett[30] have discussed a specific "black-patch delirium" in patients following cataract removal. Other investigators[4,32] have noted specific reactions to surgical orchidectomy and mastectomy. Janis[15] has considered preoperative

CHASE PATTERSON KIMBALL, M.D. • Professor of Psychiatry and Medicine, University of Chicago, Chicago, Illinois. This study was supported in part by Public Health Service grants MH-7228 and MH-11668 from the National Institute of Mental Health and grant 68-778 from the American Heart Association.

Reprinted from *American Journal of Psychiatry,* September 1969, **126**, 348–359. Copyright 1969, the American Psychiatric Association. Reprinted by permission.

anxiety as a factor determining postoperative response whereas Knox[20] emphasized preoperative life-styles as a guide to predicting long-term postoperative adjustment. Kornfeld[21] stressed the postoperative environment as a determinant of psychological adjustment.

The present report, derived from a larger study,[18] is concerned with the observation and description of patients undergoing open-heart surgery and their responses to this procedure up to 15 months later.

Method and Materials

Fifty-four adult patients consecutively admitted for open-heart surgery in two periods (April to July 1966 and October 1966 to March 1967) were interviewed on the day prior to surgery. The investigator identified himself as a member of the cardiopulmonary team who was specifically interested in determining some of the experiences of patients undergoing surgery and in following them during their hospitalization and periodically thereafter. The investigator suggested that it was necessary to get to know the patient better and to find out what his life and disease course had been.

The interviews, lasting 45 to 90 minutes, were conducted in an open-ended, nondirective manner after a method developed by the psychiatric–medical liaison group at the University of Rochester.[6,7,16,26,28] The interview material was either written up as recalled by the interviewer (16 cases) or recorded on tape (38 cases). Subsequent to the interviews, the data were reviewed with the purpose of identifying the following: (1) the presence or absence of anxiety, how it was manifested and handled, and whether it was expressed or denied; (2) the "life-style" of the individual, the adequacy of his ability to handle other "life crises," and the adequacy of his handling of the stresses of the imminent operation; (3) the patient's orientation to the future, his expectation of surgery, and his anticipation of goals, future roles, and relationships.

On the basis of these items, it was possible to set up several groups that could subsequently be used to correlate with postoperative responses.

Postoperative observations and responses were made on a daily basis. These contacts, which lasted from 5 to 30 minutes, included unobtrusive observation of the patient as he was attended by the staff, an evaluation of his mental status, and an attempt to obtain a verbal description of how he was feeling. In addition to these primary data, notes and records were reviewed, the nursing and medical staffs were consulted, and relatives were often interviewed in an attempt to obtain a comprehensive perspective of the patient's reactions.

Prior to the patient's departure from the hospital, he was interviewed at greater length to learn how he felt about the experience in retrospect. Thereafter, most of the patients were followed at the time of checkup visits to the cardiac clinic at 1- to 3-month intervals up to 15 months. At these times 20- to 30-minute interviews assessed the adjustment the patient was making, his physical status, and his general resolution of the operative and hospitalization experience.

Eight patients were observed in greater depth and over a longer period of time. Three were seen postoperatively in short-term intensive psychotherapy because of emotional problems that were intensified by the surgical experience. One patient was seen for many weeks before and after surgery for exploration of long-standing emotional problems. Four patients were seen for many weeks before and after hospitalization on the rehabilitation unit where they had been referred because of neurological complications. One patient was seen on the psychiatric unit following rehospitalization for treatment of a depression.

Initially, the study was conducted in two parts. A preliminary investigation of 16 patients was done in the spring of 1966. The data from these interviews were analyzed, and correlations were made between postoperative responses and preoperative assessments. At this time the work of other investigators was reviewed. In the fall of 1966 a second series of 38 patients was interviewed and followed along modified lines developed on the basis of a review of the methods originally employed. These patients were grouped as indicated in the next section, prior to surgery. For the purposes of this report, the data from the two series are combined. Demographic and illness characteristics are recorded in Tables I and II and are discussed in another paper.[18]

Results

Groups

On the basis of the preoperative interview, four groups were identified. Statistics relating to these groups are included in Table III.

Table I.   Demographic Characteristics ($N = 54$)

Characteristic	Number
Age (years)	
Range	18–72
Average	45
Median	46
Sex	
Female	33
Male	21
Race	
White American	38
First-generation American	13
Immigrant	2
Negro southern-born American	1
Religion	
Protestant	36
Catholic	17
Jewish	1
Current marital status	
Married	42
Single	1
Divorced	8
Widowed	3
Social class	
Professional	4
Blue-collar	6
Skilled	5
Semiskilled	22
Unskilled	17
Education	
Grade school or less	16
High school, 2 years or less	15
High school graduate	15
College or technical school, 2 years or less	4
College graduate	3
Graduate professional school	1

Group I ("Adjusted").   This group comprised patients whose general level of functioning in the past, in the immediate period preceding the hospitalization, and at the time of surgery was assessed to be intact, purposeful, and realistic. In general, the patients had coped adequately or successfully with previous life stresses including their cardiac disease. Business and domestic affairs had been successfully conducted. Surgery was viewed as desirable, necessary, and potentially life-saving. Usually these patients were able to express a moderate uneasiness, fear, or anxiety about the procedure, but their defenses to cope with these apprehensions appeared adequate and intact. They did not deny the

Table II.   Illness Characteristics of 54 Patients

Characteristic	Number
Valvular lesion	
Rheumatic	
Mitral	32
Aortic	13
Mitral/aortic	3
Mitral/tricuspid	2
Congenital	
Atrial septal defect	2
Aortic	2
Age at initial episode of rheumatic fever	
Under 12	24
Illness like rheumatic fever, under 12	6
12–22	6
Adult	2
Other:	
Rheumatic fever not known or remembered	12
Nonrheumatic congenital lesions	4
Previous cardiac surgery	
1 closed commissurotomy	11
2 closed commissurotomies	2
1 open valvulotomy	2
1 closed commissurotomy, 1 open valvulotomy	4
Total	19
Other illnesses	
None	31
Episodic: Cholelithiasis	7
Hysterectomy	6
Appendectomy	3
Total	16
Chronic: Schizophrenic	2
Conversion	2
Duodenal ulcer	1
Arthritis	1
Idiopathic thrombocytopenia	1
Total	7

Table III. Characteristics of Groups

Postoperative-period characteristic	Group				
	"Adjusted" I 13	"Symbiotic" II 15	"Anxious" III 12	"Depressed" IV 14	Total 54
Early					
Unremarkable	6	5	0	4	15
Catastrophic	2	3	6	2	13
Euphoric	1	4	1	1	7
Altered states of consciousness	3	3	2	1	9
Dead	1	0	3	6	10
Intermediate					
Phase I, anxiety	0	0	4	2	6
Phase II, general reaction	12	15	9	8	44
Phase II, complication	2	6	3	3	14
Dead	0	0	0	2	2
Posthospital (3–15-month follow-up)					
Improved	9	1	3	1	14
Unchanged	3	8	3	2	16
Worse	0	5	2	1	8
Dead	0	1	1	3	5
Total Dead	1	1	4	11	17

possibility of their dying at the time of surgery. However, they expressed confidence that the surgery would not only be successful but would also enable them to pursue carefully identified objectives and plans in the future.

These patients expressed many object relationships in their past and present life and looked forward to the fulfillment and continuation of these after surgery. These relationships included continuing and fulfilling role functions or jobs, carrying on meaningful relationships with spouses and/or children, plans for trips, and other forms of pleasure. While manifesting some apprehension, these patients appeared confident, controlled, and direct in expressing their feelings regarding the operation as well as in reviewing their life and disease histories.

Group II ("Symbiotic"). These patients had "adapted to" their illness state and were living in a "symbiotic" relationship to it on the basis of secondary gains achieved usually over a lifetime of illness. In their past life they had demonstrated considerable dependence on a parent that often had been transferred onto a spouse. There was a high incidence of failure to separate from a parent, as seen in the need of many of these patients for a continuing close relationship with a mother or father. Many demonstrated unresolved grief of many years' duration for a deceased parent. Cardiac decompensations and, where traceable, the onset of the initial episode of rheumatic fever could be correlated with major stressful life situations (e.g., loss of a parent, spouse, or child; marriage; change of life).

In this group cardiac symptoms were experienced in situations where the patient felt threatened. These patients looked to the operation as a means of maintaining a status quo that may have been recently threatened. They did not view the future as holding anything different for them from the present or the past. They stressed the need for a long recovery period during which they expected to be cared for by a family member. Otherwise, specific objects or goals for the future were not delineated.

As a group these patients tended to deny apprehension about the operation and were varyingly successful in controlling expression of that emotion. However, by direct breakthrough during the interview, manifest behavior (e.g., increased motor activity), attempts at skirting discussion of the operation, dream material, or on the basis of interviews of relatives, anxiety could be recognized not only as being present but also as partially acknowledged and dealt with.

Group III ("Anxious"). This group comprised patients whose previous lives were characterized by a persistence and adequacy in coping with the stresses of life. To a large extent, symptoms and signs of the illness were minimized or denied, and the patients persisted in an active and productive life. At the time of surgery they showed a hope for relief and improvement of a deteriorating physical condition that they could scarcely deny any longer. At the same time, they manifested much uneasiness concerning the approaching procedure but for the most part were unable to verbalize this. They tended to deny anxiety, and used a variety of defenses in an attempt to control it, such as focusing on other events in their lives, displacement, and projection. These patients appeared rigid, hyperalert, at times suspicious, motorically hyperactive, sleepless, and without appetite. They sometimes had difficulty in relating to or talking with personnel except in very stilted, general terms that placed a distance between them and their illness. Their orientation to the future appeared appropriate. They looked foward to resuming former roles and relationships, but they had no other goals or objectives.

Group IV ("Depressed"). These patients presented a varying picture of previous coping ability with life stresses. Some had a lifelong saga of disappointments and hardships and had over a prolonged interval first "given in" to their disease state and ultimately "given up."[27] Others had had a relatively successful previous life, but in the face of a recent onset or exacerbation of their cardiac symptoms had experienced a simultaneous worsening of their psychological adjustment. At the time of surgery all of these patients appeared clinically depressed. For the most part they denied having anxiety about the procedure, and there was no evidence to suggest that they were experiencing anxiety. Their motivation for surgery was characteristically verbalized as: "They [the doctors] thought I should have it." Their expectations of surgery varied from "It won't change anything" to "I won't survive." Their orientation to the future was poor. They were able to identify few object relationships that had held or would hold meaning for them in the future. The opportunity of jobs or role fulfillments was not identified. The future was poorly conceived and, if planned at all, was expressed in vague, unrealistic terms. For many patients the future appeared as an abyss of hopelessness.

Responses

Postoperatively, periods characterized by specific kinds of responses were identified as follows:

1. The Early Period. This period included the immediate postoperative interval lasting five to seven days and corresponded to the time spent in the intensive care unit (ICU). Four discrete responses characterized this period.

Unremarkable. After a transient delirium (as defined by Engel and Romano)[9] lasting up to 36 hours postoperatively, patients falling into this category were oriented in all dimensions. They were obviously uncomfortable and made no particular efforts to deny this. They were cooperative in accepting treatment and were observed struggling to help themselves.

Catastrophic. In the immediate postoperative period, these patients lay immobile. Their faces appeared as affectless masks. The eyes were usually closed, but when open they appeared to be staring vacantly. They were passively cooperative and responsive to the ministrations of the nurses and physicians attending them. They were oriented in all dimensions and replied appropriately, although monosyllabically, to questions directed to them. There was no attempt at spontaneous convervation or elaboration.

Under close observation over a prolonged period, this state appeared to be one of hyperawareness and hyperalertness. In response to any sudden noise in the room there was a direction of attention by the patient, manifested by a flicker of the eyelids and directed gaze or movement of an extremity. This lasted four to five days and ceased abruptly. Thereafter, patients were amnesic for this interval. It was observed in several patients that, at a moment of overwhelming anxiety long after hospitalization, they may recall an episode known to have occurred during this period. Impressionistically, patients showing this "catastrophic" response appeared "as if" they were afraid to move for fear of waking up to find themselves dead or severely mutilated.

Euphoric. Patients demonstrating this response were bright, alert, and responsive within 24 hours after surgery. They greeted the staff enthusiastically as though the operation had been "nothing at all." They were radiant, confident, and demonstrated considerable bravado. In the immediate postoperative period there were fewer complications in this group than any of the others, i.e., fewer hematomas, pneumonias, pyrexias, arrhythmias, and electrolyte imbalances. This group tended to lose their tubes early and to return to the general nursing units on the third or fourth postoperative day in contrast to the usual fifth to seventh day of transfer. They were fully oriented, and their behavior was otherwise appropriate.

Altered states of consciousness. In general these states were characterized by a prolonged period of delirium observed in the immediate postoperative period and extending over several days to several weeks with a gradual improvement in cognitive functioning during this interval. This was a classic delirium and diminished cognitive functioning and fluctuations in levels of awareness; it was associated with electroencephalogram slowing and diminished amplitude. It was sometimes difficult to delineate a specific underlying cause of the delirium.

Patients who fell into this group were divided into two subcategories. Subcategory *A* included three patients with classic delirium, some of whom had hallucinations and paranoid ideation. These patients varied in their awareness of the alien nature of these phenomena. Historically, most of the patients observed in this subgroup reported episodes compatible with previous cerebral emboli. In subcategory *B* were six patients who were unresponsive or comatose for varying periods following the operation and who demonstrated neurological signs indicating a focal lesion. On their return to consciousness, many of these patients demonstrated a hemiparesis, which generally improved. Such residua lasted beyond the immediate postoperative period into later stages of the hospitalization and were accompanied by prolonged cognitive deficits.

Dead. Eight patients died at the time of surgery and two within 48 hours.

2. *The Intermediate Period.* This period included the remainder of the hospitalization and commenced with the transfer of the patient from the ICU to the general nursing unit. Descriptively, three different phases were identified which are roughly the same for all survivors, regardless of their earlier or later responses. On their return to the floor, many patients experienced considerable *anxiety* and demonstrated much *apprehension.* They expressed this in various terms, e.g., "It's like being pushed out of the nest. Now you're on your own.

You have to fly or. . . ." or "Up there [ICU] you are never alone. If anything goes wrong, there are doctors and nurses right there. Down here, you don't get any more attention than anyone else."

With most patients this phase was short-lived and readily resolved. It was often associated with physiological accompaniments of anxiety. In four cases, arrhythmias were observed for which specific organic etiological factors could not be delineated. Other patients during this phase expressed annoyance about the inconveniences imposed upon them in a four-bed room or the reduced attention from the nursing staff. The most rapid adjustment was made by those patients with a euphoric response and the slowest, by the catastrophic reactors.

The major portion of this part of the hospitalization was characterized by a second phase that clinically appeared as *depression*. The patients became increasingly withdrawn, were less interested in relating with the nurses and physicians, and ignored relatives and other visitors. Later during this phase the patients had complaints about their physical condition and/or the environment. At some point there was a sudden shift that often followed an interval of several days during which the patients did little more than sleep. Then there was a gradual recathexis of the environment that characterized the third phase of the intermediate period, in which the patient began to anticipate the posthospital period and make realistic plans.

During this phase, occasional untoward complications developed. Pulmonary emboli and cardiac arrhythmias were common. Those patients identified during the early period as "euphoric" demonstrated a number of complications, e.g., conversion reactions, gastrointestinal hemorrhages, and pyrexias of undetectable etiology.

The last phase of the intermediate period was one of considerable anxiety on the part of some patients. It was not unusual for some to feel that they needed more time in the hospital "to adjust," despite the fact that their physical course had progressed smoothly. The patient had many questions concerning what he or other members of his family expected of him on his return home. There was concern about medications, diets, work, and sexual activity. Some patients *realized* for the first time that they were going to have sodium warfarin (Coumadin) and that prothrombin times would be required at regular intervals. This sometimes came as a sudden realization to the patient that the operation had not "cured" or "rejuvenated" him. Sodium warfarin and prothrombin times for him became the badge of his infirmity. At this time of preparing for a "return to life," the patient began to contrast his preoperative fantasies with postoperative reality. His ability to resolve these set the stage for the posthospital period.

3. The Posthospital Period. For the purpose of this review, it included the period 3 to 15 months following surgery. This was a period of readjustment and, often, rehabilitation. It was a time of realization, of attempting to establish a continuity between the present and the past, which were separated by the sometimes "unreal" and always dramatic interlude of surgery. Evaluations during this time were made on the basis of whether the patient was functioning on an improved, same, or worse level as pertaining to his job, domestic life, and satisfaction with himself as contrasted to his presurgical adjustment.

Correlations

On the basis of results organized into the above groups and responses, it has been possible to obtain general correlations between specific groups and specific responses (Table III).

Group I ("Adjusted") patients demonstrated an unremarkable course in the early postoperative period, a relatively benign intermediate period, and an overall improvement in long-term response.

Patients in group II ("Symbiotic") tended to respond to surgery immediately with varying responses. A number of patients experienced altered states of consciousness with specific residual neurologic manifestations. The intermediate period was often prolonged to five or six weeks. Long-term responses were unchanged or worse from the preoperative level of functioning.

Group III ("Anxious") patients reacted with a catastrophic response in the early period. One-quarter of these patients died at surgery. In the intermediate period there was a greater number of cardiac arrhythmias as compared with the other groups. An evaluation of long-term responses identified these patients as functioning at varying levels when contrasted with the preoperative level.

Group IV ("Depressed") patients did poorly. Mortality was higher in each postoperative period than in any of the other groups. The survivors in group IV showed either no improvement or a deterioration in their previous level of functioning.

Discussion

Groupings

By focusing attention on an evaluation of several characteristics in the preoperative interview, namely the patient's: (1) expression and handling of anxiety regarding the operation, (2) previous general level of adjustment, and (3) orientation to the future, patients may be divided into four groups which, when correlated with postsurgical results, are seen to have prognostic implications. The concept of grouping as a predictive instrument is similar to that devised by Kennedy and Bakst,[17] but also incorporates some of the observations and thoughts of other authors, notably Knox,[20] Meyer,[24] Abram,[1] and Kornfeld.[21]

We have found four groups adequate for the population under observation and less cumbersome to work with than the six suggested by Kennedy and Bakst. The latter, however, evaluated patients earlier in the course of their workup for cardiac surgery and included a population that did not go on to have surgery. Many of these nonsurgical patients had characteristics similar to candidates in our group II ("Symbiotic"). Although our groups have general characteristics that overlap with those of Kennedy and Bakst, we feel that our description of an emphasis on one salient characteristic of each group makes them more easily identifiable.

Abram's grouping on the basis of how patients handle the anxiety generated by the imminence of surgery (based on Janis's[15] work) presumes that anxiety is present in all patients. This has not been our experience with patients falling into group IV ("Depressed"), although it would seem to apply to groups I ("Adjusted"), II ("Symbiotic"), and III ("Anxious"). It may be argued that the depression observed in patients in group IV ("Depressed") is a defense against an anxiety not consciously acknowledged. However, stressing anxiety or the denial of it for this group does not seem clinically helpful for the identification of patients, although it may be worthy of theoretic and therapeutic consideration.

It is possible that in the group appearing clinically depressed, this phenomenon indicates an entirely different psychological and physiological adaptation of the organism to stress as suggested by Engel, Reichsman, and Segal[8] on the basis of their Monica studies and by

Weisman and Hackett[31] in their concept developed in "Predilection to Death." When group IV is juxtaposed with group III ("Anxious"), the contrast in affect and the absence of at least manifest anxiety is inescapable. Group II ("Symbiotic") is reminiscent of the poor responders or "hysterics" identified by Knox[20] on the basis of looking at patients who had unfavorable, as opposed to favorable, adjustments to surgery. In this group, "hysterical" personality traits were more frequent than in the other groups. There was also a higher incidence of postoperative psychophysiological and neurological complications.

The prognostic value of these groupings is dramatically demonstrated when we consider mortality in group III ("Anxious") and group IV ("Depressed"). Attempts to correlate these groups with severity based on the cardiologist's functional rating, duration of heart disease, or age of patients in each group failed to demonstrate significant differences. Patients in group IV ("Depressed") were characterized by a past, present, and projected future of weak or absent object relationships in terms of spouses, parents, children, and jobs. In contrast, in group II ("Symbiotic") such relationships were often ambivalent. In group I ("Adjusted") these relationships, especially with spouses, appeared marked by distance. A study of the significance of object relationships as a single determinant in determining response to stresses has been suggested by Greene.[12,13]

Personality characteristics of patients with valvular heart disease as they relate to grouping and responses have been a concern of another aspect of this study.[18] At this stage of our data analysis, it appears that while there are many personality traits common to individuals in all groups, certain ones are more characteristic of one group than another, e.g., dependency in group II.

Specific Postoperative Responses

1. The Early Postoperative Period. In discussing the various responses in this period, it is pertinent to refer to the observations of Kornfeld and associates regarding the ICU, particularly in regard to the genesis of the phenomenon identified as cardiac delirium or psychosis by Blachly.[3] Kornfeld's group noted the onset of this as commencing several days after surgery and often ceasing upon the removal of the patient from the ICU to a regular nursing floor. Their investigation delineated the peculiar nature of the ICU and considered the possible significances of this environment in the etiology of "cardiac psychosis."

As we have observed in our study, postsurgery delirium lasting up to 36 hours can be detected in some degree in all patients. It may vary from transient deficits and alterations in cognitive functions to gross impairment associated with hallucinations and paranoid ideation. The latter phenomenon was observed in our series most often in patients who had a history compatible with previous cerebral emboli or had neurologic dysfunction presumably on an embolic basis following surgery. The content of the prolonged delirium was usually identified as ego-alien by the patient. In those cases where the patient actually believed and responded to the content of the delirium, a review of the previous personality style indicated a greater predilection to suggestion.

It is notable that none of our patients exhibited the blatant, prolonged, and classical picture of cardiac psychosis described by Blachly and Kornfeld. We have observed classical examples of the phenomenon identified by these investigators in patients not included in this series at Strong Memorial Hospital and other medical centers, but we have not had the opportunity to study these patients in detail. The infrequency of psychoses in the present study may be related to the preparation of the patient for surgery and the general relationships that prevail between staff and patient at Strong.

All evaluations for surgery are carried out by the cardiopulmonary unit, and most communications with the patient are directed through the chief of his unit. Traditionally, it has been the policy of the unit to observe patients over several months prior to surgery unless this is contraindicated by the severity of the disease. A lengthy medical history that includes pertinent social data is solicited. The patient is given considerable information about his disease and the methods of investigation to be used.

One week prior to surgery the patient is admitted to the hospital and during the subsequent interval is seen daily by the cardiopulmonary and surgery team while various minor procedures are performed. Catheterization has usually been performed during a prior admission. This week-long interval serves as a period for adaptation and information gathering by the patient. A nurse from the ICU visits the patient to acquaint him with what the postoperative experience may be like and to answer any questions that he may have. The patient usually visits the

ICU prior to surgery. Following surgery, the same intensity of contact with the patient is maintained by the staff. The probable therapeutic significance of our interview for the patients in this study has caused us to become engaged in an examination of this hypothesis.

The catastrophic response appears to be a specific psychobiological reaction to the assault of surgery, similar to Cannon's[5] fright response in which, to a varying extent, the elements of catatonia are present. Perhaps this serves as a means of binding anxiety that persists into the postoperative period and that the patient has difficulty in resolving initially because of his cognitive defects. The hyperalertness identified in this state might be explained on the basis of inability of the patient with delirium to screen and select environmental stimuli. These patients give the impression that they are afraid to move out of fear that something dreadful might happen.

Kurt Goldstein[11] has drawn attention to a catastrophic reaction in patients with chronic organic brain lesions that occurs when the individual is confronted with a novel task requiring abstraction. This phenomenon would appear stimulus-specific and irreversible in contrast to the acute state identified by Meyer, which has a remittent course and which does not seem to be initiated by confronting the patient with a task he is unable to do. Rather, it appears as a continuation of the anesthetic experience.

Rheingold[25] identified such a response as having its prototype in the early mother–child relationship, suggesting that this may be more characteristic of the individual's specific defense system against trauma. Abram explains this response as a psychological response to a fear of death and as the anlage of the more extended and distorted cardiac psychosis of Blachly. Meyer[23] sees this stage as one of great vulnerability in which the susceptible patient is exposed to the unfamiliar stimuli of the ICU while still partially paralyzed from antiacetylcholine inhibitors. In our series, the catastrophic response does not appear to serve the patient adversely in the early postoperative period, but it may portend his subsequent difficulty to master anxiety during the intermediate period.

The euphoric response has not been previously identified in the literature. It is a dramatic one and appears to indicate a form of denial par excellence. It is matched by rapid physiologic improvement. In the intermediate period, however, these patients experience psychological and physiological reactions, possibly suggesting a somatic expression of repressed conflicts and/or nonverbalized affect.

A higher incidence of embolic phenomena resulting in cerebro-vascular accidents occurred in group II ("Symbiotic"). It can merely be observed that this occurrence enforces the dependent role previously enjoyed by the patient, and it may be speculated that predilection to increased clotting may be a correlate of predetermined psychobiologic interaction.

The highest incidence of deaths among the depressed (group IV) during and immediately after surgery, while striking, is not unknown. Patients who appear helpless or hopeless frequently show other signs of the 'giving up-given up" state suggested by Engel and Schmale.[10] These individuals may be incapable of erecting the necessary physiological defenses to cope with stress (Selye[29]).

It would be of interest to attempt a correlation of biological changes with the response patterns noted. On the basis of extensive observations of patients undergoing heart surgery, Blachly[2] has hypothesized specific organic processes as a cause for the acute psychological disturbance he calls postcardiotomy delirium or psychosis. Correlating an array of intriguing data with postoperative behavioral aberrations, he suggests as the cause of these disturbances the production within the body of a specific catecholamine. This may be a commonly occurring amine that, when produced in excessive amounts, is "toxic" in its own right. Either of these is viewed as a hallucinogenic agent. Should such a substance be routinely found in patients exhibiting disturbed postoperative behavior, the question would remain whether the amine was an essential cause of a behavioral state or simply one of many aberrant factors to be demonstrated in a patient's failure to psychologically master stress.

We would suggest that all of these responses appear to be on the basis of a complicated interassociation of psychological and physiological events. In our study we have attempted to view the operation and its meaning for the patient in the context of his whole life experience including the surgical and parasurgical events.

2. The Intermediate Postoperative Period. In considering this period, we are impressed by the frequency with which patients experience discomfort and anxiety on leaving the ICU to return to the general nursing units. This is in contrast to the experience of other investigators, notably Kornfeld. An explanation for this discrepancy may be in part related to the preparation of our patients for the ICU and the nature of the unit at Strong. It is important to emphasize that return to the general nursing unit from the ICU can be a time of stress and anxiety for the patient that may be overlooked by the staff. We have noted several episodes of arrhythmias occurring in patients expressing apprehension about their transfer from the ICU. Occasionally, an extra day or two in the ICU may convince the patient of his readiness to make the move.

The second phase of the intermediate period has been identified for all survivors as one of depression and withdrawal. A similarity between this and what Engel[6] has identified as "conservation–withdrawal" seems appropriate. This is a time in which the patient simultaneously experiences a "letdown" (which was expressed by one patient as, "I knew I was going to be all right now; I could give in to my fatigue") and attempts to withdraw, restoring his vitality generally by sleep. Such a response may be discouraging to the attending staff who, on observing improved physiological functioning, are confronted by a patient who appears depressed and withdrawn. This may be a necessary experience for the patient—a time for physiological and psychological adjustment and healing. The latter response may also symbolize a period of grieving for their suffering and what might have occurred—death.

As the patient emerges from the withdrawn aspects of this period, he may be preoccupied with conflicts identified in the preoperative interview that suggest his continued introspection and grief. In the last phase of the intermediate period, the patient prepares himself for the return home and his need for reassurance regarding his fears is indicated by his many questions. Such apprehensions may have to be drawn out of the patient or the relatives by giving them time for expression.

3. The Posthospital Period.   This need to express and confide persists long into the posthospital period. In the latter period, the physician may have to assist his patient in resolving the disappointments he may experience over the actual result of the operation. The unrealistic fantasies expressed by many patients in viewing the operation as one of rejuvenation, resolution of sexual maladjustments, or as a means of achieving long-fantasied success are perhaps present to some degree in all patients. The price of these, when unrealized, is a depression that may extend to the whole family and may result in the patient's failure to adjust to the demands of the family and environment and to his own internal demands.

Conclusion

In this report we have indicated how patients coming for open-heart surgery may be grouped on the basis of factors identifiable in a preoperative interview and how, on the basis of the patients' postoperative response, correlations may be made between grouping and response. Patients manifesting considerable preoperative anxiety or depression have a greater chance of not surviving surgery and a greater morbidity after surgery than other patients. For others, the operation threatens to upset the balance that the disease has come to hold in their adjustment to life, and for this group there is a higher incidence of morbidity as well as a failure to realize an improvement in their life adjustment following surgery. Some of the factors operating in the intrapsychic and environmental fields of patients around the surgical period have been discussed in relationship to particular responses exhibited by patients. On the basis of this study, several questions have been raised that are currently under investigation:

1.   Are there more objective ways than the interview in which individuals may be preoperatively evaluated for the presence of anxiety, depression, and poor coping responses?

2.   Are there specific biological correlates that may be identified for the groups and responses cited in this paper?

3.   Would those patients who were identified, due to psychological factors, as poor risks at the time of surgery benefit from limited psychotherapeutic intervention?

4.   What are the possible models for such intervention?

Acknowledgments

This work was done with the guidance of Dr. Arthur H. Schmale, Jr., while the investigator was a member of the medical–psychiatric liaison group, departments of psychiatry and medicine, University of Rochester School of Medicine and Dentistry. Dr. Paul Yu, chief, cardiopulmonary unit, department of medicine, and Drs. Earle Mahoney and James DeWeese, department of surgery, encouraged and assisted the author in the facilitation of this study. Research groups in the departments of psychiatry and medicine offered helpful criticism at various phases of the project. Drs. John Romano and Lawrence Young, chairmen respectively, departments of psychiatry and medicine, offered valuable suggestions. Drs. George Engel and William Greene of the liaison group assisted in bringing into sharper focus many of the observations reported.

References

1. Abram, H. S. Adaptation to open heart surgery: A psychiatric study of response to the threat of death. *American Journal of Psychiatry* **122:**659–688, 1965.
2. Blachly, P. H. Personal communication.
3. Blachly, P. H., & Starr, A. Post-cardiotomy delirium. *American Journal of Psychiatry* **121:**371–375, 1964.
4. Bowman, K. M., & Crook, G. H.: Emotional changes following castration. In L. J. West & M. Greenblatt (Eds.), *Explorations in the physiology of emotions. Psychiatric Research Reports, American Psychiatric Association* **12:**81–96, 1960.
5. Cannon, W. B. Bodily change in pain, hunger, fear, and rage, New York: Appleton and Co., 1915.
6. Engel, G. L. Psychological development in health and disease. Philadelphia: W. B. Saunders Co., 1962.
7. Engel, G. L., Green, W. L., Reichsman, F., Schmale, A., & Ashenburg, N. A graduate and undergraduate teaching program on the psychological aspects of medicine. *Journal of Medical Education* **32:**859–871, 1957.
8. Engel, G. L., Reichsman, F., & Segal, H. L. A study of an infant with a gastric fistula: I. Behavior and the rate of total hydrochloric acid secretion. *Psychosomatic Medicine* **18:**374–398, 1956.
9. Engel, G. L., & Romano, J. Delirium, a syndrome of cerebral insufficiency. *Journal of Chronic Diseases* **9:**260–277, 1959.
10. Engel, G. L., & Schmale, A. H., Jr. Psychoanalytic theory of somatic disorder: Conversion, specificity, and the disease onset situation. *Journal of the American Psychoanalytic Association* **15:**344–365, 1967.
11. Goldstein, K. On emotions: Consideration from the Organismic point of view. *Journal of Psychology* **31:**37–49, 1951.
12. Greene, W. A. Role of a vicarious object in the adaptation to object loss: I. *Psychosomatic Medicine* **20:**344–350, 1958.
13. Greene, W. A. Role of a vicarious object in the adaptation to object loss: II. *Psychosomatic Medicine* **21:**438–447, 1959.
14. Hollender, M. H. A study of patients admitted to a psychiatric hospital after pelvic operations. *American Journal of Obstetrics and Gynecology* **79:**498–503, 1960.
15. Janis, I. L. Psychological stress: Psychoanalytic and behavioral studies of surgical patients. New York: John Wiley & Sons, 1958.
16. Kehoe, M. The Rochester scheme. *Lancet* **2:**145–148, 1961.

17. Kennedy, J. A., & Bakst, H. The influence of emotions on the outcome of cardiac surgery: A predictive study. *Bulletin of the New York Academy of Medicine* **42**:811–845, 1966.

18. Kimball, C. P. The experience of open heart surgery: Personality characteristics of the patient undergoing open heart surgery. 1969, in preparation.

19. Kimball, C. P. The experience of open heart surgery: A review of the psychological literature. 1969, in preparation.

20. Knox, S. J. Psychiatric aspects of mitral valvotomy. *British Journal of Psychiatry* **109**:656–668, 1963.

21. Kornfeld, D. S., Zimberg, S., & Malm, J. R. Psychiatric complications of open-heart surgery. *New England Journal of Medicine* **273**:287–292, 1965.

22. Lindemann, E. Observations on psychiatric sequelae to surgical operations in women. *American Journal of Psychiatry* **98**:132–139, 1941.

23. Meyer, B. C., & Blacher, R. S. A traumatic neurotic reaction induced by succinylcholine. *New York Journal of Medicine* **61**:1255 1261, 1961.

24. Meyer, B. C., Blacher, R. S., & Brown, F. A clinical study of psychiatric and psychological aspects of mitral surgery. *Psychosomatic Medicine* **23**:194–218, 1961.

25. Rheingold, J. C. The mother, anxiety and death: The catastrophic death complex. Boston: Little, Brown and Co., 1967.

26. Romano, J. Teaching of psychiatry to medical students. *Lancet* **2**:93–95, 1961.

27. Schmale, A. H., Jr. Object loss, "giving up" and disease onset: An overview of research in progress. *Symposium on medical aspects of stress in the military climate*. Washington, D. C.: Government Printing Office, 1965. Pp. 433–443.

28. Schmale, A. H., Jr., Greene, W. A., Jr., Reichsman, F., Kehoe, M., & Engel, G. L. An established program of graduate education in psychosomatic medicine. *Advances in Psychosomatic Medicine* **4**:4–13, 1964.

29. Selye, H. The concept of stress in experimental physiology. In J. M. Tanner (Ed.), *Stress and psychiatric disorder: The proceedings of the Second Oxford Conference of the Mental Health Research Fund*. Oxford, England: Blackwell Scientific Publications, 1960. Pp. 67–75.

30. Weisman, A. D., & Hackett, T. P. Psychosis after eye surgery: Establishment of a specific doctor–patient relation in the prevention and treatment of "black-patch" delirium. *New England Journal of Medicine* **258**:1284–1289, 1958.

31. Weisman, A. D., & Hackett, T. P. Predilection to death. *Psychosomatic Medicine* **23**:232–256, 1961.

32. Yamamoto, J., & Seeman, W. A psychological study of castrated males. In L. J. West & M. Greenblatt (Eds.), *Explorations in the physiology of emotions. Psychiatric Research Reports, American Psychiatric Association*. **12**:97–103, 1960.

10

Rehabilitating the Stroke Patient through Patient–Family Groups

JUDITH GREGORIE D'AFFLITTI
and G. WAYNE WEITZ

The intermediate service of the West Haven Veterans Administration Hospital is designed as a rehabilitative setting for medical patients who have completed the phase of diagnosis and early treatment. In our nursing and social work with recuperating stroke patients and their families on this service, we noticed that although many patients were engaged in a program of physical, occupational, and speech therapy, they and their family members were frequently having great difficulty with the emotional acceptance of the patients' disabilities. This was clear from the patients' depressive affect and inability to express their feelings about their illness, with the concurrent inability of families to exchange reactions with the patients about the stroke and the ways in which this was going to affect their family life. For example, patients were often very frightened that any disability would mean that they could not function at home again. Family members sometimes shared this fear, and families and patients could not communicate their concerns. Because of

JUDITH GREGORIE D'AFFLITTI, M.S.N. ● Consultant, Nursing Service, Veterans Administration Hospital, West Haven, Connecticut, and Clinical Instructor, Dept. of Psychiatry, Yale University School of Medicine. G. WAYNE WEITZ, M.S.W. ● Brooklyn State Hospital, Division V Outpatient Services, Brooklyn, New York.

Reprinted from *International Journal of Group Psychotherapy,* 1974, 25(3), 323–332.

this poor communication, there often was a strained relationship between patient and family, and realistic discharge plans could not be made. In addition, the patients did not use the appropriate community supports that would have allowed the most effective community adjustment, i.e., rehabilitation centers, visiting nurse associations, and vocational retraining centers.

The importance of interpersonal relationships in the rehabilitation of chronic disease patients is noted in the medical and psychiatric literature. Litman[5] reported that 75% of his patients looked first to their families for support and encouragement and second to the hospital staff. Also, there are some indications that if patients can anticipate reentry into a functioning family unit, this influences their decision to engage themselves in a therapy program. Bruetman and Gordon[2] discuss rehabilitation in terms of a concurrent restoring of the patient's physiologic and environmental equilibrium. They see the family's having great impact on the patient's motivations and expectations. Robertson and Suinn[8] state that there is a relationship between the stroke patient's rate of progress toward recovery and the degree of empathy between the patient and his family members. Specifically, they indicate that stroke patients improve more rapidly when there is predictive empathy, i.e., the ability of patients and family members to foresee each other's attitudes. Finally, Millen[6] states that optimum rehabilitation of stroke patients occurs only when there is physical and psychological stimulation. Frequently, stroke patients grouped together can influence one another toward working out problems, while providing a mutual source of encouragement as well.

With these ideas in mind, we believed that we might be helpful to our patients and their families by having them participate in a patient–family group. It was hoped that the group process would facilitate communication so that the illness and feelings about it could be discussed more freely and that this would lead to a more realistic perception by the patient and his family of the amount of disability and the limitations imposed by it. Plans could then be initiated and implemented that would be consistent with these limitations, and the group could support individual members toward more independent functioning.

We began our group with two major goals: first, to encourage patients and families to talk and to share their feelings about the stroke in order to promote a constructive adjustment to the illness; second, to encourage the patient and his family to use the appropriate community resources and supports available to them. From our experience, it seemed that patients who had contacts outside the family after discharge were less likely to become depressed and regress in their physical and social functioning.

In order for the group to be viewed as part of the total rehabilitation effort of the Intermediate Service, our project needed the support of the director of the service and of the staff members. This was accomplished through our joint contact with the director, followed by his introduction and our presentation of the purposes and goals of the planned group at a staff meeting. This presentation enabled the staff to understand how the group would be structured and how its activities would complement rather than subvert or interfere with those of the medical, nursing, and rehabilitation staff.

There were four criteria for participation in the group: (1) The patient had to have had a stroke, although he might have additional medical problems. (2) He had to be competent mentally and verbally to participate in a group. (3) He had to have a family member who was willing to participate. (4) His final destination from the hospital had to be his home.

These strictures were not intended to imply that the needs of the severely damaged patient or the patient without a family or the patient who would have to be placed out of a home setting were any less important than those of the group selected, only that the problems of such patients cannot be dealt with appropriately in a patient–family group and need to be approached by other methods of intervention.

The group met for an hour and a half weekly for three months. Members were to participate for this time even if they were discharged. To date, four consecutive groups have been conducted. The authors worked as coleaders for the group sessions and shared the outside administrative responsibilities, i.e., referrals and contacts with community agencies, preadmission interviews, and contacts with staff members. Each group had three to five patients, each with his accompanying family participants. These included spouses, brothers, sisters, children, and sometimes friends. The selected patients were predominately male because the agency is a Veterans Administration Hospital. A variety of ethnic and cultural backgrounds were represented. There was a wide patient age range, 34 to 76 years. Most of the patients and family members approached the group with interest and enthusiasm; however, the group was not appropriate for all situations.

For example, Mr. A. discontinued attending because no family member would join him, and he felt anxious and uncomfortable without family support. Mrs. C. showed her resistance by attending sporadically and arriving late; soon it became clear that she and her husband had marital problems which predated his stroke, and because she covertly planned placement of her husband in a nursing home, she had difficulty identifying with the other group members. Mr. C. felt uncomfortable about attending without her.

Problems of Group Organization

We encountered some unique problems organizing the patient–family group in a medical setting. Routine issues, such as selection of a meeting place and the physical preparation of the patients for the meetings, required special effort. We finally obtained the use of a quiet classroom. We needed the cooperation of the nursing staff on the units to have the patients up, fed, and toileted in time for the meeting. Although the staff verbalized interest in the group and a desire to help with it, their behavior sometimes indicated difficulty in accepting this new program. On some units, staff members continually forgot which patients needed to be ready and at what time. We tried to minimize this problem by keeping staff informed of the patients' group participation and progress. However, our patient–family group seemed to raise questions for staff members about their own involvement and competence with the patients. Since general medical ward atmosphere is often geared to the suppression of uncomfortable emotions, it was difficult for patients and staff members to accept such a group.

Another difficult organizational problem was the establishment of a contract with the patient and his family. Through trial and error, we learned that the patient should be approached first with an explanation and an invitation to join the group. Then if he expressed interest, permission to contact a family member was given to one of us or the patient would make the contact himself. If the patient was not first consulted and given the opportunity to be in control of the decision, he would be resentful and resistive to participating in one more thing being imposed upon him.

In meeting with the patient and his family to discuss the group contract, we discovered that they could not accept the view that the illness produced a family problem. This seemed too frightening at a time when the family was mourning and shifting roles. Their anxiety was bearable only if the patient's *stroke* was seen as the focal problem. Most people were willing to participate in a group which had as its purpose the sharing of problems and ideas related to the stroke and to the home care of the person with the stroke. The following is the statement of contract we found most successful in the initial meeting with patient and family, and in the initial group meeting:

> It is often difficult for patients and their families to adjust their lives to a chronic disability, especially when it's time for the patient to come home from the hospital. We've found it can be helpful if people with these kinds of problems talk together about them. The purpose of this group is for discussion of the concerns you are and will be facing.

We experimented with an open and closed group structure, and found the latter more comfortable and apparently more productive. In the open group, as people left we replaced them with new members. This meant that the group was often disrupted by comings and goings and the issues of getting to know new members. Consequently, establishing a sense of group stability was particularly difficult. A cohesion developed in the closed group that allowed us to go further in the work of facing and living with the losses produced by the stroke.

In both types of group, we attempted to have patients continue participating in the group after discharge from the hospital. In most cases, however, people did not continue after discharge. They said it was too difficult physically to get the patient from home to the hospital. One patient did tell us he felt that "everything would be all right" once he got home, and he did not want to come back and tell us if things were not going well. We can only speculate that those first weeks at home are very difficult for the patient and family to face and share. Perhaps it is the first real confrontation with the change in physical and family functioning and the realization that everything is not "all right" in the sense that it is not the same as it was before the stroke. Additionally, the patients viewed the return to the hospital after discharge as a threat which seemed to heighten their fears and desires of being an inpatient again.

One last problem was in establishing a meeting time that was convenient for family participation. This varied with the composition of the group. If the participating family members did not work, they preferred meeting in the afternoon. If they worked, a time following the patient's evening meal seemed preferable.

Group Issues and Reactions

Once the group was organized and group work begun, it became clear that the group members were mourning and trying to learn to live with their losses. The patient had lost some parts of bodily control and functioning. This resulted in loss of some independence, a change in self-concept, and a consequent loss of self-esteem. The patient feared total loss of control over himself, loss of his family because they might regard him, as he regarded himself, as an inadequate and useless burden, and the ultimate loss, death. The family also feared the total loss of a loved one as they had once known him and as he had once functioned in the family. The changes in the patient forced changes in the functioning of the rest of the family as they attempted to fill the places left vacant by the patient.

The patients and families struggled with their grief in the group, and this struggle can be seen in the framework of Engel's[3] process of grieving.

Shock and Denial

In every meeting the group members expressed their disbelief and wished the loss away. "How could something like this happen so fast? What caused it? It can't be real. Some nights I'm sure when I awaken in the morning it will be gone as quickly as it came. I just can't believe it!"

"I'm getting better every day. Soon I'll be good as new. This arm will be fine if I just exercise it enough. You can do anything with will power, you know. I'll be back working and fishing in a few weeks."

"My husband's going to be fine, no problems. They're holding his job for him and he'll be back at work soon. I was worried when it first happened, but I'm not worried anymore."

Developing Awareness

Although it did not often appear overtly, anger was expressed by the group members. "Why did this happen to me? What did I do to deserve it? Hospital staff don't take good care of me. The physical therapists don't tell me how to get this arm moving. The nurses wake me too early in the morning. The doctor never comes to check me."

Occasionally, a patient would cry for the limbs that wouldn't move or the job he'd never work at again.

The family members felt resentment toward the patient for being ill and thus a burden, but guilt over this resentment prevented its direct expression. Instead, the family was often overprotective of the patient. "I wouldn't think of leaving him at home alone. . . ." "It took me three hours to get him dressed this morning" (patient able to dress himself on the unit in the hospital).

Restitution and Resolution

A great deal of group time was spent sharing together what life used to be like. This is the way in which they began to resolve the losses. The men shared tales of their military experiences, of their work and pastime activities. The family members talked of the things they used to enjoy together and do for each other. There was a feeling of trying to recapture the "good old days." Sometimes this reminiscing led to an attempt to reconcile the past and present. "I know we won't be able to go out as much, but do you think we could go out to dinner sometimes?"

"Maybe I can't do my old job, but there are some things around the house I could manage."

"I can't fish anymore, but the boys could put me in the boat and take me with them anyway."

In the first stage, reminiscing can be seen as part of avoidance and denial; in this stage, it is adaptive and part of the resolution of the loss. The patients and their families moved in and out of these phases and feelings of grief throughout the three months of group participation. Although phases exist concurrently, the overall movement is toward resolution. Engel says that successful mourning takes a year or more; however, in these three months, the work was well begun.

The group members also spent a lot of time discussing the more concrete aspects of being at home again. What kind of equipment was needed in the house for the patient to live comfortably? Could he get up a flight of stairs to the only bathroom? How do you manage to get the patient in and out of a car? Can the patient be left alone in the house at any time? The group supported one another in facing problems, and such focusing on concrete details served the function of decreasing anxiety and allowing families to deal with the emotional aspects of restructuring their lives.

Problems and Reactions of Leaders

It was difficult to lead a new kind of group in a somewhat nonsupportive setting. Although the literature reports a few group experiences with medical patients or their families (Strauss et al.;[9] Piskor & Paleos;[7] Bardach;[1] Heller[4]) we could find no precedent for a patient–family group of this nature.

We had the supervision of a psychiatrist whose expertise is group work and this was most useful. He helped us examine our structure and process, and encouraged us to experiment with new tactics when necessary. Most importantly, he supported us in our reactions to the helpless–hopeless feelings in our patients. A stroke is a catastrophe. The damage is highly visible. We found that we had strong wishes to "do something" for these patients and their families in a concrete way. These wishes made us vulnerable to their complaints that we were not doing enough and susceptible to their feelings of helplessness. In the beginning we tried to compensate for these problems by being active and directive leaders. We initiated conversation in most silences and often focused on individuals instead of allowing group involvement with issues raised by individuals. Both of these techniques served to suppress anger from group members about not being helped to recover permanent losses. Also, we often responded directly to questions for which there was no answer that could resolve the real issue for the patient. For example, members repeatedly asked for information about the specific causes of a stroke and specific cures. Our concrete answers seemed unsatisfactory because the real questions were: "Why me? What did I do to deserve this? Am I going to have to live this way?" With experience and supervisory support, we came to understand that the real work of the group was in the patients' experiencing these hopeless–helpless feelings. Our role was to be less directive and more supportive of the group members so that, through our empathy and acceptance, they could express their feelings and work with them toward a more productive and independent emotional state.

Outcomes

There were several important outcomes of the group meetings. First, to a greater or lesser extent, nearly all patients and their families shared difficult feelings. Through such openness, the participants often recognized that negative feelings about the stroke were not so frightening or threatening. For example, Mr. J. often felt depressed about his damaged body and inability to work at his former place of employment. At times, he started to cry, but his wife became anxious and made statements such as, "We can only think cheery thoughts." When Mr. J. was encouraged to express more of what he really felt to the group, he experienced a sense of relief, and the group helped his wife to tolerate her husband's tears and depression.

As the lines of communication became more open, families and patients began to be more realistic about their expectations. For example, Mrs. R. was secretly frightened that she would be tied to a life of drudgery once her husband was discharged from the hospital because she thought he would need constant supervision and care. When Mr. R. began to plan rehabilitation activities for discharge, she saw that he was not as helpless as she had thought. Other wives supported this idea through their experiences.

At other times, the outcomes were much more concrete and often revolved around decision making. Mr. and Mrs. L. had a two-level house which was inconvenient for Mr. L. because his wife worked and the facilites he needed were on both floors. After several group discussions, they were able to make the decision that they no longer needed the large house. They sold it and rented a ground-level apartment before Mr. L. was discharged.

As medical and rehabilitation evaluations became known to the patients and their families, they often shared the information with the group. From these discussions came the guidelines for using community supports. Mr. and Mrs. W. had lived a life of near isolation for eight years after Mr. W.'s first stroke. Both were unrealistically frightened of the stroke and remained in their third-floor flat almost constantly. Although they were never able to resolve their fears completely in the group, this time they were able to make more realistic community plans for discharge. Mr. W. was able to involve himself for several hours weekly in a work activities program of the local rehabilitation center, thus allowing Mrs. W. some time of her own.

A final outcome was perhaps less tangible, but certainly no less important. This was the increased knowledge and sensitivity of ourselves and floor staff to the reactions of stroke patients and their families to this illness. Although the floor staff were sometimes resistive to our group, they could see that there were changes in patients and families which could be related to their involvement in the group. For example, some patients were less withdrawn on the units and some families were more willing to accept the patients on weekend pass. We saw directly the negative and positive influences a family can have on the acceptance and adjustment a stroke patient makes to his limitations.

Conclusion

We have described a group method for helping stroke patients and their families adjust to this chronic disability through a shared mourning of their losses. The purpose of the article is to describe the methodology and technique of such a group so that others might be encouraged in similar endeavors. Although research needs to be done to evaluate such groups, we feel that the patient–family group described has been a positive force in the rehabilitation of stroke patients and their families toward a more independent and satisfying adjustment.

References

1. Bardach, J. L. Group sessions with wives of aphasic patients. *International Journal of Group Psychotherapy* **19**:361–365, 1969.
2. Bruetman, M. E., & Gordon, E. E. Rehabilitating the stroke patient at general hospitals. *Postgraduate Medicine* **49**:211–215, 1971.
3. Engel, G. L. Grief and grieving. *American Journal of Nursing* **64**:93–98, 1964.
4. Heller, V. Handicapped patients talk together. *American Journal of Nursing* **70**:332–335, 1970.
5. Litman, T. J. An analysis of the sociologic factors affecting the rehabilitation of physically handicapped patients. *Archives of Physical Medicine and Rehabilitation* **45**:9–16, 1964.
6. Millen, H. M. The positive approach to the care of the stroke patients. *Michigan Medicine* **69**:887–890, 1970.
7. Piskor, B. K., & Paleos, S. The group way to banish after-stroke blues. *American Journal of Nursing* **68**:1500–1503, 1968.
8. Robertson, E. K., & Suinn, R. M. The determination of rate of progress of stroke patients through empathy measures of patient and family. *Journal of Psychosomatic Research* **12**:189–191, 1968.
9. Strauss, A. B., Burrucker, J. D., Cicero, J. A., & Edwards, R. C. Group work with stroke patients. *Rehabilitation Record* 30–32, Nov.–Dec., 1967.

V

The Crisis of Illness:
Severe Burns

Burns are among the most common injuries suffered by children and adults, and serious burns are among the most traumatic. With new grafting techniques and better understanding of infection hazards and nutritional needs, even people with severe burns covering as much as 40% of their bodies now survive. The people, with their families, face an exceedingly painful treatment program, a long hospital stay, the possibility of permanent disfigurement, and many other stressful circumstances which, combined with the trauma of the injury itself, frequently provoke an emotional crisis.

While hospitalized the burn patient must handle many distressing feelings and experiences. In a major early study Hamburg, Hamburg, and de Goza[1] examined these stresses and outlined some of the adaptive skills which patients use. In the acute period the threat of death is the patients' primary concern. They are anxious about how long their suffering will last, about the welfare of their families while they are hospitalized, and about the extent of permanent damage and disfigurement. For young children the pain of modern debridement and grafting techniques and the lengthy separation from parents are particularly distressing.[2,3] The loss of family and work roles, the helplessness and enforced dependence on total nursing care, and fears that their appearance will make them repulsive to other people all have a serious impact on individual self-esteem. The coping mechanisms described by Hamburg and his colleagues include constriction (tight control over feelings), repression or suppression of feelings, denial either of the injury or of serious consequences, regression, reworking or rumination over stressful events, religiosity, rationalization, and withdrawal. In the recovery stage, once survival seems certain, the patient has three major tasks: the mobilization of hope, the restoration of self-esteem, and the restoration of interpersonal relationships.

While these tasks are important during hospitalization, they are also central to the success of long-term readjustment by burn patients. In the first article N. J. C. Andreasen and A. S. Norris discuss the processes involved in the reestablishment of psychological equilibrium after burn patients are released from the hospital. After severe burn injuries, permanent scars and/or disabilities represent significant changes which must be integrated into an acceptable self-image. As interpersonal relationships are tentatively restored, patients gradually gain assurance that their appearance is not as shocking and repulsive to others as they fear. This progressive desensitization is often accomplished by denial of the seriousness of the disfigurement or of the importance of physical appearance as a determinant of personal worth and acceptability, or by displacement of anxiety to some other aspect of appearance, such as the woman with a badly scarred face who maintained that overweight was her main worry. Achieving a sense of control and self-direction is a significant step away from the dependency of hospital routines and toward rebuilding a healthy sense of self-esteem.

Seeing some positive value and purpose in the experience through rationalization (for example, viewing it as an opportunity for personal growth) or through religion (for example, accepting it as part of God's design) can be helpful in accepting the injury and its painful consequences. Two other ways in which people have dealt with especially upsetting experiences are amnesic dissociation and reworking. Andreasen and Norris found that despite the trauma of the injury, the long and painful treatment, and the permanent scarring and disability, 70% of the patients they studied eventually achieved a satisfactory adjustment.

In the second article Gene Brodland and N. J. C. Andreason focus on the experiences of the family of the burn patient. They found that the relatives go through two stages, much as the patients do. In the acute stage, when the patient's survival is in doubt, the family is shocked and disbelieving. Ambivalent hopes that the patient might die and be spared the pain and disfigurement are repressed; they are only allowed to come to the surface if the patient actually does die. Delirious or regressive (complaining, demanding, childlike) behavior by the patient often confuses and upsets family members.

In the second stage, when the focus shifts from survival to recovery and rehabilitation, family members react to the patient's pain, repeated grafting procedures, and general discomfort with feelings of frustration and helplessness. They recognize the importance of being supportive and encouraging to the patient, but must deal with their own fears of permanent scarring and disability. Some of the distress relatives experience can be relieved if medical personnel take the time to explain treatment and care procedures, and what to expect from the patient. Brodland and Andreasen also suggest that group meetings of families can give relatives a forum for their questions, an opportunity for sharing their feelings, and support and understanding for their own problems.

References

1. Hamburg, D. A., Hamburg, B., & de Goza, S. Adaptive problems and mechanisms in severely burned patients. *Psychiatry,* 1953, **16**(1), 1–20.
2. Long, R. T., & Cope, O. Emotional problems of burned children. *New England Journal of Medicine,* 1961, **264,** 1121–1127.
3. Martin, H. L. Parents' and children's reactions to burns and scalds in children. *British Journal of Medical Psychology,* 1970, **43,** 183–191.

11

Long-Term Adjustment and Adaptation Mechanisms in Severely Burned Adults

N. J. C. ANDREASEN and A. S. NORRIS

Hundreds of thousands of people suffer from thermal burns each year in the United States. Prior to the development of modern treatments such as sulfamylon, silver nitrate, and sophisticated supportive measures, those with severe and mutilating burns usually died. Now many of these patients survive. To be burned is an intensely traumatic experience—catastrophic, painful, deforming, debilitating, and even dirty, because of the invariable presence of infection. Further, the burn victim, unlike most other victims of trauma, must continue to wear the badge of his trauma for the rest of his life.

In spite of the high incidence and prevalence of burn injury, few researchers have investigated its psychological aspects. Most of the work has concentrated on adjustment during hospitalization.[3,5-9,11,13,14] Studies of long-term adjustment are less common. Investigating the victims of the Cocoanut Grove fire 11 months after the disaster, Adler[1] stated that about half the victims had emotional problems, usually in the form of increased nervousness or anxiety neurosis. A study of 10

N. J. C. ANDREASEN, M.D., Ph.D. ● Assistant Professor, Department of Psychiatry, University of Iowa College of Medicine, Iowa City, Iowa.

Reprinted from *Journal of Nervous and Mental Disease,* 1972, **154**(5), 352–362. Copyright 1972, The Williams & Wilkins Co. Reproduced by permission.

children and their parents seen an average of 5 years after initial injury indicates an even higher incidence of complications, with significant problems being noted in 9 children and 8 parents.[12] No such long-term study of psychiatric sequelae has been done on adults, although MacGregor et al.[10] have included a few burn victims in their studies of facial deformity. Accordingly, we felt a more complete follow-up investigation was needed.

We have discussed in a previous study the incidence and types of psychiatric complications.[2] These were much less frequent than has been suggested by previous investigations mentioned above. Thirty percent of our patients were found to have emotional problems secondary to their injury, with the commonest types being traumatic neuroses and chronic depressions. Twenty percent were classified as mild, while the other 10% were considered to be moderate in severity. By 1 to 2 years after the initial trauma, most of the patients examined were functioning at their preinjury levels in terms of work, interpersonal relationships, family relationships, and recreation.

This study explores the dynamics underlying these adjustment successes and failures. In it we raise and seek to answer three questions about the burn patient: (1) What problems in adjustment does he face after discharge from the hospital? (2) What mechanisms does he use in dealing with these problems? (3) What factors predispose to or prevent the development of psychiatric complications?

Materials and Methods

Epidemiologically, the population suffering from burns includes a higher proportion of the elderly, the very young, and the chronically ill or debilitated than contained in the general population. We wished to restrict our study to healthy young adults in their productive years as we believed that more could be learned about coping mechanisms by evaluating the adjustment of burn patients during the years when social and personal demands were strongest. Accordingly, patients were selected for inclusion in the study on the basis of the following criteria: (1) age 18 to 60 at the time of burn, with preference for inclusion given to those between 20 and 40; (2) follow-up from 1 to 5 years after burn; (3) greater than 20% total body surface burn, with preference given to those with greater body surface area or facial burns; (4) general good mental and physical health prior to injury.

Thirty-three patients who fulfilled these criteria were contacted by a letter which briefly described the nature of the study. Twenty came for interviews. Those who failed to participate did so for a variety of reasons; five simply did not reply, three agreed to come but did not appear, three had moved without leaving a forwarding address, and two had unavoidable conflicting commitments. Since in most cases reasons for failure to participate are unknown, one can only speculate about the extent to which and the way in which the sample may be skewed. Failure to participate did seem to be related to several factors. These included a greater number of years since discharge, less severe burns and less need to return to the hospital after discharge for follow-up or surgical revisions, and being male. We suspect, therefore, that many of those who failed to participate did so because the trip was inconvenient for them or because the project did not seem relevant, rather than because they had significant problems that they wished to avoid admitting to or confronting. Among those who did come, several were found to have problems of the sort we had wished to avoid such as alcoholism or a history of psychiatric disorder prior to injury. Our sample included 11 men and 9 women with an average age of 35 and an average total body surface burn of 37%; they ranged from 1 to 5 years after burn, with the mean being 2 years.

Each patient was interviewed according to a standard format, which included history of injury, history of hospitalization, adaptation since discharge, past psychological history, and mental status. In most cases similar material was also covered in a separate interview with the patient's accompanying relative. Each patient took a Minnesota Multiphasic Personality Inventory, and current color photographs were obtained. Photographs taken at the time of injury and during subsequent hospital visits, review of ward charts, and sometimes discussions with the nurses and surgeons who cared for the patient provided additional sources of information. In order to introduce a quantitative measure of deformity and adjustment, each patient was asked to make a subjective estimate of these parameters in himself on a 1 to 4 scale (1 = no deformity or good adjustment, 4 = severe deformity or very poor adjustment); the interviewer also made an independent estimate of these parameters. Results are summarized in Table I.

Table I. Patient Characteristics

Patient	Age	Years after burn	Per-cent burn	Areas injured	Estimated deformity (Patient/examiner)	Estimated adjustment (Patient/examiner)	Emotional problems on follow-up
C. B.	33	3	45	Face, neck, upper extremities, back	3/3	2/2	Mild: (1) traumatic neurosis; (2) depression
T. H.	61	2	20	Face, neck, back, upper extremities, right thigh	2/2	1/2	None
B. H.	59	2	30	Face, upper extremities, legs	2/2	2/1	None
G. L.	39	1	75	All extremities, chest back	2/3	1/2.5	Mild: depression
A. T.	48	2	20	Chest, back, perineum	1/2	1/1	None
D. A.	29	3	40	Face, neck, abdomen, parts of both extremities	2.5/2	1/1	None
V. R.	32	4	30	Face, neck, chest, upper extremities	2/3	1/1	None
L. T.	27	2	60	Face, neck, chest, upper extremities	3/4	2/2.5	Mild: traumatic neurosis

D. M.	39	4	40	Face, neck, chest, back, upper extremities	1/2	2/1	None
B. M.	34	5	30	Face, upper extremities	2/2	1/1	None
G. V.	19	2	37	Face, all extremities	3/2	2.5/3	Moderate: (1) traumatic neurosis; (2) depression
J. K.	31	1	90	Almost entire body surface	4/4	2/2	Mild: depression
G. L. S.	32	1	45	Hands, face, perineum, lower extremities	2/2	1/1	None
P. E.	27	3	35	Hands, face, neck, part of chest and legs	3/2	2.5/3	Moderate: (1) traumatic neurosis; (2) marital problems
M. E.	34	4	20	Face, upper extremities	1/1	1/1	None
S. S.	28	1	22	Face, upper extremities	1/1	1/1	None
F. S.	35	1	40	Face, neck, trunk, upper extremities	2/2	1/2	None
W. M.	28	1	25	Back, part of all extremities	2/2	1/1	None
M. P.	19	1	20	Face, neck, chest, upper extremities	1/2	1.5/1	None
J. H.	45	3	20	Face, neck, upper extremities	1/2	1/2	None

Problems after Discharge

Severe burns require prolonged hospitalization, the mean duration of hospitalization for patients in this study being 79 days. When he leaves the hospital, the burn patient has physically surmounted the inferno of his initial trauma and the prolonged period of intense pain that follows as his body gradually heals. At discharge he must adjust to the additional demands of regaining a normal mode of existence with a maimed body and a mind full of terrifying memories. The problems he faces are several. In the first place, he must deal with some very real threats to his ego identity for he has in some respects become a "different person" with a distorted appearance and possibly an altered future occupational role. Secondly, he often experiences emotional reactions such as depression and anxiety which he finds puzzling and disturbing.

Altered Self-Image and Identity Crisis

In his work with adolescents, Erikson[4] has developed the concept of an "identity crisis." He sees this as a "normative development" experienced by all adolescents, a development which may become pathologically aggravated in particular stressful circumstances. Although he never defines the term specifically, he uses identity to refer to "a subjective sense of an invigorating sameness and continuity" (p. 16), while a crisis is "a necessary turning point, a crucial moment, when development must move one way or another, marshaling resources of growth, recovery, and further differentiation" (p. 14). He sees this concept as a general one, applicable to a large social group as well as an individual and to an adult as well as a child. Although he did not follow up the interest, himself applying the concept in child psychology, his earliest work on "identity crisis" was on adult trauma victims—shell-shocked World War II veterans. He noted that they "had through the exigencies of war lost a sense of personal sameness and historical continuity" (p. 17), which he then described as a loss of ego identity.

The concept of identity crisis is quite helpful in understanding the adjustment problems of the burn patient. Like the adolescent approaching the demands of adulthood, he is at a turning point in his life and must confront new demands which may seem quite overwhelming. Like the adolescent too, but far more dramatically, he must confront them with a self- and body image that are changed and changing. Nearly all the external or objective factors that contribute to his self-image have been altered by his traumatic experience. His body image must be redefined to take into account scarring, deformity, and weakness. Because he is unable to resume work for some time, he also lacks an occupational identity. Interactions with other people, whether family or friends or strangers, are altered because they now respond to him as an invalid or as a person who is obviously odd or different. He thus faces an identity crisis that could potentially overwhelm him with feelings of isolation, estrangement, hopelessness, and nihilism.

Altered Appearance. Confrontation of this problem actually beings during hospitalization, as the patient gradually begins to observe the changed appearance of his skin during dressing changes. With support from friends, relatives, and hospital personnel, however, patients learn to minimize their appearance and concentrate on "just getting well."

This rather tenuous and fragile balance may become disrupted when the patient returns home. Most patients still have some dressings over incompletely healed areas at time of discharge, and open areas still appear quite red and raw; contractures of the face and hands may further distort the patient's appearance. One young mother, eager to see her children again after 3 months in the hospital, had her worst fears about her repulsive appearance confirmed when her 5-year-old drew back in horror and said, "Yuk, Mommie, you look awful." Strangers may express a revulsion that is still more painful and intolerable in that it manifests hostility founded on unconscious dread of the different or deformed. One patient overheard a cafeteria employee comment to a co-worker, "I don't know why people who look like that go out in public and make us look at them." Patients also frequently object to the pity or the curiosity they see in the eyes of strangers, since these emotions also single them out as different even if they do not express hostility. With time the scars fade and the patients become less conspicuous, but their original body image can never be totally restored. All suffer some narcissistic damage that must somehow become psychically compensated.

Altered Interpersonal Relationships. Resumption of a familiar role within the family situation could potentially help support the burn patient in his identity crisis, but all too often the sense of identity loss may be reinforced, especially during the first few days or weeks.

Because of the prolonged hospitalization, young children often fail to recognize their parents and ignore them or draw back with surprise and fear at attempts to cuddle. Children may hold back from running to greet a mother or father and spontaneously displaying affection because a well-meaning relative has told the child that touching will cause the parent pain. Thus the long-awaited homecoming and reunion may temporarily increase the sense of identity loss. Fortunately, the child's need for mothering or fathering is usually great enough to predominate eventually over any other idea or feeling, and the returned parent is able to resume his old role, his position within the family becoming the strongest single factor in his recovery of a sense of continuity and sameness.

The patient is in a somewhat different position with respect to his spouse. Usually the patient's husband or wife has been with the patient during hospitalization. In general the relationship with the spouse reinforces a sense of continuity and sameness, since the husbands and wives of burn patients tend to remain remarkably loyal and patient, demonstrating a depth of love and reassurance often previously unrecognized by either partner. However, problems nonetheless do occur, usually in the sexual sphere. Women find this adjustment difficult because of the premium placed on their physical attractiveness. Very few of the younger women interviewed were able to enjoy sex fully, commenting that they no longer felt physically attractive or sexually desirable, even in spite of assurances from their husbands that their appearance made no difference. In some, capacity to experience orgasm was reduced, while others continued to reach climax but with less subjective enjoyment. They tended to prefer to undress in seclusion or even in the dark, to react to assurances about their continued attractiveness with disbelief, and to be hypersensitive to any remark that might be interpreted as critical of their appearance. Only two men had sexual problems. One remained sexually impotent for 1½ years after being burned but eventually recovered his sexual capacity. Another, who had incurred severe perineal burns, became convinced that these had rendered him sterile and, without seeking any objective verification from a physician, assumed that he would be unable to father children.

Confronting strangers can be difficult, for they do not know how the deformity was obtained and respond at best with curiosity and at worst with hostility. Because they do not have a significant emotional investment in the patient, they do not feel any urgent need to handle him tenderly or carefully. Sensing this, patients are naturally hesitant to go out in public where they may have to submit to stares, questions, or rude remarks. One woman was taunted by neighborhood children who called her "scar-face" after she disciplined them. Several have been refused jobs because "their appearance wasn't suitable for meeting the public." Patients tend to be particularly self-conscious about going into restaurants or out on bathing beaches. They may adopt a clothing style that will cover as much of the scarring as possible, some going to such extremes as always wearing turtle necks, head scarves, or a hand covering.

Physical Handicaps. After they leave the hospital, most patients will have a prolonged period of convalescence before they are able to resume normal levels of work. Many face the prospect that they may never be able to resume normal levels or that they will have to return to a different type of work. Ability to work productively or to enjoy favorite recreations are also significant components of identity sense. The young woman with bandaged or severely contractured hands discovers not only that her child no longer recognizes her but that she finds it difficult to rebuild the relationship through mothering. Someone else still must change his diapers, feed him, and lift him out of his crib. The man discovers that he can no longer hold a wrench or a screwdriver or that he must learn new ways to do so. His skin is more fragile, more easily abraded, and more sensitive to extremes of cold and heat.

Psychological Reactions

The problems described above are realistic, objective, and concrete. Patients may at least feel they can partially resolve them through conscious effort and with the passage of time. However, they also experience a variety of more subtle and intangible emotional disturbances precipitated by the stresses of confronting these realistic problems.

Separation Anxiety and Regaining Independence. A hospital situation enforces dependency and is handled most comfortably when the patient accepts the proffered invitation to regress. Many patients become quite anxious prior to discharge, recognizing that they must now become independent again. On return home, concerned relatives, especially mothers, may encourage continued dependency and offer the patient considerable secondary gain. Rather surprisingly, considering the severe trauma incurred by patients in this series, all resisted chronic dependency and refused to become chronic invalids. A few weeks or months after discharge, they began to work actively toward the greatest measure of independence possible.

Traumatic Neurosis. During their first few weeks at home, most patients experience an intense reaction of insomnia, crying spells, excessive sensitivity, emotional lability, and marked anxiety. Some have terrifying nightmares during which they relive their past trauma, and they also tend to relive their past experiences with ruminative reworking during the day. Symptoms gradually diminish without treatment, becoming much less troubling after several months and absent after about a year. If they must return to the hospital for reconstructive plastic surgical procedures, however, patients tend to have a return of their symptomatology just prior to readmission.

Phobic Neurosis. Although most patients are quite naturally afraid of fire, none describes a phobic reaction concerning fire alone. Rather, they tend to fear circumstances which remind them of their initial injury, sometimes at an unconscious level. For example, one man who was unable to sleep at night finally discovered that he awakened whenever he heard his gas furnace turn on and this reminded him of being burned. His insomnia disappeared as soon as he moved to a home with a different heating system. Others are phobic at a more conscious level and avoid closed spaces such as elevators, basements, or second stories, which are difficult to get out of, generalizing from the specific area where they were trapped. If forced to go into such a feared area, they experience a severe panic reaction. Like the traumatic neurosis, the phobic neurosis is at its height during the first year after discharge and usually clears spontaneously without treatment.

Grief Reaction. Some patients lose husbands, wives, or children in the accident which caused their own injury. During hospitalization their minds are focused on their own survival and their own pain. Because of their regression and withdrawal into self, their grief reaction occurs only in mild form while in the hospital. Its full impact is delayed until their return home. Here a familiar face is now missing, and the realization of their loss now achieves its full impact. The pain of the loss of another is thus added to loss of continuity and sameness.

Adjustment Mechanisms Used after Discharge

The majority of the patients studied (70%) adapted quite well to the multiple problems facing them. The development of a successful adjustment is dependent on the patient's ability to absorb these multiple shocks to his sense of continuity and sameness and eventually to rebuild his sense of identity so that he feels proud of what he has become. Those patients who thus resolve their identity crisis tend to use a fairly consistent pattern of adaptive mechanisms.

Adaptive Mechanisms

Progressive Desensitization. Badly scarred patients tend to look quite grotesque to people who are not accustomed to seeing burn victims. Early after his injury, the patient himself is painfully aware of this and reacts to looking at himself or letting others see him with anxiety. His anxiety is based on a primitive fear of damage to his narcissism. His way of dealing with it is also rather primitive, although quite effective. The patient's self-administered therapy, arrived at intuitively and with some encouragement from his family, takes the form of a behavioristic desensitization. It is usually completed after the first year and usually begins with his family, who gradually reassure him through demonstrations of love and need that they care only about his "real self," the internal "good self" which has not been and cannot be touched by his trauma. As the patient resumes work and social contact, this process continues. Although a few people express their revulsion overtly, most attempt to support the patient, and thus he is able to rationalize away occasional remarks and embrace the more prevalent implication that he is not as repulsive as he fears. At first, in his painful self-consciousness, he goes out in public expecting everyone either to stare hostilely or turn away in horror; he is surprised and pleased to discover that most people react to him simply as another person. The process is reinforced as he gradually redevelops his identity and self-esteem through the additional mechanisms described below and through the subsidiary mechanism of displacement. The latter is particularly common in patients with badly scarred faces who, when asked about their appearance, express concern about relatively trivial deformities. A man with a badly scarred and contractured face felt that this was no handicap to him but expressed severe disappointment that he had lost his left ear, although it had been replaced by a prosthesis. A woman with a markedly deformed face felt that the chief problem in her appearance was that she was overweight. Indicative of the extent to which desensitization works is the fact that 7 patients out of 20 gave their deformity a lower rating than the examiner did. Thus their progressive desensitization permitted them to use denial, a mechanism that one would a priori expect to be difficult for the burn patient to use. By the time progressive desensitization is completed, the patient has learned to conceptualize his identity primarily on the basis of internal or nonphysical values and his body image is blurred, ignored, or denied.

Rationalization and Religiosity. "Why did this happen to me?" is a natural question for the burn patient to ask. Rather than responding with the self-pity or anger that one might expect, a surprising number tend to reply, "This occurred to me to make me a better person." They see their experience as a trial by fire or a purgatory through which they have passed, having proved themselves and improved themselves by surviving. One man indicated that prior to his injury his primary dedication was to drinking heavily and chasing women. He left the hospital thoroughly sobered up, began to look upon his life as a gift which he ought to be putting to better use, resolved to "work for the solid things" and to live for others as well as himself, and then by both his and his wife's accounts successfully acted on his resolution. Such a "conversion," not uncommon in the patients interviewed, helps to provide the foundation for the improved, internalized self-image which the patients must develop to resolve their identity crises. They may explain their experience as God's will, as a means of improving their family relationships or permitting them to see a goodness in others of which they were not previously aware. They almost invariably describe themselves as drawn closer to their spouses, as more trusting of them and aware of their loyalty and devotion, and as appreciative of being given a second chance to show their love for their partner. Having nearly lost their lives, their awareness of their role within the family and the extent to which they are needed by their spouse or their children is intensified.

Mastery and Control. The handicapped patient takes a great deal of pride after discharge in rehabilitating himself. Many exercise long and hard and drive themselves to return to their former strength. Patients often make a symbolic gesture soon after returning home to demonstrate that their independence and essential selfhood is not lost. His first evening home, a farmer got on his tractor and drove it around his 120 acres. Another man attended his 10-year high school reunion the day of his discharge with bandages covering the left side of his face. As their strength improves, patients throw themselves intensely into work, working longer hours than they did previously, thereby both reinforcing their self-esteem and displacing their attention from more anxiety-provoking areas. Active mastery thus becomes another significant way of recovering their sense of identity and increasing their sense of self-worth and internal strength.

Dissociation or Reworking.   Terror at the time of being burned and prolonged suffering while in the hospital are central facts in the experience of every person who has been burned. He can handle them by either dissociation or by reworking. Many patients were unable to recall what happened during large blocks of time subsequent to their injury, and this information had to be provided by their accompanying relative, who usually indicated that the patient appeared to suffer terribly during this block of time. Although Adler[1] speculated that such amnesia was correlated with improved adjustment to the injury, there was no close correlation in this study. Patients who recalled their experience in intimate detail appeared to function as well as those who were amnesic. They simply used a different method for handling the traumatic memories. By rethinking, ruminating, and ventilating, they gradually removed the painful affect from the experience and thus learned to exert a personal control over it. One might speculate that such a process of working through the resolution should produce a better adjustment than the dissociative method, but in fact this did not appear to be so either.

Maladaptive Mechanisms

*Withdrawal and Regression.*The burn patient may be tempted to use mechanisms that decrease his emotional suffering but do not further his painful struggle forward toward a "normal life." One might anticipate that some patients would develop an almost psychotic picture, with autistic withdrawal, regression, heightened sensitivity handled by a projection or denial of affect, etc. In fact, however, none did. Two patients, both women with grotesque facial scarring, did have markedly abnormal Minnesota Multiphasic Personality Inventories (MMPI) with "floating" sawtooth scales following an 8-6-7-2 pattern, which in a noninjured person would imply a severely decompensated paranoid schizophrenia with considerable depression and anxiety. Except for some increase in sensitivity and anxiety about interpersonal relations, which did not prevent them from carrying on day-to-day activities or markedly restrict their interpersonal contact, neither displayed any symptoms of the sort suggested by their MMPI patterns. Like these two, other patients admitted to being shyer, more sensitive, and more easily hurt because of self-consciousness about their deformity. They may avoid recreational activities such as swimming, be embarrassed about undressing to try on clothes in a store, or even be uncomfortable about undressing in front of their spouse. However, by and large this mechanism is most conspicuous by virtue of its absence.

Depression. One might also hypothesize that depression would be a common reaction in the burn patient. He has suffered a severe personal loss in that he has lost a portion of himself through bodily damage, and usually this loss is on conspicuous display. Such narcissistic damage does indeed produce depression at some time during hospitalization, and a few patients continue to show depressive symptoms several years after discharge. The depression tends to be mild in degree and neurotic in type with predominantly affective rather than physiological components. Six patients showed depression scales over 70 on the MMPI but none was over 80, and not all of these appeared clinically to be depressed. Among those who did, the most frequent complaints were of decreased interest or drive, intermittent blue spells, and a tendency to cry easily.

Factors Influencing Adaptation

Most patients successfully resolve their identity crisis by redefining their self-image in terms of such nonphysical and intangible attributes as courage, perseverance, living for others, increased religious faith, etc. Their belief that, in spite of physical losses, they are really better and more mature people than prior to their injury is confirmed by accompanying relatives and is probably correct. The mean estimated adjustment of patients is 1.4, while that of the examiners is 1.6, further verifying the impression that adaptation is generally good. Capacity to adapt or failure to do so is influenced by a variety of factors.

Amount of Deformity. In their studies of congenital facial deformity, MacGregor et al.[10] have noticed a tendency for those patients with lesser deformity to be more psychologically distressed by it than those with greater deformity. Although patients in our series differ in that deformity occurs during adulthood, some of our findings bear out these impressions. Two patients (10%) were felt to have moderately severe adjustment problems. Neither had any noticeable facial scarring, and both estimated their deformity at 3 while the examiner's estimate was 2. Many other patients had similar amounts of deformity and did not have similar adjustment difficulties, however, and therefore one cannot identify a close correlation between minimal deformity and maximal adjustment problems. On the other hand, two patients (10%) were felt to have marked deformity, as indicated by an examiner's estimate of 4, and yet these patients were among the 30% who were felt to have adjustment problems, although their problems were felt to be mild. Patients with very grotesque deformities incurred during their adult life can probably rally enough defenses to achieve a moderately successful adjustment, but no mechanism seems adequate to permit the patient to absorb completely the shock to his identity.

Immaturity and Narcissism. The patients noted to have adjustment difficulties disproportionate to their deformity were relatively young and very good-looking. They described themselves as having always placed a high value on physical attractiveness, feeling their own good looks contributed significantly to prior personal success and judging the worth of others by appearance primarily. "I would never go out with a girl who wasn't good-looking," one of them commented. One may speculate that their problem in accepting minimal deformity could arise either from their youth, in that they had not as yet had time to establish firmly a sense of personal identity broadly based on personal achievement as well as personal beauty, or that it could arise from a generally immature and narcissistic life-style, which is threatened by deformity at any age and always predisposed to the development of psychiatric complications.

Male vs. Female. While the male to female ratio of patients in the study was 11 to 9, the ratio of patients developing complications was 4 women to 2 men. Our society places a higher premium on attractiveness in women that it does in men. It also gives women fewer opportunities to base their identity sense on productive work or recreational skills. Women may, therefore, be more prone than men to experience a sense of identity loss as a result of physical deformity, and these data support this possibility.

Ventilation.   Some patients interviewed wept as they recalled the pain and suffering that they had experienced, even when the initial trauma occurred 4 or 5 years ago. Some of these had traumatic neuroses, but others had no significant emotional problems. What they all shared was a tendency to feel they should be brave and stoical, to be embarrassed about their tears, and to repress expression of emotion as much as possible. Quite naturally, physicians and nurses on burn units encourage patients to be stoical, since the staff gets considerable gain from being spared the sight of the patient's suffering. Relatives may also become distressed when the patient cries during hospitalization, in part because direct confrontation of the depth of the patient's suffering is painful to them and in part because they also may place a high premium on emotional control and apparent courage. The patient is thus deprived of the valuable safety valve for his emotions provided by ventilation. Remaining repressed, these distressing feelings of sorrow and pain continue to trouble him unconsciously although they rather readily achieve conscious expression when he weeps as he recalls them.

Refusal to Permit Desensitization.   Although most patients, with the help of their relatives, almost intuitively force themselves to go through the process of progressive desensitization as described above, a few do not and these patients tend to be markedly handicapped in their interpersonal relationships. One young man whose scarring was limited to his torso and legs was so self-conscious about it that he never appeared other than fully clothed in front of anyone except his parents or his physicians. He wore long trousers and a T-shirt when waterskiing, and in his college dormitory he walked fully clothed to the shower and undressed only after the shower door was closed. He always wore a bandage covering his scarred hand. Because he had no opportunity to observe the reactions of others to the appearance of his scars, he became convinced that they were much more unsightly than they actually were. Reinforced for two years, permitted and even encouraged by his family, his desire to keep his scarring hidden had reached almost obsessional proportions.

Conclusions

When he leaves the hospital, the burn patient is painfully conscious that he has in some respects become a different person facing new and different stresses. His basic adjustment problem is learning how to rally new coping and defense mechanisms that will help him resolve this crisis within his sense of identity and maintain his sense of continuity and sameness. He does this by readjusting his value system so that greater emphasis is placed on internal nonphysical qualities. Most patients eventually emerge from this crisis with renewed self-esteem based on their demonstrated ability to triumph over external limitations.

References

1. Adler, A. Neuropsychiatric complications in victims of Boston's Cocoanut Grove disaster. *J.A.M.A.*, 1943, **123**, 1098–1101.
2. Andreasen, N. J. C., Norris, A. S., & Hartford, C. E. Incidence of long-term psychiatric complications in severely burned adults. *Annals of Surgery*, 1971, **174**, 785–793.
3. Cobb, S. & Lindemann, E. Symposium on management of Cocoanut Grove burns at Massachusetts General Hospital. *Annals of Surgery*, 1943, **117**, 814–824.
4. Erikson, E. H. *Identity: Youth and crisis.* New York: W. W. Norton. Pp. 16–19.
5. Hamburg, D. A., Artz, C. P., Reiss, E., Amspacher, W. H., & Chambers, R. E. Clinical importance of emotional problems in the care of patients with burns. *New England Journal of Medicine*, 1953, **248**, 355–359.
6. Hamburg, D. A., Hamburg, B., & deGoza, S. Adaptive problems and mechanisms in severely burned patients. *Psychiatry*, 1953, **16**, 1–20.
7. Holter, J. C., & Friedman, S. B. Etiology and management of severely burned children. *American Journal of Diseases of Children*, 1969, **118**, 680–686.
8. Lewis, S. R. Goolishian, H. A., Wolf, C. W., Lynch, J. B., & Blocker, T. G. Psychologic studies in burn patients. *Plastic and Reconstructive Surgery*, 1963, **31**, 323–332.
9. Long, R. T., & Cope, O. Emotional problems of burned children. *New England Journal of Medicine*, 1961, **264**, 1121–1127.
10. MacGregor, F. C., Abel, T. M., Brut, A., Lauer, E., & Weissmann, S. *Facial deformities and plastic surgery: A psychosocial study.* Springfield, Illinois: Charles C Thomas, 1953.
11. Martin, H. L. Parents' and children's reactions to burns and scalds in children. *British Journal of Medical Psychology*, 1970, **43**, 183–191.

12. Vigliano, A., Hart, L. W., Singer, F. Psychiatric sequelae of old burns in children and their parents. *American Journal of Orthopsychiatry*, 1964, **34,** 753–761.
13. Weisz, A. E. Psychotherapeutic support of burned patients. *Modern Treatment*, 1967, **4,** 1291–1303.
14. Woodward, J. M. Emotional disturbances of burned children. *British Medical Journal*, 1959, **1,** 1009–1013.

Adjustment Problems of the Family of the Burn Patient

GENE A. BRODLAND and N. J. C. ANDREASEN

Patients who have been severely burned experience an intense and varied trauma involving catastrophic injury, severe pain, possible cosmetic or functional deformities, and a threat to their sense of identity and worth. Hospitalization is usually prolonged. During this time, the family of the burn patient often remains with him to comfort and console him. Because most of the attention of the medical staff is focused on the suffering patient, the family members remain in the background and few people are aware of their suffering and emotional needs. Yet, just as the patient himself must adjust to his injury, so the family must go through a complicated process of understanding, accepting, and adjusting to the illness and distress of the loved one.

The adjustment problems of the adult burn patient have been the subject of only a few studies, and the problems of his family have drawn still less attention.[1] Studies done in England have examined the grief reactions of parents of fatally burned children and pathology in the parents which may have contributed to behavioral problems in surviving children.[2] One follow-up study of 10 children and their parents, an

GENE A. BRODLAND, M.A., A.C.S.W. • Assistant Professor, Department of Psychiatry, Southern Illinois University School of Medicine, Springfield, Illinois. N. J. C. ANDREASEN, M.D., Ph.D. • Assistant Professor, Department of Psychiatry, University of Iowa College of Medicine, Iowa City, Iowa.

Reprinted from *Social Casework*, 1974, **55**, 13–18. Published by the Family Service Association of America.

average of 4½ years after injury, discovered recognizable psychological disturbance (usually depression) in 8 of the mothers and none of the children.[3] This morbidity is high, and it suggests that further examination of the reactions of families is needed.

The observations presented in this article are based on a study done over a period of approximately 1 year on the burn unit at the University Hospitals in Iowa City. A total of 32 adults and their families were evaluated psychiatrically on admission and were interviewed daily thereafter until the time of discharge. Initial evaluation was based on complete psychiatric and social histories and mental status examinations. The patients ranged in age from 20 to 59 with a mean of 36, in total body surface burn from 8% to 60% with a mean of 29%, and in duration of hospitalization from 2½ weeks to 3 months with a mean of 1 month. Patients outside the age range of 18 through 60 or with severe mental retardation were excluded.

The relatives of the burn patient appeared to go through an adjustment process, similar to that of the patients, involving two stages. The first stage was one of acute shock and grief analogous to the acute physical and emotional trauma experienced by the patient himself. In the second or convalescent stage, the relatives had overcome shock and disbelief; they rationalized and accepted the fact of the injury and its accompaniments and began to assist the patient in the process of recovery.

Initial Reactions of Relatives

The family's first reaction on arriving at the hospital is usually relief that the patient has not died or been burned more severely. Rationalizations that "it could have been worse" provide an affirmative basis from which to begin coping with the stress that they face. In this first stage, the relatives express little concern about the potential scarring that might take place. Their primary concern is for the recovery of the patient, no matter what his appearance on recovery. The following case history illustrates the initial reaction of many families in the first stage of hospitalization.

> Mr. S, aged 23, was severely burned in a car–truck accident. Having been pinned in the truck cab which caught fire, he sustained third-degree burns over 45% of his body. He was transferred to the burn unit 2½ weeks after being burned and

remained hospitalized for 2½ months. His wife, who visited him daily, expressed her feeling that the scarring which might result was not important. She said she "would be happy if he could get well no matter what his condition is, so the kids will have a father." She demonstrated a considerable amount of quiet desperation; tears were often evident when she expressed her feelings.

Despite expressions of relief that the patient has not died, the fear that the injury might ultimately prove fatal lingers with many relatives. Sometimes this fear is expressed overtly. Interwoven with these feelings is a well-repressed wish by some relatives that the patient would die and thereby avoid the pain and frustration that lie ahead of him. Relatives of patients who die as a result of burns support this idea; when informed that a loved one has died, they often comment, "It is probably a blessing for he won't have to suffer any more now." Such feelings are usually suppressed because of the guilt they could arouse. The case of Mrs. K illustrates this reaction.

Mrs. K, aged 24, was burned in a natural gas explosion in her home. Her husband suffered more severe burns and subsequently died. Her comments following his death indicate a degree of relief. She said, "I will miss him and it will be hard without him. He won't have to suffer for months and months. I'm glad God took him soon. I know he wouldn't want to live being terribly burned as he was. His death was a blessing." Mrs. K probably would not have said this before his death but as she rationalized in an attempt to face reality, these feelings were allowed to come to the surface.

During this early period, the relatives and the patients form feelings of trust or mistrust toward the medical staff. When a patient suffers from pain and fear, he and his relatives have to decide whether everything is being done medically to insure his comfort and recovery. Occasionally, patients and relatives question the competence of the staff and feel that the patient is the object of experimentation. The extended waiting period prior to skin grafting is often seen as abandonment and may lead to feelings of mistrust. Such feelings were expressed to the psychiatric social worker more often than to the medical staff. Relatives were concerned that by expressing angry feelings toward the staff they might jeopardize the patient's relationship with the staff.

Mr. L sustained a steam burn while working on a construction job. After skin grafting failed to take, the patient became suspicious and remarked that the resident doctor was practicing on him as if he were a "guinea pig." He requested that the social worker arrange for a transfer to a private doctor or to another hospital. He did not want to talk to the nurses or the staff doctor about his change, because it might cause hard feelings. It was determined later that his problem centered on the lack of communication between the resident and the patient. The problem was resolved when the resident made conscientious efforts to explain the treatment procedures more fully to the patient.

Soon after admission, a number of extensively burned patients experience confusion and disorientation as a result of an acute brain syndrome that often accompanies burn trauma. Many relatives found this reaction stressful. Sometimes a patient was verbally abusive or assaultive, and relatives had a difficult time in deciding whether this behavior represented his true feelings or whether it was the result of delirium. Relatives were frightened by this sudden "mental illness" and needed reassurance that delirium is a common occurrence in burn patients and that once the burn begins to heal, the delirium passes.

> Mr. R, a 28-year-old farm hand, was burned over 60% of his body in a natural gas explosion. About a week and a half after admission to the burn unit, he became delirious. During his periods of confusion, he thought of a period during his second year of marriage when his wife had had an extramarital affair. Mr. R angrily expressed the belief that this affair was still going on. His bewildered wife thought that this problem had been resolved 8 years before. Mrs. R needed reassurance that his accusations were a result of his delirium. After Mr. R recovered, he denied any feelings of suspicion toward his wife.

Another source of difficulty for relatives is the psychologic regression that is often observed among the burn patients. Patients who have been quite self-sufficient in the conduct of their daily lives before being hospitalized often become complaining, demanding, and dependent during hospitalization. The family, unaccustomed to this behavior, becomes alternately confused and angry. They want to respond to the patient's needs but are confused by demands that seem so out of character. Relatives become angry when the patients do not give them credit for their efforts and continue with their childlike behavior.

Reactions after Initial Crisis

During the second phase of adjustment, the family is assured that the patient will survive and begins to consider the process of getting well. The family members begin to recognize that they and the patient still have many weeks in the hospital ahead of them. The patient and his relatives usually have no prior knowledge of the treatment and procedures required for recovery; now they begin to ask questions of physicians and nurses about the process of healing, dressing changes, grafting procedures, and so on. Often relatives of other patients on the ward are important sources of information, just as they are sources of reassurance. The family of the patient must prepare themselves psychologically for an extended stay in the hospital. From a practical standpoint, family members must make arrangements for their own physical well-being during this period and establish "a home away from home." This often involves spending days at the hospital and nights in a nearby motel.

The pain the patient suffers is a primary problem at this time, and it often results in a sense of helpless frustration in the relatives. The patient seems to become increasingly cognizant of his pain once the threat of death has passed. He then begins to verbalize the pain, at times in tones of desperation. The helplessness which relatives feel in handling this pain produces conflict. On the one hand, they try to do everything within their power to aid the patient by making him physically comfortable and providing emotional support. On the other hand, relatives sometimes feel the staff could relieve pain more adequately by the administration of analgesic medication. The relative often is in a precarious position, trying to maintain a good relationship both with the patient and with the medical staff. Few persons understand fully the principles followed in the use of pain medication. The following example illustrates the development in one relative of mistrust of the staff.

> Mrs. B was burned when she and her family were trapped upstairs in their burning home. She broke her arm when she jumped from a second-story window to escape the flames. Because of the burns, the staff were unable to put her arm in the correct cast. The arm was very painful. Because of her complaints of pain and her mother's frustration in attempting to alleviate the pain, the mother confronted the nurse with the accusation that the staff was neglecting her daughter by not giving her enough pain medication. Once the problems inherent in using potent analgesics for long periods of time were explained in detail, the patient's mother was much relieved and could again be supportive to the patient.

Another source of pain occurring during this period is the process of autografting. The donor site, from which the skin for grafting is taken, often is more painful than the burn site itself, causing great distress to the patient. Further, the patient must lie quietly after the grafts have been placed, increasing the sense of helplessness felt by both patient and relatives. The fear of doing something that might disturb the graft is a significant cause of anxiety.

The frequent trips to the operating room for skin grafting are yet another source of anxiety. The fear of anesthesia must be faced each time the operative procedure approaches; the patient is anxious about being put to sleep and having to relinquish control. This anxiety is often sensed by the relatives.

Reactions during Recovery

Still later in the recovery period, the problem of pain is supplanted by one of itching, which creates a problem for the relatives who try to help the patient to tolerate each new stress. It often seems that total recovery will never arrive and that one discomfort is simply succeeded by another.

Another major problem faced during the recovery phase is fear of deformity. Most families initially expect grafting to restore fairly normal appearance. What medical personnel consider an excellent job of skin reconstruction is often viewed by the lay person as almost grotesque. Thus, patient and family tend to be disappointed by the results of grafting and to find a gap between their expectations and those of medical personnel. During this stage of recovery, the patient begins to prepare himself for facing the outside world by realizing that scarring and deformity may have made him unattractive and unacceptable to others with whom he has previously associated. He becomes hypersensitive to initial reactions and wonders what reactions he will find himself meeting the rest of his life. Relatives have similar fears.

The relatives' reactions are the first ones that the patient observes, and his distress is increased when he sees revulsion. A fairly typical case of family reaction was noted in a follow-up study of burn patients.[4] A young mother who had been hospitalized for 3 months eagerly anticipated seeing her children. She was greeted by her 5-year-old with "Yuk, Mommie, you look awful." Adult family members, on the other hand, tend to recognize intuitively that they need to be supportive and to help the patient establish a denial system. Yet, providing a reassurance that they do not always sincerely feel is often quite stressful for them. Only with time and thoughtful support on the part of doctors, nurses, and relatives can the patient resolve his feelings about disfigurement and come to realize that angry red scars eventually fade and that his appearance will gradually improve.

Sometimes relatives carry an additional burden because of their feeling that they have contributed to or caused the accident in which the patient was injured. Even when the relatives have had nothing to do with the injury, some feel guilty; they explain this feeling on the basis of not having foreseen the possibility of the accident and not having taken steps to prevent it. Eventually, the relative resolves his guilt feelings and achieves a rationalization that relieves him of full responsibility for the accident—for example, that the accident happened because it was God's will, because it would draw the family together, or because of the carelessness of others.

Notable throughout the recovery period is the difficulty that relatives have in dealing with the patient's need to express his feelings. They find it difficult to strike a balance between letting the patient describe his feelings about being burned and possibly handicapped and providing adequate emotional support. Sometimes relatives attempt to discourage the patient from expressing feelings of grief or fear and try to be constantly supportive and optimistic. In preserving their own comfort, they sometimes unwittingly deprive the patient of a necessary safety valve.

There are also relatives who become overwhelmed by the emotional stress of sitting at the bedside of a loved one and sharing his suffering. Many are reluctant to leave the bedside in the early stages of recovery, fearing that something might happen while they are gone. Occasionally, relatives become too depressed or anxious and must be asked to leave the ward temporarily to regain their emotional equilibrium. Remaining at the bedside of a burned patient is an unusually draining experience for his relatives. Much like a young child, the burn patient tends to focus only on himself and provides little support in return, leaving little opportunity for relatives to converse or receive support from others.

Recommendations from This Study

A burn injury is a traumatic experience for the uninjured relatives, as well as the patient himself. The families of the burn patients face multiple stresses and adjustment problems. They go through essentially the same phases of adaptation as the patients, for they must cope with anxiety about death, communication difficulties with the medical staff, fear of deformity, and the boredom of a prolonged hospital stay, as well as enduring the trauma of watching a loved one suffer. In some respects, their suffering may be greater than that of the patient. Although they do not suffer pain directly, they must stand by in helpless frustration, their guilt over the fact that the injury occurred at all further enhanced by their guilt about the anger which they must inevitably feel sometimes. Although they do not fear death or deformity for themselves directly, they must face these threats more immediately than the patient. Few patients are informed of their prognosis soon after admission and, if they were, their minds would be too clouded by trauma to comprehend it fully; however, relatives cannot be shielded from this information, and they must receive it when their minds are usually in a state of heightened sensitivity and alertness.

Relatives may provide valuable assistance on wards by helping to feed the patient, by providing companionship for him, and often by encouraging and assisting him with exercise and physical therapy. Nevertheless, nurses and physicians provide primary care, and the role of relatives must inevitably be simply a supportive one. This role is a difficult one to fulfill in such an emotionally draining situation unless the person providing the support receives support from others for himself. On the burn unit, this need was often met by the relatives of other patients. Although there was no formal effort by the staff to enhance such relationships, relatives often pooled their information about treatment methods, compared notes on the condition of the patient, and consoled one another when things were going badly.

Hospital burn units could learn a lesson from this phenomenon and formalize it in several ways. Relatives could be helped greatly if hospitals prepared a simple pamphlet to be given to them on arrival, explaining simple facts about injuries from burns and the operation of the unit. It should state the visting hours established and describe the daily routine, the purpose of unfamiliar treatment methods such as the use of silver nitrate and sulfamylon, the rationale behind the use of milder and preferably oral analgesics, the usual course of recovery from a burn injury, the nature of the grafting procedures usually done, and so forth. A glossary of unfamiliar terms—*autograft, zenograft, debridement,* for example—should be included. Because of the complex nature of this type of injury, burn treatment units are often run quite differently from other hospital facilities, and relatives cannot carry over any prior hospital experience. For example, they find it difficult to understand the infrequent use of potent analgesics, although this practice usually becomes acceptable when they realize that the long-term use required in a burn injury might lead to dependence or addiction. On the affirmative side, on some burn units, rules about visiting hours are flexible and most relatives are permitted to remain with the patient as long as they wish.

A second way of providing communication and understanding among relatives would be the establishment of group support meetings. A group composed of family members or close friends of patients currently on the burn unit could meet at a regularly scheduled time once or twice weekly. The group would remain in existence, although the membership changed as the patient population changed. Ideally, this group would be conducted by a pair of group leaders—a psychiatric social worker and a nurse or physician who are members of the burn unit treatment team. A physical therapist, a dietitian active on the burn unit, and a psychiatrist familiar with the problems of adjustment to chronic illness would be other potential members or guest visitors.

The establishment of such a group would serve several purposes. It would demonstrate to the beleaguered relatives the interest and concern of the hospital staff, sometimes prone to leave relatives out of the picture because of their concern for primary patient care; regular group meetings would make efficient use of the professionals' time and experience. The meetings would also serve to educate relatives about problems of burn trauma, particularly when discharge draws near. Family members often take on primary responsibility for the patient at discharge and they greatly need adequate information about wound care, the need for continuing physical therapy, and the problems of emotional and social adjustment. The group discussions would provide relatives with an open forum for raising questions and for airing complaints. They would provide emotional support by strengthening the bonds formed between family members and alleviate some feelings of fear, frustration, futility, and boredom. Such a group would not be designed as therapy, but as a means of sharing strength and information. Limited experience with such group meetings on burn units indicates, however, that often staff members also receive information and support from them.

A final way for social work staff to be effective on a burn unit is perhaps the most obvious. Families of patients often suffer significant financial expenses, and even after the patient is discharged the period of rehabilitation is prolonged. Family members and patients need to receive information about funds available to assist in the high cost of hospitalization, funds for care of dependents, and opportunities for vocational rehabilitation. An experienced and sensitive social worker can often provide subtle emotional support by demonstrating his concerned involvement as he offers his resources of information and interest to the family.

References

1. Andreasen, N. J. C., Noyes, R., Hartford, C. E., Brodland, G. A., & Proctor, S. Management of emotional problems in seriously burned adults. *New England Journal of Medicine,* **286,** 65–69 (January 13, 1972); Hamburg, D. A., Artz, C. P., Reiss, E. Amspacher, W. H., & Chambers, R. E. Clinical importance of emotional problems in the care of patients with burns. *New England Journal of Medicine,* **248,** 355–59 (February 26, 1953); Hamburg, D. A., Hamburg, B., & deGoza, S. Adaptive problems and mechanisms in severely burned patients. *Psychiatry,* **16:**1–20 (February 1953).
2. Martin, H. L., Lawrie, J. H., & Wilkinson, A. W. The family of the fatally burned child. *Lancet* **295:**628–29 (September 14, 1968); Martin, H. L. Antecedents of burns and scalds in children. *British Journal of Medical Psychology,* **43,** 39–47 (March 1970); Martin, H. L. Parents' and children's reactions to burns and scalds in children. *British Journal of Medical Psychology,* **43,** 183–91 (1970).
3. Vigliano, A., Hart, L. W., & Singer, F. Psychiatric sequelae of old burns in children and their parents. *American Journal of Orthopsychiatry,* **34,** 753–61 (July 1964).
4. Andreasen, N. J. C., Norris, A. S., & Hartford, C. E. Incidence of long-term psychiatric complications in severely burned adults. *Annals of Surgery,* **174,** 785–93 (November 1971).

The Crisis of Illness: Chronic Conditions

Acute illness, as we have seen in earlier sections, can precipitate significant emotional as well as physical crises. Chronic disease or disability, where a full return to a pre–illness "normality" is not likely, requires a long-term adjustment somewhat different from that for acute illness episodes. A new equilibrium must be evolved which reflects permanently altered circumstances such as increased dependency and new limitations in functional abilities.

The onset of chronic disease can be sudden and require immediate drastic changes, as with multiple sclerosis, or more gradual changes, as with arthritis. Faith Perkins's[8] account of her experience with osteoarthritis provides an interesting example of a personal coping strategy. She took refuge in her work and other activities, using them to distract her from the pain and from her anxiety about the effects of her illness. She sought emotional support from relatives and friends at critical times (for example, by arranging for a close friend to accompany her when she had hip surgery). Other significant methods of dealing with her fears and her increasing disability included arming herself with information about the course of her disease and possible treatments, and identification with the millions of other arthritis patients who were facing problems similar to hers.

Chronic disability, a residual effect after an injury or disease, creates adjustment problems similar to those for chronic illness.

Changes in self-image, dependency conflicts, and effects on interpersonal relationships are involved in both cases. The first task is to accept the disability as final and irrevocable and make the difficult transition from being "sick" to being "different."[2] Only after that is accomplished can the necessary grieving and reintegration be done. Major social readjustments are also necessary. Blind people, for example, must deal with the strong stereotyping the sighted try to impose on the blind and the tension and uneasiness which result when these stereotypes prove inadequate.[3] Finally, it is essential to find a balance between absolute denial of any need for help, which can lead to frustration and anxiety, and excessive regression, whereby the person does not achieve his full potential and uses his illness or disability as an excuse. Those who can master their own anxiety and who enjoy the support of the significant people in their lives usually learn to accept their limitations, and recognize and use their remaining abilities effectively.

Chronic illness can have an especially profound impact on a child's physical and emotional development. Parents and siblings are also affected by the experience. Many aspects of chronic illness can be sources of stress: episodes of acute illness (for example, hemophiliac bleedings), the disablement of the child (as in the crippling of hemophiliac arthroses), special treatment procedures (such as the brace for scoliosis), the different-from-normal life-style with its sense of isolation and its implication of inferiority, the intensification of the dependence–independence conflict, and the long-term prognosis (as in cystic fibrosis, which is progressive and fatal). The resources with which children deal with these stresses are determined in large part by their developmental stage and the support available from parents and medical personnel.

In the first article Ake Mattsson provides an overview of childhood adaptation to long-term physical illness. He outlines the general stresses (such as pain, separations from the family, and the restriction of activity during hospitalization) and those related to particular types of illness (for example, fear of losing control in convulsive disorders, fear of suffocation in respiratory diseases). Mattsson describes cognitive coping functions, which enable a child to understand the nature of his illness and the purpose of various treatment procedures, and motor activities, which are an important outlet for energy and tension, especially for a young child whose verbal abilities are not fully developed (see Downey[1] for a child's personal view).

The transition from passive dependence to self-reliant independence is a critical issue in every child's development. When chronic illness occurs before independence is firmly established, it pulls the child back into dependent patterns he is trying to leave behind. Examples of difficulties surrounding this issue include the knowledge a young diabetic has that his very life depends on regular insulin injections from his parents, the inclination of some parents of hemophiliacs to encourage passivity in hopes of safeguarding their child from physical trauma, continual dependence on doctors, and frequent experiences in hospitals where nurses take over the management of many bodily functions. Parents and children both must learn to accept the reasonable limits to independence which circumstances dictate, while encouraging and struggling for the maximum development within those limits.

The role of the parents and other family members in promoting a healthy adaptation by the child is crucial. Family members must deal with ambivalent feelings and be supportive without excessive overprotection or rejection. When the illness is genetically based as in hemophilia and cystic fibrosis, parents carry an extra burden of guilt with which they must come to terms. Constant anxiety about acute episodes of illness or about the possibility of the child's death is a major threat to the parents' mental well-being and to their ability to help the sick child.

Mattsson and Agle[6] describe several coping mechanisms used by parents of hemophiliacs, including isolation of distressing feelings, especially during a crisis, mental self-preparation by thinking through anticipated events, and identification with other parents of hemophiliacs. Suzanne Massie, the mother of a hemophiliac, described her way of coping as a "constant, disciplined effort to push into the far corners of my mind all the terrible ifs" (Massie & Massie,[5] p. 140). Religiosity (for instance, seeing the illness as part of "God's plan") is another source of comfort and strength for many people (see Kolin et al.;[4] Massie & Massie[5]).

Cystic fibrosis, one of the most serious childhood diseases, presents children and their parents with a severe psychological challenge. Daily therapeutic procedures are essential for survival but cannot alter the ultimate course of the disease—progressive deterioration and an early death. The financial burden, the frequent disruption of family activities, and the deferment of parental and sibling needs to those of the patient are an integral part of the CF experience. Patients are seldom permitted to escape the harsh realities of their illness and enjoy the appearance of normalcy, as their equipment (for example, the mist tent in the bedroom) or their symptoms (cough, flatulence, retarded physical and sexual development) usually intrude and set them apart again. Recent improvements in the detection and management of CF have advanced the physical struggle significantly, but it is also important to consider the emotional adjustments which must be made in order for the quality of life to reflect and justify the physical effort expended.

Alan Tropauer, Martha Neal Franz, and Victor Dilgard discuss the psychological adaptation of cystic fibrosis patients and their families in the second article. Most of the children had a fair understanding (for their ages) of the disease process and prognosis; they had learned to limit their goals accordingly—control of symptoms rather than hope for a total cure. Patients also use the process of identification, especially with medical personnel, to relieve their anxiety about medical procedures, their role as dependent patients, and so on. Through this kind of identification (whether in fantasy or in future ambitions) the patient becomes the actor, the helper, rather than the passive and inadequate recipient of care.

Tropauer, Franz, and Dilgard also explore the nature of adaptive behavior on the part of family members of cystic fibrosis patients. Faithfully carrying out therapeutic measures such as postural drainage relieves the sense of helplessness somewhat, although for some parents there may be a reciprocal increase in the level of responsibility and guilt felt when setbacks or crises occur. The demands on time and energy which these measures make (and the need to make corresponding sacrifices in other areas) engender strong feelings of anger and resentment. Since it is usually unacceptable to direct these feelings at the patient they are often displaced to an unsupportive spouse, previous doctors, non-CF families or some other target. The prognosis, however, with its mixture of uncertainty and inevitability, is particularly stressful to the family. McCollum and Gibson[7] suggest that long-term adaptation is largely a matter of finding a balance between anticipatory mourning and denial of the fatal prognosis.

With some illnesses the treatment is a greater source of distress than the symptoms. To a certain extent this is true of hemodialysis for chronic renal disease (see part VIII) and of corrective open-heart surgery (see part IV). It also applies to less severe cases of scoliosis (a disease causing progressive abnormal spinal curvature usually occurring in growing girls especially in the preadolesent and adolescent stages) which is the subject of the third article. Beverly Myers, Stanford Friedman, and Irving Weiner interviewed 25 girls and their mothers to determine how they adjusted to the diagnosis of scoliosis and the prescription of the Milwaukee brace and special exercises for its treatment. They found that after an "initial storm" of protest and distress the majority accepted the prescribed regimen, although their faithfulness in wearing the brace and carrying out the exercise program varied. The girls and their mothers had to cope with three major threats: the threat of deformity and disability as a result of the disease, the threat of the treatment (the brace marks the girls as different at an age when conformity is very important), and the disturbing feelings associated with the first two.

The authors divide the coping process into intrapsychic defenses and motor-behavioral activity. Psychological mechanisms include denial of the threat of permanent deformity, displacement of angry feelings to safe targets, and rationalization. Motor-behavioral activity serves to reduce the threat and increase feelings of effectiveness, for example, wearing the brace and doing the exercises faithfully. As the years go by and some improvement is seen it becomes increasingly difficult for girls to maintain their commitment to wear the brace. The majority, however, do keep up the treatment, especially in cases where the girls and their mothers thoroughly understand the nature of the illness and the purpose of the brace and exercises, where they make an active decision to follow the treatment program, where the prognosis is optimistic, and where family and medical staff are understanding and supportive.

References

1. Downey, T. J. All my times in the hospital—A child remembers. *American Journal of Nursing,* 1974, **74,** 2196–2198.
2. Feldman, D. J. Chronic disabling illness: A holistic view. *Journal of Chronic Disease,* 1974, **27,** 287–291.
3. Franks, D. D. Adjustment to acquired blindness. *Kansas Medical Society Journal,* 1971, **72,** 238–243.
4. Kolin, I. S., Scherzer, A. L. New, B., & Garfield, M. Studies of the school age child with meningomyelocele: Social and emotional adaptation. *Journal of Pediatrics,* 1971, **78,** 1013–1019.
5. Massie, R., & Massie, S. *Journey.* New York: Alfred A. Knopf, 1975.
6. Mattsson, A., & Agle, D. P. Group therapy with parents of hemophiliacs. *American Academy of Child Psychiatry,* 1972, **11,** 558–571.
7. McCollum, A. T., & Gibson, L. E. Family adaptation to the child with cystic fibrosis. *Journal of Pediatrics,* 1970, **77,** 571–578.
8. Perkins, F. *My fight with arthritis.* New York: Random House, 1964.

13

Long-Term Physical Illness in Childhood: A Challenge to Psychosocial Adaptation

AKE MATTSSON

Robert Louis Stevenson, a victim of pulmonary tuberculosis, once wrote, "Life is not a matter of holding good cards, but of playing a poor hand well." Children with a chronic physical disorder who have successfully mastered the physical, social, and emotional hardships associated with their illness well illustrate his point. This paper intends to review the common forms of emotional stress experienced by the child with a long-term illness and by his parents. It also describes the major adaptational techniques enabling the sick child and his family to achieve a satisfactory psychosocial adaptation.

Long-term or chronic illness refers to a disorder with a protracted course which can be progressive and fatal, or associated with a relatively normal life span despite impaired physical or mental functioning. Such a disease frequently shows periods of acute exacerbations requiring intensive medical attention. Long-term childhood disorders may cause significant and permanent interference with the child's physical and

AKE MATTSSON, M.D. • Professor of Psychiatry and Pediatrics, University of Virginia Medical Center, Charlottesville, Virginia. Supported in part by U.S. Public Health Service Grant No. 2T01MH12904.

Reprinted from *Pediatrics*, 1972, 50, 801–811.

emotional growth and development. This is in contrast to acute non-life-threatening illnesses in which both physical dysfunctioning and attendant emotional upset usually are of a limited duration and do not as a rule interfere with the child's overall development.[1,2]

The prevalence of chronic conditions in childhood is staggering if visual and hearing impairments, mental retardation, and speech, learning, and behavior disorders are included. Such a scope yields an estimate of 30% to 40% of children up to the age of 18 suffering from one or more long-term disorders.[3] Even if only serious chronic illnesses of primary physical origin are included, American and British surveys still report that 7% to 10% of all children are afflicted.[4,5] The most common physical conditions are asthma (about 2% of the population under age 18), epilepsy (1%), cardiac conditions (5%), cerebral palsy (5%), orthopedic illness (5%), and diabetes mellitus (1%). Less frequencies pertain to cleft palate, bleeding disorders, anemias, blindness, and deafness.

The following classification of long-term childhood disorders is based on consideration of ontogenetic stages and nature of pathogenic factors:

1.   Diseases due to chromosomal aberrations (e.g., Down's syndrome, Klinefelter's syndrome, Turner's syndrome)

2.   Diseases as results of abnormal hereditary traits (e.g., spherocytosis, sickle cell anemia, hemophilia, cystic fibrosis, muscular dystrophy, osteogenesis imperfecta, diabetes mellitus, inborn errors of metabolism; certain forms of "congenital malformations" such as microcephaly, clubfoot, cleft palate, dislocation of the hip, blindness, and deafness)

3.   Diseases due to harmful intrauterine factors (e.g., infections such as rubella, congenital syphilis, and toxoplasmosis with their attendant malformations; damage from massive radiation, various drugs, prenatal hypoxia, and blood type incompatibilities)

4.   Disorders resulting from perinatal traumatic and infectious events including permanent damage to central nervous system and motor apparatus

5.   Diseases due to serious postnatal and childhood infections, injuries, neoplasms, and other factors (e.g., meningitis, encephalitis, tuberculosis, rheumatic fever, chronic renal disease; physical injuries with permanent handicaps; tumors and leukemia; orthopedic diseases;

convulsive disorders; atopic conditions; mental illness and mental retardation of organic etiology)

Psychologic Impact of Long-Term Illness

Children with long-term physical disorders are subjected to a multitude of emotionally stressful situations, often of a recurring nature. Acute illnesses pose similar psychologic threats which usually prove less harmful due to their shorter duration.[1,2,6-10] The common causes for emotional stress associated with long-term illness are:

Malaise, Pain, Various Physical Symptoms, and Reasons for Illness

Uncertainty as to why pain and suffering occur is a psychic stress to anyone. The preschool child in particular has little ability to comprehend the causality and nature of an illness and tends to interpret pain and other symptoms as a result of mistreatment, punishment, or "being bad." In a child's mind nothing happens by chance, and he looks for reasons for an event such as an illness in the immediate past.[11,12] Children up to the ages of 8 to 10 often attribute illness and injury to recent family interactions, e.g., they got sick because of their disobedience or because the parents failed to protect them. They might then blame themselves or other family members for causing the disease. These distorted interpretations of their bodily changes often become perpetuated by their reluctance to ask questions and vent their irrational fears about why they became ill. Other examples of children's crude cause-and-effect reasoning relative to illness are: A young colitis patient blamed his illness on having "eaten something dirty"; a child with cardiac disease had "run too much"; a diabetic girl had "eaten too much candy"; a hemophilic boy developed a hematoma because his "skin was so thin."

Young patients afflicted with a hereditary illness will usually learn of the likely genetic transmission before or during adolescence. Under whatever circumstances this knowledge is obtained by the child, it is potentially traumatic to the child–parent relationship. Many such children voice hostile accusations against their parents, as they try to master the anger, sadness, and anxiety aroused by their recognition of the hereditary nature of their disability.

Hospital Admissions, Nursing, and Treatment Procedures

The often frequent and lengthy hospital admissions for the chronically ill child involve separations from his family, school, and set of friends. He is expected to adjust to an unfamiliar, regimented hospital environment, with a confusing array of health specialists and frightening, often painful medical procedures.[7,13,14] Again, it is the preschool child that tends to suffer most from these stressful separations from the trusted family setting. Such repeated episodes can be destructive to the child unless a strong "therapeutic alliance" between his parents and the medical staff provides him with a plenitude of visiting and care by the mother, a homelike ward setting, and ample information and preparations regarding procedures.[8,10,13,15]

Any ill person who receives nursing care at home or in a hospital experiences feelings of helplessness, embarrassment, and irritation. To be "treated like a child" during an illness is often more upsetting to a young patient than to an adult.[6,7,11] A bedridden child, unable to dress and feed himself and to use the bathroom without help, resents the loss of such recent gains in his development. The less ill he feels, the stronger his resentment. Anger, humiliation, and anxiety about the backward pull toward a state of helpless dependency are frequently observed, and the hospital staff and the parents may become targets of defiant protests. Some children regress to more babyish behavior without much protest and need considerable help to regain achievements in motor and social functioning after an illness.

Injections, infusions, immobilization, surgery, and other procedures arouse anxiety beyond the discomfort involved, because they reactivate the universal childhood fears of bodily mutilation and disfigurement and the illogical views of medical procedures as a punishment for actual or imagined misdeeds. Such fantasies generally cause less problems for the older grade school child, because his strides in cognitive development enable him better to comprehend the causal and temporal relationship of an illness or injury.[12] Most sick children find immobilization and restriction of activity emotionally stressful. They rely on freedom of movement to discharge tension, to express dissatisfaction and aggression, and to explore and master the environment. Sudden or prolonged motor restraint of a young child can cause him to panic, develop temper tantrums, and become a serious management problem. At other times, he might show the opposite reaction of withdrawal into an apathetic, depressed state. The child with poor ability or lack of opportunity to verbalize his feelings is more prone to show marked behavioral reactions to forced restraints.

Changes in the Emotional Climate

Family members tend to change their attitudes toward their sick child and usually become more loving and indulgent, letting up on discipline and rules.[6] Changes in the opposite direction are rare but potentially more dangerous: Some parents reject their ill child, criticize him for causing much inconvenience, and even neglect his care. Any of these changes in family attitudes can be confusing to the child as, for instance, when he has to relinquish the secondary gains of being sick.

Stress Factors Related to Special Chronic Syndromes

Certain aspects of causation, symptomatology, and medical care of many long-term illnesses pose special problems and fears to the child and his family. Some common examples of such situations follow.

Fluctuations in the control of *juvenile diabetes* frequently seem related to emotional factors.[16,17] The diabetic child, along with his family, may worry about attacks of hypoglycemia or acidosis as a result of highly emotionally charged family interaction. Some adolescents in rebellious, hostile, or depressed states abandon their diabetic regime as angry and self-destructive means to threaten or retaliate. This abandonment is often conscious, which indicates a far more serious maladjustment than the chronically ill person's common use of his ailment as an escape or a defense.

Similar to the young diabetic patient, the child with a *convulsive disorder* frequently fears loss of consciousness or uncontrollable strange behavior while suffering from a seizure. Seizures are socially stigmatizing especially when they take place at school and among peers. The epileptic teen-ager feels uniquely frustrated, as he cannot obtain a driver's license until after several years without seizures. This prolongs his dependence on the parents for providing transportation in regards to many school and leisure activities.

Children with *serious respiratory disease,* such as asthma[18-20] and cystic fibrosis,[21] commonly harbor fears of suffocation, drowning, or dying while asleep. The asthmatic child often finds that his wheezing will evoke anxious, indulgent, and sympathetic responses from his family, whose members may feel responsible for contributing to his attacks of labored breathing and discomfort.

The child with cystic fibrosis has to cope with such embarrassing symptoms as flatulence and stool odor, with the complex management of postural drainage and nebulization, and with the growing awareness that his illness is hereditary and progressive, carrying a poor prognosis.

Chronic bleeding disorders, such as hemophilia, often cause the young child to be concerned about fatal bleeding resulting from physical trauma and certain medical procedures, e.g., venous puncture. Emotional distress might increase the likelihood of bleeding in face of minor physical trauma or even lead to "spontaneous" bleeding episodes without apparent trauma.[22,23]

The child with a *chronic heart disease* of infectious or congenital nature often has minimal signs of a serious condition and may find it difficult to comprehend the nature of his illness and the reasons for restrictions, extensive work-ups, and surgery. Furthermore, the knowledge of an affliction of one's heart seems especially frightening due to the common ambiguous and symbolic references to "the heart" in everyday language.[24,25] An active psychoeducational preparation for heart surgery is of special importance since states of marked apprehension and depression may complicate cardiac surgery in childhood and adolescence.[26]

An increasing number of children with *chronic renal disease* are treated with hemodialysis and kidney transplantation. Several unique features pertain to these procedures.[27,28] The life-perpetuating kidney machine often creates frightening fantasies in the child, such as fears of bleeding to death or of the machine assuming control of him. The use of immunosuppressive drugs causes Cushingoid appearance and interferes with the child's growth, already stunted by preexisting uremia. Consequently, these young patients often feel isolated and apart. This may be particularly difficult for the teen-ager, seeking independence from his family and a sense of identity among his peers. After kidney transplantation, many children find their parents tending to overprotect them and to use threats implying possible failure of the new kidney as a means of controlling their activities. The occurrence of "kidney rejection anxiety" at times of minor physical symptoms has been observed in children as long as six years after a successful transplantation. In cases of actual kidney rejection, requiring a return to hemodialysis, the young patient, like the adult, usually responds with a depressed, withdrawn state. Children in particular then tend to blame themselves for 'destroying" the kidney given to them as a special gift, often by a family member. It should be noted, however, that follow-ups on children who have undergone renal transplantation have found many of them showing growth spurts as long as five years after surgery and a good adjustment as young adults.[29]

Children with *ulcerative colitis* and similar conditions often have unrealistic fears of certain food items harming them. Their frequent inability to control defecations cause much embarrassment. The common family preoccupation with the ill child's diet and with his stools requires energetic pediatric counseling. These children and their families often have to be prepared for a temporary or permanent ileostomy when other treatment methods fail. Such a procedure entails many realistic problems which are particularly stressful to an adolescent as he is beginning to establish intimate heterosexual friendships.[30] The counseling assistance of an older person with a successful ileostomy can be useful in supporting the young patient's self-image and confidence.

The recent interest in children and teen-agers of *short stature,* often complicated by delayed sexual maturation,[31] has shown that a major problem of the undersized child is related to his environments's tendency to baby him "as a dwarf" instead of treating him according to his chronological age. His sense of uniqueness may cause him to withdraw, leading to an inhibition of his cognitive and emotional development.[32] Some short youngsters cope by an excessive denial of their condition and become either good-natured jokers with few aggressive strivings or spunky and overly assertive individuals.

The format of this paper does not permit further illustrations of specific emotional stress factors associated with many chronic handicaps and disorders in childhood, such as mental retardation,[33] brain dysfunction and cerebral palsy,[34-37] congenital amputees,[38,39] orthopedic conditions,[40] cleft palate,[41] and cryptorchism.[42] Helpful reviews of the psychological implications of long-term sensory, motor, visceral, and metabolic conditions in young patients are given by Prugh,[8] Apley and

MacKeith,[10] Vernon et al.,[14] Kessler,[43] and Green and Haggerty.[44] The unique emotional burdens associated with fatal illness in childhood and adolescence have recently been reviewed by Friedman[45] and Easson.[46]

Additional Psychologic Threats

The child with a serious, chronic disease has to cope with threats of exacerbations, lasting physical impairment, and, at times, a shortened life expectancy. Other common concerns of his and his family relate to mounting medical expenses and the interference of his illness with schooling, leisure activities, vocational training, job opportunities, and later adult role as a spouse and a parent. In learning to live with a disability that demands continuous medical attention often away from home, the growing child is expected to assume responsibility for his own care and accept certain limitations in his activities.

The final outcome of the child's attempts at mastering the continuous stress associated with his disability cannot be assessed until young adulthood. Each progressive step in his emotional, intellectual, and social development changes the psychologic impact of the illness on his personality and on his family and usually equips him with better means to cope.[37,47] Changes in the disease process and in familial circumstances will also affect the adaptational process.

Coping Behavior and Adaptation in Children

Several authors have used the conceptual framework of coping behavior to describe the responses of children and parents to such severe stress situations as serious illness, separation, and the threat of death.[23,48-51] This term denotes all the adaptational techniques used by an individual to master a major psychologic threat and its attendant negative feelings in order to allow him to achieve personal and social goals. Coping behavior, then, includes the use of cognitive functions (perception, memory, speech, judgment, reality testing), motor activity, emotional expression, and psychologic defenses. (Defenses represent unconscious processes aiming at reappraisals and distortions of a threatening reality to make it more bearable.[48,52]) Successful coping behavior results in adaptation, which implies that the person is functioning effectively.

Many studies on long-term childhood disorders report a surprisingly adequate psychosocial adaptation of children followed to young adulthood.[7,8,10] These well-adapted patients have for years functioned effectively at home, in school, and with their peers, and with few limitations other than those realistically imposed by their disease and its sequelae. Their dependence on their family has been age-appropriate and realistic, and they have little need for secondary gains offered by the illness. From age 6 to 7, these children's use of such cognitive functions as memory, speech, and reality testing provided them with a beginning understanding of the nature of their illness. This allowed them to accept limitations, assume responsibility for their care, and assist in the medical management. This appropriate appearance of a sense of self-protection served the vital function of self-preservation and precluded the development of helpless, inactive dependence on their environment.[53] While slowly accepting his physical limitations, the well-adjusted child finds satisfaction in a variety of compensatory motor activities and intellectual pursuits, in which the parents' encouragement and guidance assumes great importance.

In addition to cognitive flexibility and compensatory physical activities, the appropriate release and control of emotions is an essential coping technique. The expression of anxious, sad, impatient, and angry feelings at times of exacerbations, and of confidence and guarded optimism during periods of clinical quiescence is characteristic of well-adapted children with a chronic illness.

In terms of psychologic defenses, most of these patients use denial as well as isolation in coping with their emotional distress caused by pain, malaise, and interrupted plans. They also show an adaptive use of denial of the uncertain future, which enables them to maintain hope for recovery at times of crisis, for more effective medical care, and for a relatively normal, productive adult life. Identification with other young and adult patients afflicted with a chronic handicap is a helpful defense for many children. Learning about and associating with others who are successful in dealing with similar problems can effectively support the development of a positive self-image as a socially competent and productive individual. Many of the well-adapted young patients display a certain pride and confidence in themselves as they become successful in mastering the ongoing stress associated with their illness.

The nature of the specific illness appears less influential for a child's successful adaptation than such factors as his developmental level and available coping techniques, the quality of the parent–child relationship, and the family's acceptance of the handicapped member.[8,10,12] Regarding the latter point, the parents' ability to master their initial reaction of fear and guilt, and their tendency to overprotect the child, has received much emphasis.[8,23,54-57]

Children and adolescents with prolonged poor adjustment to their chronic disorder tend to show one of the three following behavioral patterns.[8,22,23] One group is characterized by the patients' fearfulness, inactivity, lack of outside interests, and a marked dependency on their families, especially their mothers. These youngsters present the psychiatric picture of early passive dependent states and their mothers are usually described as constantly worried and overprotective of them.

The second group contains the overly independent, often daring young patients, who may engage in prohibited and risk-taking activities. Such youngsters make a strong use of denial of realistic dangers and fears. At times their reality sense is impaired and they seem to seek out certain feared situations, challenging the risk of trauma. Since early childhood, many of these rebellious patients have been raised by oversolicitous and guilt-ridden mothers. Usually at puberty, they rebel against the maternal interference and turn into overly active, defiant adolescents.

A third, less common pattern of maladjustment is seen in older children and adolescents with congenital deformities and handicaps. They appear as shy and lonely people harboring resentful and hostile attitudes toward normal persons, whom they see as owing them payment for their lifelong sufferings.[58] Usually these patients were raised in a family that emphasized their defectiveness and tended to isolate or "hide" them in an embarrassed fashion. They came to identify with their family's view of them and developed a self-image of a defective outsider.

These illustrations of prolonged maladaptation to a chronic illness differ from more temporary situations, where the disease and its management become the vehicle for conflicts between the patient and his parents, siblings, friends, or school. Overt or covert refusal to cooperate in the medical regimen can be used as an effective weapon by a resentful young patient. Practically all children with a chronic disability will occasionally try to take advantage of their disease in order to avoid unpleasant situations, as for instance a disciplinary action or a school test.

Emotional Stress and Coping Behavior of Parents

When a serious, long-term illness afflicts a child, the intial reaction of his parents usually includes acute fear and anxiety related to the possible fatal outcome of the disease. A closely associated stage is that of parental disbelief in the diagnosis, particularly if the obvious signs of illness have subsided.[55] The parents might then complain about being poorly informed by the physician and occasionally "shop around" for additional medical opinion, which will disprove the initial diagnosis. Beyond those denying, often uncooperative attitudes of the parents, feelings of mourning the "loss" of their desired normal child and feelings of self-blame in regard to their ailing child usually begin to emerge.[24,54] When the parents become aware of and can verbalize these feelings, they are able to accept the reality of the serious disability and its impact on the whole family.

A crucial factor in determining the parents' acceptance is their ability to master resentful and self-accusatory feelings over having transmitted or in some way "caused" their child's disorder.[23,54-57] Those parents who remain highly anxious and guilt-laden about their ill child tend to cope with their emotional distress by overprotecting and pampering him, and by limiting his activities with other children. Such prolonged parental overconcern, usually more prominent among mothers, can often be related to one of the following predisposing factors:[47,59] The child suffered a life-threatening condition at birth or as an infant, from which the family did not believe he would recover; the child is afflicted with a hereditary disorder present among relatives; the child's illness reactivates emotional conflicts in the parents stemming from the past death of a close relative; or the child was unwanted, causing a mixture of loving and rejecting feelings, particularly in the mother.

Any child being raised by oversolicitous, controlling, and fearful parents senses the parental expectation of his vulnerability and likely premature death.[59] He may either accept this tacit view and assume passive–dependent characteristics, or he may rebel against the parents' concerns and become a daring, careless youngster, who seems to challenge their notions of his fragile condition.

The factors mentioned here as common determinants of prolonged parental overconcern also may lead to parental rejection or neglect of a disabled child and to extreme parental denial of the severity of the illness. These latter types of reaction are infrequent compared to the former one of overprotection. Again, strong unresolved feelings of guilt for their child's illness are often present in such detached and uncooperative parents.[10,23] They may talk angrily about all the inconvenience their child's ailment causes the family, and they often blame crises and complications on the child or the medical staff. In addition, they frequently "forget" instructions about the home care and are inconsistent in guiding their child. Such a child, when sensing the parental rejection, will often respond with both despondent and defiant attitudes, which greatly jeopardize his clinical condition.

Parents who have successfully adapted to the challenge of raising a chronically ill child will enforce only necessary and realistic restrictions on him, encourage self-care and regular school attendance, and promote reasonable physical activities with his peers. These well-adapted parents use some common psychologic defenses in coping with the constant strain caused by their child's illness.[60] For example, they tend to isolate and deny their anxious and helpless emotions, especially during a medical crisis, which helps them to remain calm and assist effectively in the medical care. When the crisis is over, many parents experience a rebound phenomenon of feeling depressed and irritable, indicating that certain painful affects have been denied consciousness until that time when it is safer to experience them.

It is common among parents of handicapped children to show attitudes of critical superiority toward health specialists, particularly toward house officers. Some of this criticism may be valid, but one also senses that the parents are trying to ward off, by denial, their long-standing helpless feelings in this manner. They may also displace and project helpless and angry feelings about their child's condition onto various medical professionals and blame them for delays or mistakes in treating their child. Closely related to denial is rationalization, that is, the defensive use of rational explanations, valid or invalid, in an attempt to conceal some painful emotions from oneself. One commonly hears from parents of chronically ill children that the disorder has enriched the whole family, both emotionally and spiritually, and has developed their sense of compassion and tolerance. While indeed there may be some truth in such statements, these attitudes assist the parents—often the healthy siblings too—in hiding from themselves sad and resentful affects related to their unique burden.

All effectively coping parents, along with their sick children, use intellectual processes to master distressing emotions caused by the illness; that is, they rely on the coping technique of "control through thinking."[61] The parents often make it a point to learn all they can about the medical, physiological, and even the psychological aspects of the disease. Thus, they lessen their anxiety by familiarizing themselves with the likely future course of development of the child.

The association and identification with other parents of seriously ill children is helpful to many parents. Informally and in group discussions, at times conducted by a health specialist, they can share many of their distressing hardships and learn to adopt more realistic and relaxed child caring attitudes and also pass on their positive experiences to less knowledgeable parents.[33,60]

Conclusion

The successful psychological management of a child with a long-term physical illness and his family depends on two interrelated factors:[8,10,23,55,56,62] (1) the continuous "personalized" support and counseling by the physician, who should be alert to all the incompatible feelings with which both the patient and his parents are coping; these affects are normal reactions, which often will subside if given time and verbal expression; and (2) the parents' acceptance of the disease with its uncertain course and impact on the family, which implies that they have gradually mastered their conflicting emotions aroused by their child's ailment.

The parents as well as their child require repeated, truthful, and comprehensible information about the illness, its etiology, and therapeutic concepts. Whenever possible, they should be prepared for procedures and likely changes in clinical manifestations. Such preparation helps to mobilize their intellectual functions and psychologic defenses to cope with the anticipated stress. The physician should make sure that his explanations and plans are understood by the parents and the young patient, and well coordinated with the collaborative efforts of his medical, nursing, and social service colleagues. The medical team and the parents can greatly assist the ill child by encouraging him to ask questions and to verbalize distressing feelings.

The parents need instruction to develop in their child an increasing responsibility for self-care and protection. The goal of raising the handicapped child as normally as possible may be achieved by promoting reasonable activities with other children and regular schooling, modified by individual needs. Overprotection and undue restrictions, both at home and in school, should be discouraged. The father's active involvement in the child-rearing can be fostered by his assuming major responsibility for helping his ill youngster to succeed in compensatory activities and interests. In terms of the healthy siblings, the physician should assess whether they are receiving needed parental love and attention as well as acceptance of their frequent feelings of anxiety, resentment, and guilt toward their ailing brother or sister.

The physician should tactfully call attention to parental attitudes of overindulgence, lenient discipline, or neglect which can endanger the child's emotional growth. He may suggest a psychiatric consultation when he notices many unresolved conflicts in the parents responsible for prolonged overprotective, inconsistent, or rejecting handling of the child. Psychiatric intervention can also be of value for some young patients with marked difficulties in adapting to their long-term illness, such as children showing defiant, risk-taking behavior, a fearful, passive dependence, or hostile, embittered attitudes toward their environment and life situation.

References

1. Mattsson, A., & Weisberg, I. Behavioral reactions to minor illness in preschool children. *Pediatrics,* **46,** 604, 1970.
2. Carey, W. B., & Siblinga, M. S. Avoiding pediatric pathogenesis in the management of acute minor illness. *Pediatrics,* **49,** 553, 1972.
3. Stewart, W. H. The unmet needs of children. *Pediatrics,* **39,** 157, 1967.
4. Pless, I. B. Epidemiology of chronic disease. *In* M. Green & R. J. Haggerty (Eds.), *Ambulatory pediatrics.* Philadelphia: W. B. Saunders Co., 1968. Pp. 760–768.

5. Rutter, M., Tizard, J., & Whitmore, K. *Handicapped children. A total population prevalence study of education, physical, and behavioral disorders.* London: Longmans, 1968.

6. Freud, A. The role of bodily illness in the mental life of children. *Psychoanalytic Study of the Child* **7,** 69, 1952.

7. Langford, W. S.: The child in the pediatric hospital: Adaptation to illness and hospitalization. *American Journal of Orthopsychiatry* **31,** 667, 1961.

8. Prugh, D. G. Toward an understanding of psychosomatic concepts in relation to illness in children. *In* A. J. Solnit & S. A. Provence (Eds.), *Modern perspectives in child development.* New York: International Universities Press, 1963. Pp. 246–367.

9. Shrand, H. Behavior changes in sick children nursed at home. *Pediatrics,* **36,** 604, 1965.

10. Apley, J., & MacKeith, R. *The child and his symptoms.* Philadelphia: F. A. Davis Company, 1968. Pp. 209–215, 216–240.

11. Jessner, L. Some observations on children hospitalized during latency. *In* L. Jessner & E. Pavenstedt (Eds.), *Dynamic psychopathology in childhood.* New York: Grune and Stratton, Inc., 1959. Pp. 257–268.

12. Freeman, R. D. Emotional reactions of handicapped children. *In* S. Chess & A. Thomas (Eds.), *Annual progress in child psychiatry and child development, 1968.* New York: Brunner Mazel, 1968. Pp. 379–395.

13. Robertson, J. *Young children in hospitals.* New York: Basic Books, 1958.

14. Vernon, D., Foley, J., Sipowicz, R., & Schulman, J. *The psychological responses of children to hospitalization and illness. A review of the literature.* Springfield, Illinois: Charles C Thomas, 1965.

15. Mason, E. A. The hospitalized child—his emotional needs. *New England Journal of Medicine* **272,** 406, 1965.

16. Swift, C. R., & Seidman, F. L. Adjustment problems of juvenile diabetes. *Journal of the American Academy of Child Psychiatry* **3,** 500, 1964.

17. Tietz, W., & Vidmar, T.: The impact of coping styles on the control of juvenile diabetes. *Psychiatry in Medicine* **3,** 67, 1972.

18. Dubo, S., McLean, J., Ching, A., Wright, H., Kauffman, P., & Sheldon, J. A study of relationships between family situation, bronchial asthma, and personal adjustment in children. *Journal of Pediatrics* **59,** 402, 1961.

19. Purcell, K., Brody, K., Chai, H., Muser, J., Molk, L., Gordon, N., & Means, J. The effect on asthma in children of experimental separation from the family. *Psychosomatic Medicine* **31,** 144, 1969.

20. Purcell, K., & Weiss, J. H. Asthma. *In* C. G. Costello, (Ed.), *Symptoms of psychopathology.* New York: John Wiley & Sons, 1970. Pp. 597–623.

21. McCollum, A. T., & Gibson, L. E. Family adaptation to the child with cystic fibrosis. *Journal of Pediatrics* **77,** 571, 1970.

22. Agle, D. P. Psychiatric studies of patients with hemophilia and related states. *Archives of Internal Medicine* **114,** 76, 1964.

23. Mattsson, A., & Gross, S. Social and behavioral studies on hemophilic children and their families. *Journal of Pediatrics* **68,** 952, 1966.

24. Glaser, H. H., Harrison, G. S., & Lynn, D. B. Emotional implications of congenital heart disease in children. *Pediatrics,* **33,** 367, 1964.
25. Toker, E. Psychiatric aspects of cardiac surgery in a child. *Journal of the American Academy of Child Psychiatry* **10,** 156, 1971.
26. Barnes, C. M., Kenny, F. M., Call, T., & Reinhart, J. B. Measurement in management of anxiety in children for open heart surgery. *Pediatrics,* **49,** 250, 1972.
27. Abram, H. S. Survival by machine: The psychological stress of chronic hemodialysis. *Psychiatry in Medicine* **1,** 37, 1970.
28. Bernstein, D. M. After transplantation—the child's emotional reactions. *American Journal of Psychiatry* **127,** 1189, 1971.
29. Lilly, J. R., Giles, G., Hurvitz, R., Schroter, G., et al. Renal homotransplantation in pediatric patients. *Pediatrics,* **47,** 548, 1971.
30. McDermott, J. F., & Finch, S. M. Ulcerative colitis in children. Reassessment of a dilemma. *Journal of the American Academy of Child Psychiatry* **6,** 512, 1967.
31. Rothchild, E., & Owens, R. P. Adolescent girls who lack functioning ovaries. *Journal of the American Academy of Child Psychiatry* **11,** 88, 1972.
32. Money, J., & Pollitt, E. Studies in the psychology of dwarfism: II. Personality maturation and response to growth hormone treatment in hypopituitary dwarfs. *Journal of Pediatrics* **68,** 381, 1966.
33. Mandelbaum, A. The group process in helping parents of retarded children. *Children,* **14,** 227, 1967.
34. Birch, H. G. *Brain-damage in children. The biological and social aspects.* Baltimore: Williams & Wilkins Co., 1964.
35. Gardner, R. A. Psychogenic problems of brain-injured children and their parents. *Journal of the American Academy of Child Psychiatry* **7,** 471, 1968.
36. Chess, S., Korn, S. J., & Fernandez, P. B. *Psychiatric disorders of children with congenital rubella.* New York: Brunner Mazel, 1971.
37. Minde, K. K., Hachett, J. D., Killon, D., & Silver, S. How they grow up: 41 physically handicapped children and their families. *American Journal of Psychiatry* **128,** 1554, 1972.
38. Gurney, W. Congenital amputee. *In* M. Green & R. J. Haggerty (Eds.), *Ambulatory pediatrics.* Philadelphia: W. B. Saunders Co., 1968. Pp. 534–540.
39. Roskies, E. *Abnormality and normality: The mothering of thalidomide children.* Ithaca, New York: Cornell University Press, 1972.
40. Myers, B. A., Friedman, S. B., & Weiner, I. B.: Coping with a chronic diability: Psychosocial observations of girls with scoliosis treated with the Milwaukee brace. *American Journal of Diseases of Children* **120,** 175, 1970.
41. Tisza, V. B., & Gumperty, E. The parents' reactions to the birth and early care of children with cleft palate. *Pediatrics* **30,** 86, 1962.
42. Cytryn, L., Cytryn, E., & Rieger, R. E. Psychological implications of cryptorchism. *Journal of the American Academy of Child Psychiatry* **6,** 131, 1967.
43. Kessler, J. W. *Psychopathology of childhood.* Englewood Cliffs, New Jersey: Prentice-Hall, 1966. Pp. 332–367.
44. Green, M., & Haggerty, R. J. (Eds.). Part VII. The management of long-term

illness. *In Ambulatory pediatrics*. Philadelphia: W. B. Saunders Co., 1968. Pp. 441–768.

45. Friedman, S. B. Management of fatal illness in children. *In* M. Green & R. J. Haggerty (Eds.), *Ambulatory pediatrics*. Philadelphia: W. B. Saunders Co., 1968. Pp. 753–759.

46. Easson, W. M. *The dying child. The management of the child or adolescent who is dying*. Springfield, Illinois: Charles C Thomas, 1970.

47. Mattsson, A., & Gross, S. Adaptational and defensive behavior in young hemophiliacs and their parents. *American Journal of Psychiatry* **122,** 1349, 1966.

48. Murphy, L. B. *The widening world of childhood*. New York: Basic Books, 1962.

49. Friedman, S. B., Chodoff, P., Mason, J. W., & Hamburg, D. A. Behavioral observations on parents anticipating the death of a child. *Pediatrics*, **32,** 610, 1963.

50. Chodoff, P., Friedman, S. B., & Hamburg, D. A. Stress, defenses, and coping behavior: Observations in parents of children with malignant disease. *American Journal of Psychiatry* **120,** 743, 1964.

51. Mattsson, A., Gross, S., & Hall, T. W. Psychoendocrine study of adaptation in young hemophiliacs. *Psychosomatic Medicine* **33,** 215, 1971.

52. Lazarus, R. S. *Psychological stress and the coping process*. New York: McGraw-Hill, 1966. Pp. 258–266.

53. Frankl, L. Self-preservation and the development of accident proneness in children and adolescents. *Psychoanalytic Study of the Child* **18,** 464, 1963.

54. Solnit, A. J., & Stark, M. H. Mourning and the birth of a defective child. *Psychoanalytic Study of the Child* **16,** 523, 1961.

55. Tisza, V. B. Management of the parents of the chronically ill child. *American Journal of Orthopsychiatry* **32:**53, 1962.

56. Green, M. Care of the child with a long-term life-threatening illness: Some principles of management. *Pediatrics* **39,** 441, 1967.

57. Findlay, I. I., Smith, P., Graves, P. J., & Linton, M. L. Chronic disease in childhood: A study of family reactions. *British Journal of Medical Education* **3,** 66, 1969.

58. Freud, S. *Some character types met with in psychoanalytic work: I. The "Exceptions."* (1916). London: Hogarth Press, standard edition, vol. 14, pp. 311–315, 1957.

59. Green, M., & Solnit, A. J. Reactions to the threatened loss of a child: A vulnerable child syndrome. *Pediatrics* **34,** 58, 1964.

60. Mattsson, A., & Agle, D. P. Group therapy with parents of hemophiliacs: Therapeutic process and observations of parental adaptation to chronic illness in children. *Journal of the American Academy of Child Psychiatry* **11:**558, 1972.

61. Bibring, G. L., Dwyer, T. F., Huntington, D. S., & Valenstein, A. F. A study of the psychological processes in pregnancy and of the earliest mother–child relationship. Appendix B: Glossary of defenses. *Psychoanalytic Study of the Child* **16,** 62, 1961.

62. Solnit, A. J. Psychotherapeutic role of the pediatrician. *In* M. Green & R. J. Haggerty (Eds.), *Ambulatory pediatrics*. Philadelphia: W. B. Saunders Co., 1968. Pp. 159–167.

14

Psychological Aspects of the Care of Children with Cystic Fibrosis

ALAN TROPAUER, MARTHA NEAL FRANZ, and VICTOR W. DILGARD

Recent advances in detection and management of cystic fibrosis have significantly improved the affected individual's chances of survival beyond childhood years. With early recognition of the disease the patient and his family often become involved in a program of intensive treatment that continues for the remainder of his life.[1-3] The daily care at home necessitates large expenditures of time and effort for the patient and his parents. The financial burden can be considerable, resulting often in the depletion of savings and the forgoing of luxuries and vacations. Siblings frequently must defer their needs and desires as the patient becomes the focus of attention. In the more severe cases, recurrent hospitalization of the sick child for complications disrupts family routine and creates emotional crises. Finally, despite the most adequate care, the course of the disease may be inexorable, with death usually intervening in early adult life.[4]

ALAN TROPAUER, M.D. • Assistant Clinical Professor, Department of Child Psychiatry, Emory University, Atlanta, Georgia. This investigation was supported by Children and Youth Project 617, a comprehensive health care program of the Children's Bureau, Department of Health, Education, and Welfare.

Within this context, it is understandable that psychological complications and problems in adaption to the illness occur for the patient and the family. These in turn, may intensify the stress for everyone and create additional difficulties for the physician in the total management of the case.

Awareness of types of emotional strain experienced by these children and their families can be of use to the pediatrician in helping to avert potential problems which may seriously impair therapeutic effectiveness and the patient's well-being. It is the purpose of this study to convey our impressions of attitudes, feelings, and reactions experienced by a representative group of children with cystic fibrosis and by their families.

Previous Studies of Cystic Fibrosis

The intensive study by Lawler et al.[5] of 11 children with cystic fibrosis stresses the major psychological problems for the patient and the family group caused by the disease. The children were often depressed, and there was a high incidence of emotional illness among the parents. The attitude of the children toward their illness was characterized by marked anxiety and preoccupation with death.

Turk[6] has dealt primarily with the effects of cystic fibrosis on the family. She notes the emotional, material, and social deprivation experienced by those related to the patient. Breakdown in communication regarding important family issues is seen as a consequence of the disruption of the usual patterns of behavior. This frequently leads to a "web of silence," increasing the burden and sense of frustration for all concerned. The author points up the necessity for the entire family to reach an understanding of cystic fibrosis and its effects and to share this awareness with one another. Greater utilization of professional and community resources is recommended.

Methods

Twenty children with cystic fibrosis and 23 mothers (including 18 mother–child pairs) were selected for this study on the basis of their availability for psychiatric and psychological examination. They were part of a larger group of families regularly attending the Cystic Fibrosis

Clinic at Barney Children's Medical Center in Dayton, Ohio. The ages of the children ranged from 5 through 20. The parents and children were seen separately by the psychiatrist in hourly interviews. Occasionally, patients or their families were followed more extensively when it became apparent that their adaptive difficulties were interfering with the medical program.

During the psychiatric interviews mothers were questioned in detail about their child's personal and social adjustment, his reactions to the medical routine, and apparent anxieties. Their own feelings, worries, thoughts about prognosis, and major frustrations were also discussed. Reactions of siblings and the effect of the sick child on the entire family were explored, in addition to marital adjustment, family closeness and the ability to communicate about the illness. Assessment of the mother's mood, behavior, and defensive patterns used to cope with her anxiety was made.

The children were asked about their experiences in relation to the illness. Their understanding of the nature and prognosis of cystic fibrosis, their hopes and expectations, and predominant fears in relation to the disease were explored. Their perception of the attitudes and concerns of others in the family and their feelings about the overall therapeutic program were elicited. Interests, ambitions, wishes, dreams, and early memories were obtained in order to explore the child's fantasies. A summary of the relevant psychosocial data based upon these interviews is included in Tables I through III.

In addition, the patients were administered a modified form of the House-Tree-Person technique in belief that a brief projective study might provide presumptive evidence of psychological conflict. Each child was asked to (1) draw a picture of a house, (2) draw a picture of a tree, (3) draw a picture of a person, and (4) draw a picture of a person of the opposite sex.

Another primary source of information was the experience of the clinic director, who had frequent and prolonged contact with every patient and family during clinic visits and hospitalizations. This provided useful long-term observations, as well as impressions of the family's reactions under increased stress. It also furnished supplementary knowledge concerning the adjustment of other family members who could not directly be interviewed at the time because of scheduling difficulties. Table IV refers to the medical status of the individual patients at the time of this study.

Table I. Attitudes Toward Management and Family Compatibility and Communication

Patient	Attitudes toward management	Family compatibility and communication
A	Patient resents time involved, no difficulties	Family close, communicative
B	Father uncooperative, but no overt difficulties	Close family life centers on patient, free communication
C	Patient fearful without tent, morbid fantasies, family cooperative	Family close, supportive, well informed
D	Patient and family cooperative	Family close, communicative
E	Patient resents interference with play	No discussion, facts of illness concealed from patient and siblings
F	Therapy supports mother–child closeness	Husband avoids discussion, child poorly informed
G	Mother more devoted to healthy children	Family not close, all well informed, expect early death
H	Mother inconsistent, patient embarrassed by illness, both resent time involved	Open discussion, father overindulges patient
I	Patient and family cooperative	Close, indulgent family, child well informed
J	Parents rebellious and neglectful of therapy, patient mildly ashamed, resents time involved	Stormy marital situation, restricted communication
K	Parents inconsistent, patient resistive, uses illness to avoid responsibility	Parents discuss freely themselves, child "doesn't ask"
L[a]	Patient resistive to therapy, defiant, resents time involved	Lack of closeness, parents unable to share anxieties, no discussion with patient or siblings
M	Child mildly ashamed of illness, parents cooperative	Parents withheld information for years, told patient not to read about cystic fibrosis
N	Patient resents time involved	Close family, open communication
O[b]	Family uncooperative, follows program poorly	Data unavailable
P	Patient and family cooperative	Free discussion, yet nonsupportive
Q[b]	Patient resistive to therapy	Data unavailable
R	Patient feels neglected, worries about getting proper therapy	Information concealed from patient and siblings until puberty, when illness was self-discovered
S[a]	Patient ashamed, resists treatment	Lack of closeness, parents unable to share anxieties, no discussion with patient or siblings
T	Mother overprotective, father neglectful, patient resistive, ashamed, avoids therapy	Divorced family, information concealed from patient until late adolescence

[a] Siblings.
[b] No parental interview.

Table II. Family Reactions to Illness and Mother's Adaptive Behavior

Patient	Family reactions to illness	Mother's adaptive behavior
A	No difficulties	Depressed, realistic acceptance
B	Family helpful, cooperative	Moderate guilt, periodic depression, realistic acceptance
C	Other children demanding, sister with learning difficulties	Hopeful, encouraged by child's progress
D	No problems, illness draws members closer	Denial, "lucky" to have child with cystic fibrosis
E	No difficulties	Suppression, inability to share feelings, denial, periodic discouragement
F	Family life built around patient, siblings complain	Periodic depression and intense anxiety, overprotective, gives in to child
G	Financial strain, sibling resentment, much family illness, child died of cystic fibrosis (sibling)	Depressed, suppresses feelings, pessimistic and hopeless
H	Siblings helpful, understanding	Mild denial
I	Mutual cooperation and concern, no problems	Denial and suppression of thought
J	Dissension, lack of cooperation and concern, hostility and resentment	Anxious, ambivalent, hostile behavior toward patient, suppression and minimization of illness
K	Only difficulty is doing therapy consistently	Mild optimistic, inconsistent in therapy, misses appointments
L[a]	Younger siblings show resentment, vie for attention, adolescent son delinquent	Depressed, self-depreciating, much guilt
M	Financial strain, siblings cooperative, previous sibling death, sister blind	Significant denial, mild guilt over hereditary transmission
N	No difficulties	Cheerful, denial and repression of feelings
O[b]	Data unavailable	Data unavailable
P	Older sister resentful and jealous, father involved in cystic fibrosis group activities to exclusion of own family	Mildly depressed and guilty, anxious, takes tranquilizers
Q[b]	Data unavailable	Data unavailable
R	Occasional resentment of realistic difficulties, patient provocative, financial strain	Moderate guilt, periodic discouragement
S[a]	Younger siblings show resentment, vie for attention, adolescent son delinquent	Depressed, self-depreciating, much guilt
T	Parents at extremes, overprotective vs. neglectful	Overprotectiveness, recurrent depression, displacement of anger

[a] Siblings
[b] No parental interview.

Table III. Mother's View of Patient's Adjustment and Anxieties and Concerns of Patient

Patient	Mother's view of patient's adjustment	Anxieties and concerns of patient
A	Happy, well adjusted	No anxieties revealed, expects cure
B	Very shy, not enough friends, immature (may be retarded)	Confused whether sick or not, worries about dying (borderline intellect)
C	Independent, outgoing, no anxieties	Expects cure, though preoccupied with topic of lung damage, resents missing play
D	No problems	Concerned about death, and not being taken care of in later years
E	Overdependent, introverted in preschool years, now happy, occasionally moody	Poorly informed about cystic fibrosis, worries about being cured
F	Clingy, overdependent, unhappy, few friends	Pills, shots are worst part, therapy interferes with play
G	Lost initiative to make friends, sensitive about small size	Sacrifice of time and money, worries about getting treatments when older
H	Seems happy	Worst part is missing good, rich foods
I	Well adjusted and happy	Feels past crisis period, concerned with size of abdomen
J	Teased, disliked, feels unaccepted by other children	Main concern is rejection by other children, dislikes therapy, feels parents do not want to do it
K	Well adjusted, no anxieties or impairments	Annoyed with therapy, no other concerns, expects cure
L[a]	Some shame about illness	Worries about being cured, resents missing play
M	Well liked, good adjustment	Saddened by physical restriction, worries about dying, cautious optimism
N	Well adjusted	Poorly informed about cystic fibrosis, no worries, expects cure
O[b]	Data unavailable	Expects cure, periodically depressed, concerned with being teased
P	Happy, well adjusted	Worries about dying, not marrying, being skinny, and periodic isolation from friends
Q[b]	Data unavailable	Concerned with weight and easy fatigue, acute illness arouses anxiety over dying
R	Too dependent, unhappy, ashamed, few friends	Unhappy, feels deceived, concerned with size, weight, conceals fear of dying
S[a]	Too dependent on family, defiant, discipline problem, ashamed of having cystic fibrosis	Concerned with isolation from friends when sick
T	Ashamed of illness, avoids close friends, insecure	Anxious about breathing difficulties and dying, resists therapy yet aware of its value

[a] Siblings.
[b] No parental interview.

Table IV. Relevant Medical Data

Patient	Sex	Age[a]	Length of intensive treatment (yr)	Extent of disability[b]	Prognosis
A	M	6	3½	P-moderate, D-mild, mild disability	Early adult life
B	F	8	3½	P-moderate, D-mild, little disability	Over 10 yr
C	F	8½	8½	P-mild, D-mild, deafness from neomycin sulfate	Adult life
D	F	8½	3½	P-mild, D-moderate, little disability	Adult life
E	M	9	4½	P-mild, little, if any disability	Adult life
F	M	10½	4½	P-moderately severe, D-mild, moderate disability	5 yr
G	M	11	5	P-severe irreversible damage, moderately disabled	Under 5 yr
H	M	11	4½	P-moderately severe, D-moderately severe, moderate disability	10 yr
I	M	12	3½	P-moderate, D-severe, disabled by impaired muscular strength	7–10 yr
J	M	12	4	P-mild to moderate, D-early obstructive biliary cirrhosis, little disability	Early adult life
K	F	12½	3	P-mild, D-mild, no significant disability	Adult life
L[c]	M	12½	4½	P-mild, D-mild, no significant disability	Adult life
M	M	13	2	P-severe, D-severe, severe disability	Under 5 yr
N	F	14½	5	P-moderately severe with moderate disability	5–7 yr
O[d]	F	16	4	P-mild, D-mild, little disability	Over 15 yr (5–6 yr without therapy)
P	F	17	3	P-mild, D-mild, little if any disability	Adult life
Q[d]	M	18	2½	P-mild, D-mild, little disability	Over 10 yr
R	F	19	1	P-severe with cor pulmonale, D-mild, severe disability	2–3 yr
S[c]	F	19	4½	D-mild, P-severe, irreversible, moderately severe disability	5–7 yr
T	M	20	4	P-moderate, D-moderate, little disability	10–15 yr

[a] Age is to nearest one-half year.
[b] P indicates pulmonary; D, digestive.
[c] Siblings.
[d] No parental interview.

Adaptation of the Child to the Illness

Fifteen of the 18 children interviewed had a reasonably good understanding of the nature of cystic fibrosis relative to the degree of intellectual maturity. Few expected cure, hoping rather that the disease might be controlled with the proper therapy. An accurate and realistic concept of cystic fibrosis did not always ensure a cooperative attitude toward treatment, as many therapy difficulties were encountered with highly intelligent adolescents. Although information was occasionally distorted by the younger children (one 9-year-old girl believed that "fatness" in food infected her mucus), the fact that the situation was discussed with them appeared to relieve some anxiety. The destructive, unrelenting character that cystic fibrosis seemed to provide for some children was revealed in one 10-year-old boy's description of it as a disease that "gets your lungs like termites in wood."

Although there was a general absence of overt apparent depression, this did not necessarily mean that the youngsters were free from morbid thoughts and preoccupations concerning their disease. Children rarely exhibit through symptoms or signs the familiar mood and behavioral changes characteristic of depression in adults.

About one third of the mothers reported that their children had voiced concerns about dying prematurely. This would lead parents to attempt reassurance which at times had questionable value. One boy was told not to worry because "we didn't think you would make it this far." Such encouragement implies the expectation of another "miracle," while discouraging the child from verbally expressing his fears and offering him no understanding or support.

In the interviews, preoccupation with death and ultimate disability was seen more frequently with adolescents. They also worried about the restrictions the disease imposed upon their social life and the lack of acceptance by peers. Three teen-agers were particularly concerned with their small, frail appearance, secondary to the effects of the disease on growth. This tended to intensify uncomfortable feelings of being different from their friends because they had cystic fibrosis.

Young children complained frequently about interruption of play, dietary deprivations, or the physical limitations which prevented them from keeping up with others. A few expressed worry as to how they would get treatments when they grew up and moved away from home.

It seems that the younger child with limitations in his abstract thinking is concerned less with death and more with separation from his parents on whom he is totally dependent.

Patients were often quite tolerant of the arduous treatment routines when the situation was openly presented to them. This was reinforced when experiences of frequent coughing, fatigue, abdominal cramps, or odorous bowel movements arose because of neglect of the corresponding aspects of the treatment program. To some, the mist tent became a symbol of security: Its effectiveness in easing respiration, its comforting noise, and closed-in construction contributed to its value, and several children could not sleep well without it. One 8-year-old boy regarded the tent as a powerful ally that prevented bad dreams and thoughts of frightening monsters.

Although interests varied, one-third of the children had future ambitions concerned in some manner with "helping people," such as medical research, clinical medicine, nursing, or, in one case, being a life-guard. Fantasies of being the helper, rather than the recipient of help, tend to relieve anxiety by converting a passive experience into an active one, through the process of identification.[7] Thus, the sick child anxious about medical procedures or the effects of the illness emancipates himself by becoming the doctor or nurse who combats disease in others. Admiration and respect for his physician may also foster this identification. A few actively suppressed thoughts about the future. One sad, inhibited little girl hoped "to become a teen-ager," when asked her ambition.

Early memories and dreams were punctuated with themes of illness, injury, and hospitalization. Some of this can be attributed to the setting and type of interview of current experiences. One 19-year-old boy, hospitalized with intestinal obstruction, recalled recurrent dreams of painful objects sticking him in the stomach. It is conceivable that dreams of drowning, feeling trapped, being sprayed with something that puts one asleep, or being eaten up might have some symbolic association to cystic fibrosis and related anxieties about breathing, restriction, and the sense of slow decay.

Exploration of animal wishes and fantasies revealed longings to be wild or free in nine children. Pleasurable aspects of such choice included lack of restriction, eating whatever one wished, and having an abundance of free time. Passive longings were seen in five children who would have preferred to be soft, cuddly, domestic animals who are fed and taken care of. One very debilitated girl with severe pulmonary involvement, requiring significant attention, loudly proclaimed her desires for complete independence and self-management. Concomitantly, her animal fantasy was to be a sacred cow in India where "everyone would bow down to me and feed me." Such fantasies illustrate the intensifying effect that chronic disease has in the developmental conflict between independence and dependency.

Behavioral difficulties mentioned by mothers included disciplinary problems, excessive dependency, oversensitivity, and shame about cystic fibrosis in their children. Such concerns were more frequently seen in families where the parents lacked the ability to face the situation openly and rely upon one another for emotional support.

In over 75% of the cases, the children's drawings reflected feelings of inadequacy or insecurity, or both. Anxiety was experienced by many of the patients regarding the image of themselves in relation to their environment, and inner tensions were frequently associated with conflicts within the home. A minimum of 70% of the patient's human figure drawings showed two or more indicators often obtained from children considered to be emotionally disturbed.[8,9]

Tables I through IV indicate that, in this study, the manifestations of the child's anxiety were not solely related to the severity of the illness and disability. It is also apparent (Tables I through III) that comparison of the patients worries and concerns with the mother's view of her child's adjustment reveals contradictions in several cases. One explanation may be that the child's anxiety, though discernible, may not be sufficient to overtax his coping ability and affect his observable behavior. However, it appeared in other cases that the mother's own emotional state or maladaptive defenses rendered her relatively insensitive to perception of her child's feelings.[10]

Children with acute or chronic illnesses will experience anxiety at some level of consciousness.[11] Its effects depend upon the child's emotional reserves, his coping mechanisms, and the degree of support he sustains from his immediate environment. It is not the existence of anxiety per se that handicaps the sick child and intensifies his invalidism, but rather its degree and his methods of dealing with it. Neurotic symptoms, inhibitions, immaturity, behavior problems, and resistance to therapy are signals of the patient's inability to contend with inner stress, and warrant further exploration.

Patterns of Defense and Adaptation Seen in the Mothers

Only three of the mothers appeared clinically depressed, as evidenced by psychomotor retardation, self-depreciation, and a mood of hopelessness, pessimism, or saddened resignation. However, eight others admitted frequent periods of dejection and discouragement over the child's illness, often related to clinical exacerbations. The combined sense of uncertainty and inevitability was very disheartening. Encouraged to treat the child "normally" and to adhere to daily therapy routines in order to prolong his life, the parents are nonetheless faced with the inescapable fact that their child's life-span is limited, no matter what they do.

Guilt was prevalent, frequently felt by the mothers when their children had setbacks. At these times they questioned the adequacy of their care and vaguely felt they "could have done more." One woman would not permit anyone else to give her child treatments. The parent of an adolescent girl experienced intense feelings of guilt when she had to forgo giving postural drainage therapy because of the daughter's cardiac decompensation.

In the intensive treatment of cystic fibrosis, much importance is attached to the active role the mothers and fathers must take in helping the child prolong and maintain a useful life. In other chronic diseases, parental participation has been reported as helpful in relieving guilt through expending personal effort, with the consolation that the parent has done everything possible for his child.[12] For some people, however, this may lead to an unrealistic overevaluation of the effects of their efforts and powers. Under such conditions, clinical exacerbations can engender self-blame and intensify existing guilt.

In some instances, experience with family sickness in childhood, death of another child from cystic fibrosis or concurrent family illness had a decided influence on the parents' attitude and behavior.

One unfortunate woman had lost a child previously with cystic fibrosis, her husband suffered from cardiac disease, and another daughter had a severe eye condition in her youth. The mother conveyed the attitude that she had "written off" her remaining son with cystic fibrosis in order to devote her emotional reserves to those who were going to live.

Another mother greatly resented devoting time to the treatment of her mildly sick youngster and would not tolerate his expressions of dependency. She revealed that in her adolescent years she had been grossly irritated with a nervous, hypochondriacal mother. In addition, her father was chronically ill with bone cancer for a prolonged period in which he remained at home.

Methods of handling the guilt, anxiety, frustration, and emotional depletion varied considerably. Both overprotective and overtly rejecting behavior was seen. Sometimes mothers used treatment as a way to exclude others from their relations with the child. Missing clinic appointments frequently, neglecting important aspects of home care, or permitting the child to resist his treatments appeared to be consistent with rejecting attitudes in a few cases.

Some women felt that they were "chosen," in a sense, to carry such a burden because of their inner strength. Anger and resentment toward the patient was transferred at times to unsupporting husbands, careless parents of other children with cystic fibrosis, or those people with healthy children "who don't appreciate their kids."

Other mothers defended themselves against feelings of despair by consciously suppressing the realities of the child's condition, with the admonition that they "couldn't go on" if they let themselves "dwell on things."

Unconscious denial of the gravity of the illness often prevailed, regardless of prognosis or disability. Two mothers whose children each had a prognosis of less than five years illustrate this. One stated that she expected complete recovery and the other felt that her child would live "longer than a normal child" with the proper therapy.

Past experiences sometimes reinforced this denial. One woman who had a Rh negative blood factor and delivered several children without complication against medical advice, blithely related her expectation of complete recovery for her cystic child.

Tables I through III illustrate the prevalence of denial, guilt, and recurrent depression among the mothers. These reactions are not infrequent in parents of chronically sick children, particularly if the prognosis is uncertain.[5,7,13] It is difficult to determine what type of parental behavior could possibly be "normal" under such circumstances.

Perhaps the most useful gauge of successful adaption is the ability of the mother to continue functioning in a supportive role for the child, despite internal conflicts and psychological distortions of reality. Her problems become disabling to herself or the child when they either retard communication, interfere with educating the child about his illness, or prevent her from perceiving his needs and feelings.

It is our impression from this study that most mothers retained the ability to perform their role effectively despite significant emotional conflicts and personal suffering.

Effects of Cystic Fibrosis on the Family

Even when the total family adaption to cystic fibrosis was considered successful, siblings often complained about their relative deprivation and sacrifice. Younger children frequently demanded "their time," had somatic complaints, or pretended at having cystic fibrosis in order to gain parental indulgence. In the more defensive families, where suppression of feelings and avoidance of discussion were operative, resentment was more open and pronounced.

School adjustment difficulties, learning problems, and delinquency in siblings were attributed by both patients and their mothers to the strain imposed by the chronic illness and its aggravating effect on family rivalries. Mothers complained about the fathers' lack of participation in administering therapy, of disinclination to discuss feelings, or involvement in cystic fibrosis organizational groups to the exclusion of family interests. In some cases the closeness of the family bond was enhanced through sharing of grief or concern. In other instances the intensity of the experience aroused latent hostilities. The patients were unusually attuned to resentments in others, whether expressed overtly or subtly. Parental neglect of therapy, a brother's misbehavior, an annoyed frown when they coughed were sensitively perceived as evidence of dissatisfaction with themselves and the burden that their care entailed. Two children gauged the extent of the mother's hostility by the strength of her pounding during postural drainage. Although the reference of family problems to themselves has a basis in reality, it may be magnified by the child's guilt over receiving gratification of infantile dependent needs secondary to his illness.

An 18-year-old girl, who bitterly complained about her mother's inconsiderate, neglectful attitude reflected much guilt about not being as independent as she felt she should be. Her complaints ceased after it was arranged that she get a part-time job, receive tutoring toward high school credit, and have two of her daily postural drainage treatments at the hospital.

Parents with a good understanding of the pathological condition of cystic fibrosis would usually acquaint the child with the purpose of the treatment in order to gain his cooperation. However, several children with serious cases of cystic fibrosis were not told the nature and significance of their illness before adolescence. Knowledge was concealed or distorted, leaving the child puzzled, anxious, and mistrustful of his parents. Mothers would rationalize that this spared the child unnecessary anguish, there being "no need to explain" or "dwell on" it.

Adolescents from these families were ashamed and embarrassed of having cystic fibrosis and would try to conceal tents, medication, or other evidence from their peers. Occasionally they would openly rebel against the therapeutic program to the point of seriously endangering their health. It appeared that patterns of deception and avoidance practiced by the parents became the child's style of coping with the experience themselves.

A highly intelligent 18-year-old girl with severe cystic fibrosis and cardiac decompensation was told she had bronchiectasis in early adolescence. The mother also tried to hide the fact that her diet was specially prepared. As a young adult she was extremely suspicious, often depressed, and preoccupied with death. Much anxiety was relieved after her physician carefully explained the facts of her disease to her.

A 19-year-old boy, with severe digestive involvement, often refused medication and postural drainage therapy. He was deeply ashamed of having cystic fibrosis and did not know the nature of his illness until he was 17 years old, as his parents had overprotectively deferred explanations. Similarly, he concealed the fact of his illness from his fiancée until he was admitted to the hospital with intestinal obstruction a few weeks prior to marriage.

In families where children were uncooperative with therapy or ashamed of their illness, the situation was often characterized by marital difficulties, lack of closeness and harmony, or inability of the parents to handle their anxieties by open and supportive communication with each other and their children. Within such families, the lack of empathy and incapacity to share experiences made each member more vulnerable to additional stress. This resulted in further estrangement, interference with effective medical therapy, and emotional maladjustments. Where openness and mutual support prevailed, the child's illness had little disruptive impact on the family unit.

Conclusions

The experience of cystic fibrosis has considerable emotional impact on the child and his family. As modern methods of therapy prolong life, new kinds of problems have emerged relative to the chronicity of the disease. Judicious handling of psychological crises in these families can be of inestimable value for all concerned. Some tentative conclusions gained from this preliminary study may be of use in alerting the physician to possible sources of conflict and their resolution:

1. The absence of obvious signs or complaints of emotional distress concurrent with organic disease by no means excludes the possibility that such distress exists. Chronically unexpressed feelings of anxiety, hostility, or despair can evolve into seriously maladaptive behavior patterns which prevent effective cooperation with the physician and wholehearted participation in a treatment program. Arbitrary handling of resistance to treatment tends to solidify defensiveness, since it fails to deal adequately with the underlying anxiety. When the presence of depression, guilt, rejection, denial of illness, or chronic behavioral disturbances in parent or child impair therapeutic effectiveness, social casework or psychiatric consultation should be strongly considered.

2. An intellectual understanding of the disease achieved through educational efforts does not prevent or eliminate psychological complications which originate in unconscious distortions and faulty interpersonal relationships. However, the physician's efforts in educating the youngster with cystic fibrosis helps develop a relationship which may prove quite beneficial during later emotional crises. At times, the physicians' approach may be at variance with that of some parents who make ill-advised attempts to hide the facts about the disease from their children. In such cases it is imperative to reeducate these people and secure their cooperation, lest the child be further confused and frightened by conflicting sources of information. Of particular value to adolescents and young adults with cystic fibrosis would be the opportunity to discuss with the physician their concerns about continu-

ing education, employment, marriage, and parenthood, so that realistic future plans can be made. Family members are often unable to give useful, objective advice and assistance in these vital areas because of their emotional entanglements with the patient.

3. The less communicative and less emotionally supportive members of the family are with each other, the more likely that difficulties in adjustment to the illness will arise. Under such conditions, individuals affected by the strain may derive emotional support from sources outside the family. Cystic fibrosis parent groups, religious leaders, medical caseworkers, public health nurses, and family counseling agencies can, in many cases, be of benefit.

4. Parents under stress are sometimes capable of itensifying the child's difficulties or remaining unaware of his problems in adjustment. Professional time would be well spent in interviewing children directly, in an effort to elicit their true thoughts, feelings, and anxieties in relation to the illness. With patient, direct inquiry the child often reveals his deeper concerns. The physician is thus in an excellent position to provide him with needed reassurance. It should be stressed, however, that reassurance is often destroyed by superficiality and generalization. It can only be effective if the sick child can communicate his personal anxieties in the context of a relationship characterized by empathy, mutual respect, and honesty.

5. The primary anxieties and conflicts related to cystic fibrosis vary according to the patient's age and developmental maturity. Adolescence is a particularly trying time since the relative invalidism and necessity for daily care prolongs the dependent relationship between the sick child and his parents. This is intensified when physical limitations and recurrent, acute illnesses interrupt the natural association with his friends that helps the teen-ager emancipate himself from the family and gain independence. Chronic illness may isolate the adolescent from his peers, preventing him from utilizing the group approval he so desperately needs to combat his insecurity.[10] In later adolescence, it is probable that he has already begun to think seriously about his educational and vocational goals.[14] Self-esteem and feelings of security are enhanced when he finally chooses a career commensurate with his abilities and opportunities. The teenager with cystic fibrosis, despite his abilities, may be forced to relinquish his hopes and ideals when schooling is interrupted or prolonged by poor health. Family

funds originally destined for education may be depleted by the cost of treatment. Lack of stamina can interfere with choice of work requiring considerable activity or long hours. Recurrent hospitalizations tend to create uncertainty as to the worth of consolidating any future plans at all.

Thus, the tremendous job of emerging from the adolescent years with a stable identity and a sense of purpose is complicated by conflicts unique to the experience of being chronically ill. These must be resolved successfully so that the patient be allowed maximum realization of his potential, within the confines of his physical disability. Patience, understanding, and flexibility in approach by the physician and others involved can help him develop and mature optimally during these difficult times.

References

1. Doershuk, C. F., & Matthews, L. W. *Cystic fibrosis and obstructive pulmonary disease, ambulatory pediatrics*. Philadelphia: W. B. Saunders Co, 1968.
2. *Living with cystic fibrosis: A guide for the young adult*. New York, National Cystic Fibrosis Research Foundation, 1967.
3. Stoutt, G. E., Jr. *Cystic fibrosis: A booklet for parents*. Louisville, 1962.
4. Warwick, W. J. Cystic fibrosis: Nature and prognosis. *Minnesota Medicine* **50,** 1049–1053, 1967.
5. Lawler, R. H., Nakielny, W., & Wright, N. A. Psychological implications of cystic fibrosis. *Canadian Medical Association Journal* **94,** 1043–1046, 1966.
6. Turk, J. Impact of cystic fibrosis on family functioning. *Pediatrics* **34,** 67–71, 1964.
7. Freud, A. *The ego and the mechanisms of defence*. New York: International Universities Press Inc, 1946.
8. Buck, J. N. *The House-Tree-Person Technique, Revised Manual*. Los Angeles: Western Psychological Services, 1966.
9. Koppitz, E. M. *Psychological evaluation of children's human figure drawings*. New York: Grune & Stratton Inc, 1968.
10. Glaser, H. H., Harrison, G. S., & Lynn, D. B. Emotional implications of congenital heart disease in children. *Pediatrics* **33,** 367–379, 1964.
11. Langford, W. S. The child in the pediatric hospital: Adaption to illness and hospitalization. *American Journal of Orthopsychiatry* **31,** 667–684, 1961.
12. Richmond, J. B., & Waisman, H. A. Psychological aspects of the management of children with malignant diseases. *American Journal of Diseases of Children* **89,** 42–47, 1955.

13. Glaser, H. H., Lynn, D. B., & Harrison, G. S. Comprehensive medical care for handicapped children: I. Patterns of anxiety in mothers of children with rheumatic fever. *American Journal of Diseases of Children* **102,** 344–354, 1961.
14. Gardner, G. Psychiatric problems of adolescence. *In* S. Arieti (Ed.), *American handbook of psychiatry*. New York: Basic Books, 1959, vol. 1.

15

Coping with a Chronic Disability: Psychosocial Observations of Girls with Scoliosis

BEVERLY A. MYERS, STANFORD B. FRIEDMAN, and IRVING B. WEINER

The psychosocial implications of wearing the Milwaukee brace for scoliosis have been commented upon by orthopedic surgeons. Riseborough[1] summarizes: "Patients adapt to the brace rapidly, but the initial experience may provoke an emotional storm." Harrington[2] points out that a major alteration in daily living is involved and that patient–parent cooperation is critical for successful treatment. He groups brace wearers into three types: (1) brace riders (who develop ulcers on the chin and avoid exercises), (2) habit formers (who twist their necks and hence avoid the therapeutic forces of the brace), and (3) ideal patients. This paper represents a more detailed examination of how adolescent girls and their mothers psychologically adjust to the girl having to wear a Milwaukee brace.

BEVERLY A. MYERS, M.D. ● Assistant Professor of Pediatrics and Psychiatry, Johns Hopkins School of Medicine, Baltimore, Maryland. This investigation was supported by Children's Bureau grant 148 and Public Health Service grant K3-MH-18, 542 (Dr. Friedman) from the National Institute of Mental Health.

Reprinted from *American Journal of Diseases of Children,* September 1970, **120**(3), 175–181. Copyright 1970, American Medical Association.

The effectiveness of the Milwaukee brace in the treatment of mild to moderate idiopathic scoliosis has been demonstrated over the past 10 to 15 years.[1] With early detection, the brace, in conjunction with prescribed exercises,[3] will prevent the progression of the curve in the majority of those children treated.[4] At the University of Rochester Medical Center, one orthopedic surgeon, Louis Goldstein, M.D., has extensive experience in the management of scoliosis.[5] In his treatment program, children with curves under 20° are generally observed, while the Milwaukee brace is recommended in children under 15 years (bone age) who have curves between 20° and 50°. In the 50° to 70° more mobile curves, the Milwaukee brace also is recommended, but surgery is the treatment of choice when the spinal deformity is rigid and more than 70°. The Milwaukee brace, in conjunction with prescribed exercises, initially is worn 24 hours a day (a few do not wear the brace to school). If the curve is controlled with the brace and exercise management, it is worn until the spine is mature by radiologic criteria. The duration of wearing the brace is then gradually decreased. If, during the course of this treatment, the progress of the curve is not controlled, surgery is recommended.

Method

The principal author (B.A.M.) interviewed 25 girls, 9 to 16 years of age, and their mothers. Nineteen of these 25 girls were selected randomly from the total group of patients with scoliosis seen by the orthopedic surgeon and his staff. Six girls were referred to us because they presented problems in cooperating with the treatment program.

Each mother was interviewed to explain the study and to obtain information regarding her daughter's experience in adjusting to the Milwaukee brace. General background information on the girls' behavior at home, with peers, and at school was also obtained from each mother. Approximately one month later, the girl was interviewed and three projective tests administered (Holtzman inkblot, Draw-A-Person, and Miale-Holsopple Sentence Completion tests). Most of the girls also were observed during at least one physical therapy session. Further data were obtained from their medical records regarding diagnosis and response to orthopedic table management. Table I summarizes the clinical data on the girls included in the study.

Table I.   Summary of Clinical Data

Case	Age (yr)	Duration/ wearing brace (mo)	Degrees of curvature		Problems with brace and exercises	Adjustment
			Before	Change		
1	12	10	18	−13	Not doing exercises regularly	G
2	12½	4	18	0	Overly dependent on mother	G
3	13½	6	36	0	None	G
4	13	48	40	−15	Out of brace often; problems with exercises; overly dependent on mother	P
5	12½	2	25	0	Initial refusal; later worn 18 hr/day[a]	G
6	12½	10	54	−34	None	G
7	13	12	31	−4	None	G
8	14	4	36	−9	None	G
9	15½	10	30	−15	None	G
10	12	33	29	−16	None	G
11	12½	8	54	−12	Overly dependent on mother	G
12	12	3	52	−16	None	G
13	12½	1	21	−3	None	G
14	15	33	65	−25	Out of brace often; problems with exercises	G
15	9	8	38	−20	Problems with exercises; enuresis[a, b]	P
16	13	6	25	−14	Problems with exercises	P
17	14	Data not available	40	Data not available	Refused brace; doing exercises; withdrawn[a]	P
18	13½	4	48	−8	Not doing exercises; school phobia	P
19	12½	7	60	+2		G
20	13½	16	30	−18	None	G
21	13½	24	51	−19	Problems with exercises for six months; dependent on mother	P
22	13	6	61	−24	None	G
23	10	25	34	−8	Congenital scoliosis; +33° in three weeks out of brace; wearing and doing exercises[a, b]	P
24	13	6	Data not available	Data not available	Problems wearing brace and doing exercises; mental retardation	P
25	14	Data not available	Data not available	Data not available	Muscular dystrophy; refused brace[a, b]	P

[a] Referred because of problems.
[b] Projective tests not given.

Results and Comment

General Findings

At the time the brace was recommended by the orthopedic surgeon, 15 of the 25 girls were noted to express overt distress, as manifested by tears and an expression of feeling unable to wear the brace. The setting for this "breakdown" was variable in that it sometimes occurred in the physician's office, later at home, at the brace shop to get the mold for the brace, or upon getting the brace itself. A few expressed no overt negative response to having to wear a brace per se, but cried at some initial frustration, such as having difficulty entering a car for the first time wearing the brace. The first night in the brace was spontaneously mentioned by three mothers as a frightening event for their daughters, their fears being related to falling out of bed or choking. Despite their initial distress, all but five of the girls regularly wore the brace within two to four weeks and, for the most part, were able to resume their usual daily routine.

The task of facing friends, school, and the public in a brace was difficult, but not insurmountable. The brace, in drawing attention to a deformity not previously conspicuous, altered the girls' relationships to the outside world and commonly resulted in a tendency to withdraw. Five of the 25 girls persisted in their refusal for several weeks or longer, but eventually three of these five agreed to wear the brace. Facing the public alone with the brace outside of the school was more difficult. For example, the girls preferred to go shopping with their mothers, rather than alone, and preferred not to wear their braces for church. Thus, although they were able to resume their usual school and extracurricular activities, the majority exhibited some avoidance of being seen in public in the brace.

The girls' compliance with the exercise program, an essential aspect of the treatment, was noted to be related to the nature of their relationship to their mothers. Twelve of the girls, who were judged to have a good relationship with their mothers, were able to take responsibility for doing the exercises with minimal need to be reminded. On the other hand, 11 girls, judged to be overly dependent on their mothers, relied heavily on them to carry out the exercises, as well as to help with many other aspects of their daily life. (In two cases it was not possible to judge the mother–child relationship from the information obtained.)

The treatment program went well as long as mothers did not resent this marked dependence on them. However, a previous pattern of overdependence and mutual resentment, identified in 4 of the 11, was exaggerated by the demands of the exercise program, and the conflict resulted in haphazard, intermittent attempts at the exercises.

It was our impression that those girls who displayed overt crying and what appeared to be a period of withdrawal and depression followed by a conscious decision to wear the brace and do the exercises showed a better ability to tolerate the brace than those girls who did not show this type of initial response. The active decision of both daughter and parents to follow through with the recommended program seems essential to effective results, and when either was not convinced of the need for the brace, difficulties arose. However, this impression that better cooperation and follow-through actually led to better correction of the curvature could not be measured objectively in this study.

Families' continued support and praise for their daughters was crucial in keeping the girls wearing their braces and continuing their usual activities. This support was noted to be impaired by serious personality problems in the parents or marital conflicts. Such parental problems were noted in six of nine having difficulties in wearing the brace, but were not identified in any who wore the brace without difficulty.

The support of the staff involved (orthopedic surgeon, physical therapist, bracemaker, secretaries, school nurses) was also important to the continued wearing of the brace. The physical therapist played a key role in encouraging the girls, as well as in detecting those who were having difficulties. Likewise, regular orthopedic visits facilitated coordination and communication between staff and families, as problems related to the brace could be raised and handled jointly by the orthopedic surgeon, bracemaker, and physical therapist.

Families with previous experience with the brace were able to support others who were just starting out. A visit to meet a girl currently wearing a brace was sometimes suggested and was of considerable help to a family in making a decision about their own commitment to this corrective procedure.

Stabilization or improvement in the curvature, usually achieved within the first three to six months, was gratifying to the girl and her family. However, as the months and years went on, problems appeared. The brace, viewed more as a "prison," was worn less often and exercises were done less regularly. Of the four girls who had worn the brace more than two years, three were having increasing difficulty in complying with wearing the brace 24 hours a day and doing the exercises.

An overall assessment of the adaptation, or "adjustment," of the girls studied was made with placement into one of two groups: (1) "good" adaptation (G) was defined as the ability to wear the brace and do the exercises, a good attendance record at school, the presence of positive family and peer relationships, and the identification of few or no emotional problems; and (2) "poor" adaptation (P) was defined as the presence of serious problems in wearing the brace and doing exercises, difficulties attending school, poor peer and family relationships, and the presence of behavioral or emotional symptoms. Of the 25 girls, 16 were judged to have made a good adaptation, and 9 were judged to have made a poor adjustment. It should be noted that 6 of these 9 girls were specifically referred to the authors because of behavioral problems, and, thus, this sample does not reflect a nonbiased population of girls wearing Milwaukee braces.

Coping Behavior

The process of adaptation to a brace for a disability may be viewed from the point of view of psychological stress and the coping process. Lazarus[6] defines *coping behavior* as "those means utilized by an individual to tolerate a threat without disruptive anxiety or depression." After the recognition of a threat to himself or to his motives, the individual may be observed to respond to this stress in one or more of several ways: (1) intrapsychic defense mechanisms or maneuvers in which the individual deceives himself about the actual conditions of the threat (e.g., denial, intellectualization); (2) motor-behavioral reactions to reduce the threat (including actions aimed at strengthening the individual's resources against harm, attack, or avoidance); (3) disturbed affect of varying degrees (including anxiety, anger, guilt, depression). The first two categories, intrapsychic defense mechanisms and motor behavioral reactions, comprise the *coping process,* the means by which anticipated threat or harm is reduced or eliminated.

The coping process may be judged as effective with reference to the degree to which it protects the individual from overwhelming psychological distress, regardless of whether the behavior is socially or medically desirable. Thus, for example, complete denial of the threat of a deformity may protect an individual from experiencing extreme distress, though it may also prevent him from seeking the appropriate medical help. Coping behavior also may be judged in terms of the individual's ability to carry out socially desirable goals, irrespective of the distress he experiences psychologically. Thus, for example, a mother who is able to tend to her chronically handicapped child, no matter how distressed she feels, may be viewed as coping successfully. Optimal coping, therefore, protects the individual from being psychologically overwhelmed, yet allows for sufficient recognition of the illness to seek medical help.

Coping behavior depends upon many variables, including the nature and duration of the threat, the personality resources and past experience of the individual involved, and the resources available in the environment. Coping under severe stress situations has been studied in patients with severe burns,[7] polio patients with respiratory paralysis,[8] parents of fatally ill children,[9] as well as chronic physical disabilities.[10] The following is an examination of the coping process of girls and their mothers to the girl wearing the Milwaukee brace for scoliosis.

Intrapsychic Defense Mechanisms

The process of identification, or the perception of another as an extension of oneself, was a prominent feature of all mothers interviewed. In fact, during the interview with the mothers, it was often difficult to have them describe their daughters' reaction as separate from their own. The threat to the daughter seemed to be an identical threat to the mother. This was reflected in such statements by the mother as: "I didn't think it would happen to *us*" and "How can *we* live with this." Several mothers commented on their need to make a conscious effort not to do everything for their daughters and to recognize them as separate individuals. Moreover, the girls' expressed attitudes toward the brace were usually identical to those of their mothers. Their ability to cope with the brace well (or poorly) seemed so closely tied with their mothers' attitudes that it was impossible to attribute strength to either independently. At times, the strength to cope with this chronic disability seemed to be increased by the support that was gained via this identification process, even when marked, as in the following example:

> A mother with an only daughter actually performed the exercises herself regularly with her daughter and constantly wished there was something more she could do for her. This obese girl was able to cope with the brace both at school and in public, and had even begun to lose weight. Thus, the mother's identification with her daughter aided rather than impaired the girl's ability to function independently at school (case 11).

Denial was recognized frequently as a coping mechanism in the group of mothers and their daughters. It was usually not so pervasive that it interfered significantly with the ability to follow the treatment recommendations. The process of *denying the feelings* or distress (isolation of affect) was observed in most mothers. They showed no overt distress at critical times in their daughters' course, and several mothers commented about feeling an initial "shock" or numbness when first informed about the seriousness of their daughter's deformity. This absence of experiencing the full emotional impact upon hearing the diagnosis and treatment can easily be misinterpreted as lack of concern, rather than a protective mechanism. At least some of the girls experienced the same initial "shock" which later gave way to the overt distress and tears.

Most families *denied the threat* of the deformity by minimizing the problem before seeing the orthopedic surgeon, e.g., "I didn't think it was serious." This tendency to minimize the seriousness of the handicap and the wearing of the brace protected the individual from overwhelming distress, whereas total denial of the threat can lead to rejection of medical help:

> A 14-year-old girl who refused to wear the brace, despite a 40° curve, denied the threat of scoliosis in such comments as "I don't have to look at it [her back]. . . . There's something wrong with it, but it's not that bad. I do my exercises. That's enough. . . . I just don't want to hear about them [the possible long-term effects of ignoring the scoliosis] . . . it's none of my business. . . ." This girl had difficulty in complying with the orthopedic management and was specifically referred to the authors because of her refusal (case 17).

The inability to admit the very existence of an obvious deformity is a severe distortion of reality and an indication of little personal resources to cope with threat. It is frequently accompanied by an intense expression of anger at those who attempt to point out the presence of this deformity. This degree of denial was observed only in one family, and such denial seriously interfered with the treatment plan:

> A father of a 9-year-old girl had considerable difficulty accepting her severe deformity, and, according to mother, felt "the defect doesn't exist if he doesn't think about it." He felt the brace was of no use and discouraged his daughter from wearing the brace. It took several attempts to have him talk over his daughter's management with the physician and thus support her to wear the brace. A deterioration of 33° in the curvature in three weeks out of the brace "because she was ill" may have helped convince him, yet some weeks later, the author met this girl without her brace at a store (case 23).

Intellectualization, or the process of analyzing a situation rationally, was used frequently as a means of reducing the threat. Almost all mothers rationalized by saying that "the brace is better than surgery." Understanding scoliosis and the therapeutic program greatly helped both the girls and their families in tolerating the long orthopedic program. Conversely the inability to understand, because of communication difficulties, as observed in cases due to mental retardation, deafness, or the inability to speak English, seriously interfered with the comprehension of the back deformity and compliance with the treatment program.

> A 13-year-old mentally retarded girl with epilepsy had little understanding of her deformity and the reason for the brace. She seemed to feel her mother "didn't love" her and made her wear the brace as punishment. Mother felt intensely distressed and guilty by this and found it difficult to insist that her daughter wear the brace.

Reaction formation is an action, feeling, or opinion which is the opposite to what would commonly be expected and may help the individual master a stressful situation. This process was seen in a few families where the commonly expected responses seemed to be intolerable or unacceptable. When not extreme, this process served to diminish the anticipated threat and increase the sense of mastery.

> A mother of a 13-year-old girl was persistently upset that her daughter had to wear "one of those awful things," took her daughter out to a concert shortly after getting the brace "to prove we could do it" (case 1).

Displacement is the transfer of a feeling away from the individual or situation to which it was originally attached to another individual or situation. It was impossible for some families to express anger or distress directly in response to an emotionally arousing event. For example, rather than express anger directly at the current medical staff, previous physicians were blamed for disappointments about progress. In addition, there were complaints about the school not being helpful, when in reality, the hospital was the source of the difficulty. In this way, the possible disruption of the necessary relationship with the physician and paramedical staff was avoided.

Motor Activity

Motor-behavioral interactions with the individual's environment were observed to be part of the coping process and served to reduce the threat of this deformity. Most important, obviously, were wearing the brace and doing the exercises. These activities had both direct medical benefit and also the psychological assurance that something was actively being done to deal with the threat of an increasing back deformity. By their actions, mothers also were able to help their daughters adapt to the brace. For instance, they were quite imaginative in finding clothing to make the girls feel more attractive. Parents created various adaptations to enable the girls to see down to what they were eating or writing while at a desk or table. A preparatory visit to school after hours with a parent to make desk rearrangements also was noted to be helpful. By these and other ways, the girls and their families were able to take appropriate action to reduce the threat of the deformity and of the wearing of the brace.

Avoidance of the brace itself may be the only alternative to avoidance of society and overwhelming distress. Occasionally, but rarely, the brace may be too much to ask of an adolescent girl, given her particular life situation:

> A 13-year-old girl with progressive muscular weakness as a young child had been thought by her family to have a fatal illness. Although her weakness did not progress or alter ambulation, she later had to cope with the loss of her mother. When a progressive scoliosis developed, her new stepmother was quite unable to support the girl in wearing the Milwaukee brace. The girl stated, "I don't care what the future holds. I want to enjoy myself now and the brace makes me miserable. I am going to high school next year (instead of a class for physically handicapped) and I don't want to be different from the other kids." The many prior stresses left this girl little reserve to cope with the superimposed stress of a developing scoliosis (case 25).

Projective Testing

Because of the adolescent youngster's usual concern about the appearance of his body and his heightened sensitivity to deviations from the ideal, it was expected that these girls' adjustment to their scoliosis would be reflected in their perception of their body. The projective test data were accordingly analyzed primarily for indications of disturbed body imagery and inordinate concerns about physical disability.

Fisher and Cleveland,[11-13] in their extensive explorations of the relation of body image to other personality factors, have developed two major body boundary indices that can be scored from the Holtzman ink-blot test: the Barrier index, which refers to definiteness of body boundaries, and the Penetration index, which measures a lack of disruption of a perceived discrete body exterior. A number of studies have demonstrated an association between increasing boundary definiteness, diminished likelihood of psychosis, and enhanced ability to deal effectively with difficult disturbing experiences, especially those involving body disablement.[11] Thus, higher Barrier scores have been observed to be directly related to the ability to adjust to the stress of body disablement as measured in paraplegic men and pregnant women.[14] High Penetration scores, on the other hand, are associated with schizophrenia and have also been observed in individuals several years after colostomy. Fisher[11] also suggests that Penetration scores are particularly sensitive to immediate situational conditions.

The Barrier scores of these girls wearing the Milwaukee brace for scoliosis ranged from 0 to 7 with a median of 3.6. This median value closely resembled the median Barrier score of 3 observed in normal populations of adults and adolescent girls. Indeed, the Barrier scores of the girls with satisfactory adjustment did not differ significantly from those of the girls with adjustment problems. In contrast to the normally observed median Penetration score of 1, however, these girls had a Penetration range of 0 to 10, with a median of 5.5. This median value for the whole group was comparable to the level seen in schizophrenic groups. One interpretation of this finding would be that the whole experience of wearing a Milwaukee brace, even though there is no actual penetration of the skin, constituted a threat to the perception of bodily integrity and is reflected in these high Penetration scores. With respect to recency to the traumatic event, however, no significant differences in median Penetration score were found between those girls who had recently begun to wear the brace (six months or less) and those who had worn it for a relatively long time (more than six months).

The Draw-A-Person and Sentence Completion tests did not contribute further to the demonstration of problems with body image. With only one exception (a girl with onset of scoliosis in early childhood), none of the girls drew human figures containing significant body distortions reflecting disturbed body imagery. The Sentence Completion protocols were strikingly free from references to disability, and the most that could be concluded from them was the girls, as noted above, probably had significant needs to deny their deformities.

Conclusions

The majority of the girls observed were able, after an "initial storm,"[1] to cope with wearing a Milwaukee brace and carry on their usual daily lives. This was in spite of a biased sample which included an inordinate number of girls having problems wearing the brace. In this study it was possible to identify a number of the factors existing in the girl and her family, as well as in their environment (including the medical milieu), which influenced the manner and success of coping with a chronic disability. Those factors contributing positively to the girls' ability to cope included: (1) the girls' and their mothers' intellectual understanding of scoliosis and the reason for the bracing procedure; (2) the girls' and their parents' active decision to wear the brace; (3) the family's continuing support and encouragement; (4) the relatively optimistic view of outcome with a definite termination time; (5) the support, coordination, continuity and interest of the regular visits with the medical staff.

Another possible factor may be the fact that these girls had a handicap appearing later in childhood, rather than one existing from birth. Although there are few studies comparing acquired versus congenital handicaps, it is interesting to note a study by Kimmel[15] who suggests that children with acquired orthopedic handicaps have a greater esteem for their bodies and can cope with more anxiety than can children with congenital handicaps. In agreement with this the two girls who had handicaps dating from early childhood (case 23 and 25) were observed to have especially serious problems in adapting to the brace in contrast to the majority of the others whose deformity developed much later. The minimal disturbance of body image in the majority of girls, as measured by the projective tests, may reflect the later onset of scoliosis.

Among those factors which contributed to difficulties in coping were: (1) limitations in intellectual understanding of scoliosis and the brace (e.g., mental retardation, language barriers); (2) total denial of the deformity or the threat it posed; (3) daughters' excessive dependence leading to conflict with mother, particularly around exercises; (4) marital conflicts and other personality problems in the parents leading to little support for the daughters; (5) the long duration of wearing the brace; and (6) increasing threat of surgery, indicating the failure of the brace.

There are several implications in our data for the physician and other professionals dealing with children with chronic handicaps. While each individual's manner of coping is unique and related to his personality structure and available resources, there are nevertheless certain patterns common to many. Awareness and understanding of these patterns can facilitate the effectiveness of any professional dealing with the chronically handicapped. Green and Haggerty[16] emphasize this in discussing the general principles of management of long-term, non-life-threatening illness in children, which include continuity of care, individualization of care, and awareness of parental reactions. Coping mechanisms should be viewed not only as protection from intolerable anxiety or depression, but also in terms of how such behavior contributes to, or interferes with, cooperation with the treatment program for the handicapped child.

The pediatrician, in addition to his early detection of the scoliosis, can help the family by his continuing interest and support and by his preparation of the family for referral. Some explanation of the problem and the possible means of management can facilitate understanding and hence a greater ability to adjust to the therapeutic program. This anticipatory guidance by the referring physician may be extremely helpful in that the expected psychosocial problems can be discussed with the family. Such advanced warning, if not in itself made overwhelming, promotes subsequent mastery of the task the adolescent must face in wearing the Milwaukee brace.

Acknowledgment

Louis Goldstein, M.D., chairman, Division of Orthopedic Surgery, University of Rochester cooperated in this study and made constructive comments. Margaret Morrow, R.P.T., Strong Memorial Hospital, cooperated in this study.

References

1. Riseborough, E. J. Current concepts: Treatment of scoliosis. *New England Journal of Medicine* **276**:1429–1431, 1967.
2. Harrington, P. R. Nonoperative treatment of scoliosis. *Texas Medicine* **64**:54–65, 1958.
3. Blount, W. P., & Bolinske, J. Physical therapy in the nonoperative treatment of scoliosis. *Physical Therapy* **47**:919–923, 1967.
4. Blount, W. P. Scoliosis and Milwaukee brace. *Bulletin of the Hospital for Joint Diseases* **19**:152–165, 1968.
5. Goldstein, A. L. Surgical management of scoliosis. *Journal of Bone and Joint Surgery* **48**:167–180, 1966.
6. Lazarus, R. S. *Psychological stress and the coping process.* New York: McGraw-Hill, 1966.
7. Hamburg, D. A., Hamburg, B., & deGoza, S. Adaptive problems and mechanisms in severely burned patients. *Psychiatry* **16**:1–20, 1953.
8. Visotsky, H. M., Hamburg, D. A., Goss, M. A., et al. Coping behavior under extreme stress. *Archives of General Psychiatry* **5**:423–488, 1961.
9. Friedman, S. B., Chodoff, P., Mason, J. W., et al.: Behavioral observations on parents anticipating the death of a child. *Pediatrics* **32**:610–625, 1963.
10. Wright, B. *Physical disability: A psychological approach.* New York: Harper & Row, 1960.
11. Fisher, S. A further appraisal of the body boundary concept. *Journal of Consulting Psychology* **27**:62–70, 1963.
12. Fisher, S. Body image psychopathology. *Archives of General Psychiatry* **10**:519–529, 1964.
13. Fisher, S., & Cleveland, S. E. *Body image and personality.* Princeton, New Jersey: D Van Nostrand, 1958.
14. Landau, quoted by Wiener, I. *Psychodiagnosis of schizophrenia.* New York: John Wiley, 1966. P. 132.
15. Kimmel, J. A comparison of children with congenital and acquired orthopedic handicaps on certain personality characteristics. *Dissertation Abstracts* **19**:3023, 1959.
16. Green, M., & Haggerty, R. *Ambulatory pediatrics.* Philadelphia: W. B. Saunders, 1968. P. 443.

VII

The Crisis of Treatment: Unusual Hospital Environments

Hospital environments are designed to facilitate the delivery of special medical care and to promote healing, but because of the unfamiliar equipment and procedures many patients are as upset and frightened by their hospital experience as they are reassured by the medical resources made available to them. The nurses, doctors, and other hospital personnel become familiar with its routines and build up the necessary psychological defenses (see part X) to treat it simply as a place of employment and thereby distance themselves from its distressing emotional overtones. Patients, on the other hand, must deal with these strange settings and procedures (often without sufficient explanations) at a time when their physical and emotional resources are already being severely taxed by their illness.

In the first article Donald Kornfeld provides an overview of various hospital environments and some of the problems which patients encounter within these treatment settings. Even "routine" diagnostic tests such as EKG or standard treatments like radiotherapy arouse fear among some patients, but much of this anxiety could be alleviated by the health professional through reassurance and careful explanations. Kornfeld describes some of the problems of special settings, such as the

233

sensory deprivation and decreased human contact of isolation units and the anxiety and disorientation of open-heart recovery rooms. He suggests the use of denial by patients in surgical recovery rooms to blot out that which is frightening or upsetting. He proposes several architectural and procedural changes designed to lessen patient distress and has discussed elsewhere[3] the value of other intervention measures, such as a preoperative visit by the anesthesiologist to prepare the patient psychologically by answering questions, telling him or her what to expect in the recovery room, and offering general reassurance.

Coronary care units and other intensive care facilities have been receiving some attention recently because of the unexpected difficulties which patients have experienced in these specialized environments. The setting has been shown to be a significant factor in the occurrence of postcardiotomy delirium[4] and general disorientation, and may contribute to high anxiety levels among myocardial infarction patients.[2] Unlike other critically ill people, those who have just had an MI are alert, aware of their surroundings, and communicative. They usually begin to feel better soon after their attack, so their stay in the CCU allows them time to think about the prospect of greater dependence and other changes in their life-style, about the damage to their heart, and about the reality of death. While many find the array of monitoring equipment reassuring, it is also evidence of the danger their lives are in.[5]

There are several ways to alleviate anxiety and facilitate the patient's own coping techniques. These include giving information, building up self-esteem (for example, by pointing out the patient's value to others), giving reassurance, promoting ventilation of feelings, fostering identification with those who survive, supporting a healthy use of denial, and encouraging future planning by the patient (in order to forestall any tendency toward excessive withdrawal). Technical changes such as quieter machinery and monitoring equipment which allow the patient more movement, and procedural changes such as fewer interruptions to patients' sleep and nursing efforts to orient the patient to time and place, have decreased the incidence of delirium and disorientation somewhat.[1]

In the second article Samuel Klagsbrun describes a project designed to alter the social environment of a cancer research ward. Initially, the poor morale of the ward was manifested by patients' frequent complaints of being used as guinea pigs by "uncaring doctors" and "unavailable nurses," and a high turnover rate among nurses. Klagsbrun began by organizing weekly group discussions with the nurses. Through these sessions the nurses explored their feelings toward the doctors and patients, and gradually achieved a clearer perception and acceptance of their own role in this complex interrelationship. When the focus shifted to patient management problems, the group sessions provided emotional support and information to enable them to recognize the underlying meaning of patient behavior.

The second phase of the project was an attempt to enable the patients to see themselves as functioning, productive people rather than "walking dead." Patients were encouraged to take over their own physical care, such as making their own beds and filling their water pitchers. To counteract the tendency toward withdrawal and isolation, a small dining room was set up so patients could eat communally. An activist group of patients took over a variety of ward duties and began to organize social activities. The whole atmosphere on the unit changed with an increase in self-esteem, mastery, and involvement for patients, and a sharp decline in nursing staff turnover.

As more people are treated on an outpatient basis, the clinic waiting room becomes an increasingly important setting for patients and their families. In our third article Irwin Hoffman and Edward Futterman describe the experiences of families in the waiting room of a pediatric oncology clinic and discuss the impact of psychiatric intervention on the ability of patients and their families to cope with this stressful environment. While the monthly clinic visit represents an assertion of hope and of some mastery over the illness, it also serves as a painful reminder and reawakens feelings of grief, anger, fear, helplessness, and guilt. Parents need to find an appropriate balance between maintaining hope and a strong emotional tie to the child, and accepting their impending loss and beginning the mourning and detachment process in anticipation of it. The sick child's tasks include dealing with his losses and injuries, the threat to his self-image, constant interruptions in his daily life for medical care, and general anxiety.

While the disease is in remission, denial can be a useful coping technique for a sick child and his family, but it is difficult to maintain during clinic visits. Before the intervention project parents and children in the waiting room were "locked into patterns of passivity, noncommunication, and social isolation," withdrawn into tense family groups. Since the play program was instituted, children (patients and siblings) have the opportunity to express pent-up feelings and work out their anxieties through playing. The patient is encouraged to see himself as an independent, functioning person, while siblings are offered temporary escape and relief from tension. Meanwhile parents are free to talk to other parents sharing information and their feelings, reducing their sense of isolation, and giving each other valuable social and emotional support. By encouraging a sense of individual control over the situation, by offering opportunities for the ventilation of feelings, and by increasing the emotional interaction and support available within the group, the play program enabled the patients and their families to cope better, not only with the stresses of the clinic visit but also with the general adaptive tasks which they faced.

References

1. Budd, S., & Brown, W. Effect of a reorientation technique on postcardiotomy delirium. *Nursing Research,* 1974, **23,** 341–348.
2. Cassem, N. H., & Hackett, T. P. Psychiatric consultation in a coronary care unit. *Annals of Internal Medicine,* 1971, **75,** 9–14.
3. Kornfeld, D. S. Psychiatric aspects of patient care in the operating suite and special areas. *Anesthesiology,* 1969, **31,** 166–171.
4. Lazarus, H. R., & Hagens, J. H. Prevention of psychosis following open-heart surgery. *American Journal of Psychiatry,* 1968, **124,** 1190–1195.
5. Obier, K., & Haywood, L. J. Role of the medical social worker in a coronary care unit. *Social Casework,* 1972, **53,** 14–18.

16

The Hospital Environment:
Its Impact on the Patient

DONALD S. KORNFELD

It is not enough for us to do what we can do; the patient and his environment, and external conditions have to contribute to achieve the cure.　　　　　HIPPOCRATES

With the growth of modern hospital technology, there has been increasing concern by physicians for the emotional impact of the hospital environment on patients. In the past, the hospital environment has been studied primarily by social scientists[1-5] who have examined it as a social system. Few studies, however, have been done by physicians. This probably reflects two facts:

1. Members of the medical profession develop the necessary psychological defense mechanisms which allow them to work in this environment but in doing so, prevent themselves from appreciating its effect on others.

2. Physicians have not, until recently, appreciated that clinically significant reactions to the hospital environment can occur.

While space-age electronic gadgetry has dramatized the problem, the hospital has probably always been a frightening place for patients and their families. Certainly on one psychological level patients can

DONALD S. KORNFELD, M.D. • Chief, Psychiatric Consultation Service, Columbia-Presbyterian Medical Center, Associate Professor of Clinical Psychiatry, College of Physicians and Surgeons, New York, New York.

Reprinted in abridged form from *Advances in Psychosomatic Medicine*, 1972, **8**, 252–270.

appreciate hospitalization as a reassuring thing. We all know that "modern medicine" is now able to perform "miracles," but that big building with its special sights, sounds, and smells remains for most people a very frightening place. The hospital, however, is staffed by special people who have chosen to be there. It is merely the place where they work and they pass through its doors each morning with no more anxiety than business executives and secretaries entering an office building. Obviously, it is important that a medical staff be able to work without the emotional upheavals experienced by patients. They must, therefore, develop psychological defenses to allow themselves to deal objectively with the serious problems they must face each day. As a result, most of them do not appreciate the stress of hospitalization on the average patient.

A patient's maladaptation to the hospital environment can produce important clinical changes. The cardiovascular and endocrine responses associated with anxiety are well known. More recently we have begun to identify physiological changes which may accompany depression. It is reasonable to suspect that such psychophysiological responses can influence the course of illness. However, the environment can produce effects which are more obviously a threat to a patient's physical well-being. For example, the agitated psychotic patient in the open-heart recovery room with tachycardia and rising blood pressure is in danger of compromising his cardiac status. The patient who signs out of the hospital against medical advice because she misunderstood a remark made at bedside rounds runs all the risks of delayed diagnosis and treatment. Therefore, to consider the impact of the hospital environment on patients is not mere compassion, but a medical necessity.

What is the hospital environment? Bricks, machines, people. Each, in its own way, contributes to the atmosphere of the institution and its effect on the individual patient. Hospital architecture is a specialty which has concerned itself, until recently, primarily with creating efficient space in which medical people can work. There is little written regarding the impact on patients of hospital design. Architects are, therefore, forced to extrapolate from the body of knowledge available from home and office planning. However, the hospital patient is sick and helpless, and aspects of the physical environment which are relatively unimportant when one is well can become important when one is confined to a hospital bed. The healthy client can make adjustments in his environment. He can rearrange furniture; he can move about to avoid unpleasant noises, odors, or lights. The hospital patient must, for the most part, accept the environment as given.

The Hospital Environment—An Overview

Certainly, most people do regard hospitalization with considerable apprehension. We view the hospital as a more efficient place in which to study and treat our patients; however, for the patient, the act of hospitalization implies the presence of illness too serious to be treated in a doctor's office. This fact alone can be terrifying. It means the patient must abandon his role in society and face the reality of his own mortality. Man does not usually live with this anxiety in the forefront of his consciousness. It is hard to do otherwise in the hospital where one is surrounded by serious illness and death 24 hours a day. Certainly, each patient deals with this situation in his own way but each one must come to grips with it. The question is, how does the hospital environment affect the individual patient in his struggle with this anxiety-provoking situation?

First, we must examine in more detail those aspects of the hospital situation which we see as "routine." Many of what we regard as standard procedures, to a patient, are new and very anxiety-provoking experiences. No diagnostic test is "routine" to the patient upon whom it is done. Such "standard" items as EKG machines, oxygen tents, and intravenous fluids may be new and terrifying experiences for some patients. What then of radioactive counters, cardiac catheters, arteriography and cobalt therapy machines? How much unnecessary anxiety is produced because we are unaware of these reactions. Patients often assume we are too busy to answer their "foolish questions." We must therefore, anticipate their anxiety and take the initiative, since simple explanations can usually provide adequate reassurance.

What are the effects of "routine" bedside rounds on a teaching service?[6,7] On the positive side, patients report they feel there is great benefit in having the talent of so many doctors applied to their problem. The potentially harmful effects of rounds are apparent. The presentation of the history and laboratory data along with a detailed discussion of the diagnostic and treatment possibilities may reveal information for which the patient has not been prepared. The use of euphemisms to avoid this is not very effective as patients become increasingly sophisticated. Similarly, the barrage of medical terms at the bedside can just as easily lend themselves to inaccurate assumptions. The "cancer" discussion between the attending and the intern could very well have been related to the last patient visited, but for the patient at whose bedside it occurs, this may not be so apparent. The physical exposure of patients without concern for their privacy does occasionally occur but should not require additional comment. Perhaps the most disturbing phenomenon at bedside rounds is the heated discussion regarding diagnostic and therapeutic possibilities. What a dilemma for the patient to see the physicians in apparent disagreement regarding her problem and how best to treat it. What a blow to see her doctor, a house officer, publicly chastised for some omission. We should be grateful for the mental mechanism of denial which allows most patients to deal with these situations. Certainly rounds can have a therapeutic function. The history presentation and discussion need not take place at the bedside. Most hospital wards have a room nearby where the group can assemble and discuss these matters. The patient can then be visited to have physical findings corroborated. At this time, he can be given an opportunity to ask questions and receive emotional support from the professional staff.

The entry into the hospital environment can also have very acute effects. The first psychiatric patient most interns have to treat is a little old lady who becomes disoriented at night and too often climbs out of bed and fractures a hip. She is probably suffering from an acute organic brain syndrome. Despite her chronically impaired cerebral functioning, she had been able to function adequately in her familiar home environment. In the hospital, often under the influence of sleeping medication, the darkness and unfamiliar surroundings produce a more acute disorganization of her mental faculties. The problem is often solved by canceling the sleeping medication and leaving a night light burning. A more severe form of this syndrome can exist with disorientation, confusion, agitation and, occasionally, paranoia, persisting day and night. Here the patient becomes disorganized by the strangeness of the environment and a senile psychosis occurs. While phenothiazines may give some symptomatic relief, the introduction of familiar people and objects can be helpful. Obviously, the treatment of choice is to return the patient to the familiar environment of home where rapid improvement usually occurs.

Similar response can also be seen in patients who require eye-patching.[8] This is especially true in those who are also immobilized. They may react to the diminished sensory input with delusions, hallucinations, disorientation, and agitation. The treatment of choice is early patch removal and mobilization but in the meanwhile, the introduction of frequent meaningful auditory cues can help.

Special Hospital Areas

As medicine has become increasingly specialized, a need has arisen for separate hospital units in which highly trained staff and special equipment can be concentrated to allow for efficient care. Some of these units are unique environments and the observations which have been made on their psychiatric effects will be reviewed.

Isolation Units

Our understanding of sensory deprivation effects has also provided some insight into the occasional acute psychiatric problems which occur in isolation rooms for patients with infectious disease or where reverse precautions are needed. Here the patients are in individual rooms visited only by gowned and masked staff and family. The need for the mask and gown undoubtedly reduces the number of visits. Those visits which do occur take on a strange quality as the masked figures go about their chores. Family members become less familiar and reassuring. This environment can therefore easily intensify whatever anxiety the patient may be experiencing regarding the nature and seriousness of his condition. For an occasional patient, this setting can trigger an acute psychotic reaction, often with paranoid trends. If transfer out of the unit is impossible, measures must be taken to relieve anxiety and increase meaningful stimulation. The patient's physician should attempt to explore possible misconceptions regarding the illness. The nurses should increase the frequency and length of their visits and these should be made to socialize and not just to perform tasks. The introduction of a television set and telephone can also be therapeutic. Phenothiazines can be used to provide symptomatic relief.

Holland et al.[9] have studied a group of acute leukemia patients treated in "germ-free units." These are plastic bubblelike enclosures or plastic-lined rooms in which patients are literally separated from all direct contact with anyone. They are touched only through plastic gloves at the end of plastic arms built into the walls or by individuals dressed in "space suits" wearing gloves. The average patient stayed 28 days.

Twenty percent of patients eligible for treatment in these units declined such treatment or were rejected as unsuitable. Twelve patients were studied. Eleven reported that they could have stayed longer if necessary. No acute psychiatric problems related to the environment were reported. All stated that the personality of the nurses contributed to their ability to tolerate the totally dependent situation. The most significant complaint by patients was their inability to touch or be touched directly by another human being. As one patient put it, "About a week ago, it started to get on my nerves in the bubble and not being able to feel other people and hoping I could come out soon. I felt like I couldn't stand it anymore. I just had to feel other people. I wanted to feel somebody; touch another human being. If I could have done this, I could have stuck it out longer in the bubble."

Dr. Holland observes that physical contact is an important way of providing emotional support and comfort to someone who is ill. The pat on the shoulder, the squeeze of the hand, are often so automatic that we are unaware of how often it occurs between the patient and his visitors, both staff and family. Physicians apparently cannot underestimate the continuing importance of "the laying on of hands" in the practice of medicine.

Intensive Care Units

The intensive care unit (ICU) in its various forms has come under special scrutiny. McKegney[10] has referred to an "intensive care syndrome" and called it a new disease of medical progress. These are indeed psychiatric problems which appear to be a reaction to the unique environment of the ICU itself and these phenomena will be reviewed. However, intensive care is applied in a variety of medical and surgical settings and the nature and extent of the psychiatric problems can vary. Sgroi et al.,[11] for example, report no meaningful difference in the incidence of psychiatric symptoms in a group of patients in a general medical ICU when compared with comparably ill patients treated in the ward. Above all, one must realize that in any setting in which there are very sick patients, a variety of psychiatric problems can emerge. It would be unfortunate if the concept of the ICU syndrome were overemphasized and other possible causes of psychiatric difficulties in that setting were overlooked. This is especially true of the acute organic brain syndrome (delirium) which can be the product of a variety of metabolic, cardiovascular, neurologic, or pharmacologic factors. These possibilities must be ruled out before one can assume that the patient's delirium is a reaction to the environment alone.

Open-Heart Recovery Room

The concept of an ICU syndrome developed out of reports of a high incidence (38–70%) of delirium following open-heart surgery.[12-14] The delirium developed in the open-heart recovery room (OHRR) after a lucid postoperative interval. While a variety of preoperative and operative factors appeared to contribute to the delirium, some felt that the environment of these rooms played a major contributory role.[12,14] The typical OHRR was a large open area with 5–7 beds, separated by a movable curtain. The patients were attached to EKG cables, intravenous tubing, and a bladder catheter. Although movement was possible, most patients remained relatively immobile as a result of pain and the implied limitation of motion produced by the cables. An electronic monitor with an oscilloscope was placed next to the bedside and flashed constantly. The patient was placed in a plastic oxygen tent which produced a constant background humming and hissing noise. Nurses and house officers arrived at frequent intervals to perform their chores. The room's overhead light was constantly on. There was always the possibility of an emergency with the associated activity. Thus, for the 4–6 days that most patients were there, they were subjected to an experience which combined elements of a sensory monotony experiment with sleep deprivation. This was similar to the experience of patients with polio placed in tank respirators. Having possibly had their cerebral function partially compromised by the cardiac bypass it was not surprising that these cardiac surgery patients had a high incidence of delirium. The typical patient would appear lucid for the first 3–4 days. He would then experience an illusion, for example, sound arising from an air-conditioning vent might begin to sound like someone calling him. This might then progress to auditory and visual hallucinations and frank paranoid delusions. Disorientation to time, place, and person could occur. In a typical case, the delirium would clear within 24–48 hours after the patient was transferred to a standard hospital environment where he would have a sound sleep.

On the basis of these findings, it was suggested that certain modifications in the design of these rooms and the nursing procedures associated with them might reduce the incidence of delirium.[14] The authors suggested: (1) Nursing procedures should be modified to allow the maximum number of uninterrupted sleep periods; the usual day-awake, night-asleep cycle should be maintained wherever possible. (2) Patients should be placed in individual cubicles. There they would not be awakened or made more anxious by activity occurring around other patients. (3) Monitoring equipment should be maintained, when possible, outside the patient's room. Bedside monitors could be turned on whenever needed. This would reduce the anxiety in those patients who are aware of the significance of these signaling devices and the danger implicit with any change in their pattern. (4) Patients should be allowed increased mobility by removing as many wires and cables as possible. Telemetry equipment would achieve increased mobility and allows for the use of remote monitors. (5) The constant noise of oxygen and cooling tents should be modified or removed wherever possible. (6) Each room should be equipped with a large clock and calendar. (7) An outside window should be visible to the patient to allow for orientation.

Lazarus and Hagens[15] found that modifications in the OHRR and its routines which were designed to lessen anxiety, sensory monotony, and sleep deprivation did produce a lower incidence of delirium after open-heart surgery. Heller et al.[16] also reported a reduction in the incidence of delirium in recent years. Diminished time required on the heart–lung machine may have contributed to this decline; however, modifications in the environment of the OHRR which allow for more sleep and reduce anxiety may also have played a role.

Operating Room

The operating room had been considered one area where a patient's psychological responses could be temporarily ignored. Recent reports have suggested that this may be a false assumption. The work of

Cheek[17] and Levinson[18] indicates that patients may perceive remarks made while they were apparently anesthetized. They have demonstrated through the use of recall under hypnosis that patients can recall statements made during surgery by the operating team. A remark which suggests that the patient may have been in danger seems to be most readily recalled. This type of recall is most common in patients being operated upon with regional or spinal anesthesia where the accompanying sedation still allows some awareness of what is being said. However, it can apparently also occur with patients under general anesthesia. The problem is complicated by the use of muscle relaxants which can obscure a patient's true level of awareness. Unexplained postoperative anxiety or depression have been attributed to the effects of remarks made during surgery and been successfully treated with hypnosis and ventilation therapy.[17]

Recovery Room

Until very recently little attention has been paid to the psychological responses of patients in the surgical recovery room. However, a paper by Winkelstein et al.[19] questions the assumption that patients in the recovery room are too obtunded to be aware of what goes on about them or to communicate their concern regarding their recent surgery. They interviewed a series of patients in the recovery room and demonstrated that very shortly after emerging from surgery they were able to relate quite directly with an interviewer. They were also able to recall 24 hours later much of the content of these interviews. Therefore, what many have felt to be a pharmacologically induced obtundity may very well be the use of the mental mechanism of denial to blot out the unpleasantness of surgery and the frightening sights and sounds which surround the patient in the recovery room itself. This is not to suggest that denial may not be the most effective mental mechanism to be used by an individual in such circumstances. But it should be noted that such patients are not as oblivious as may first appear to what is happening to them. This knowledge should be applied to the management of the recovery room experience for patients.

What are the frightening aspects of the recovery room? Typically, a recovery room is a large, open area in which a group of patients lie about at various levels of consciousness; an area in which one patient may be lying for 3 hours waiting for spinal anesthesia to wear off, while across the room a patient who has suddenly begun to bleed is being frantically worked upon by a group of physicians and nurses. In the same room, a patient emerging from anesthesia is screaming loudly for pain relief while another patient, awaiting transfer to her floor, lies quietly, staring off into space apparently oblivious to what goes on about her. In one corner, a patient appears to doze as two surgeons discuss the pathology found at frozen section. In another corner of the room, a child who has just had a tonsillectomy lies terrified watching this group of sick adults. The picture I have just painted is perhaps not typical of all recovery rooms but demonstrates the psychological problems which do exist there: unnecessarily exposing patients to frightening experiences by allowing them to observe all that goes on about them; inadequate analgesia for patients left with only postoperative orders to be administered upon return to their hospital floor, unnecessarily exposing patients to frightening remarks by staff who believe they are oblivious to these comments. There is especially the problem of the impact of this generally horrifying scene upon the mind of a child.

What can be done to reduce the anxiety-provoking aspects of this room? One basic change can be made in the structure of the room itself. It is possible to construct a room with a central nursing station and individual cubicles for patients. In this way, patients are not totally exposed to the sights and sounds of other patients about them. While it is true that with limited nursing staff one must provide easy access to all patients, there is still no reason why partitions cannot be built so that the patient, lying flat on his back, is not exposed to the problems on either side of him. Curtains can also be provided on an overhead track which can be used to provide complete privacy when indicated. Hopefully, someone will remember to close them at those times. There is a special danger that with increasing reliance upon electronic monitoring equipment, the recovery room could too quickly become a place in which patients attached to machines are watched from afar by nurses and medical staff. This would be most unfortunate. Patients coming out of anesthesia are in particular need of human contact for reassurance that all is well.

It is strongly recommended, whenever possible, to have a separate recovery room for children. The surgical experience is difficult enough for them without their being exposed to the recovery room of a general hospital. Some of the suggestions made for the adult recovery room could be applied here. A special preoperative preparation room could be of great value. Here a child could be adequately premedicated and perhaps have a final reassuring visit from a physician. If possible, the route by which children enter the operating suite should not take them past the recovery room. The recovery room could be constructed as suggested for adults so that patients are separated in cubicles and thus not completely exposed to whatever disturbing scene may occur in their vicinity. Children awaiting transfer back to the hospital proper could also be separated from those still recovering from anesthesia. The special pediatric recovery room also provides a group of nurses specially trained to deal with the specific problems of children, both psychological and physiological. These nurses develop an expertise in dealing with children which can be remarkably effective.

Despite all efforts to diminish the anxiety-provoking features of the recovery room, there are certain limits to what can be done. I would, therefore, recommend that patients be removed from the recovery room to their hospital quarters as quickly as possible. It was striking, for example, that even in a special pediatric recovery room frightened children would stop crying when placed on the stretcher returning them to their hospital bed. Returning to the hospital proper removes the patient from the stresses of the recovery room scene and also indicates to him that all is well. A delayed departure for some administrative reason, e.g., waiting for a nursing shift to take place, may be interpreted as a sign that some surgical problem still exists.

Summary

I am sure that there are few surprises for the average physician in what he has just read. Most of the observations have been made by psychiatrists, i.e., physicians not involved in the primary care of these patients. They were able to identify the effects of the environment because they were not initially a part of it. Their recommendations are often obvious to the physicians involved once these observations are brought to their attention. The modifications in the environment can often be readily incorporated into a hospital routine with gratifying results. Therefore, what is needed is for all physicians to increase their awareness of the potential environmental hazards which they encounter each day. What is essential is that we enhance our ability to empathize with patients, i.e., to recognize the meaning of the hospital situation for them, without our overidentifying with the patients themselves. In this way, using good common clinical sense, we can do a great deal to make the environment at the bedside, which is the most important of all, truly therapeutic.

References

1. Brown, E. L. The use of the physical and social environment of the general hospital for therapeutic purposes. I. Newer dimensions of patient care, New York: Russell Sage Foundation, 1961.
2. Coser, R. L. Life in the ward. E. Lansing: Michigan State University Press, 1962.
3. Field, M. Patients are people. New York: Columbia University Press, 1967.
4. Friedson, E. (Ed.) The hospital in modern society New York: Free Press, 1963.
5. Dichter, E. The hospital–patient relationship. *Modern Hospital* **83** (1954).
6. Kaufman, M. R., Franzblau, A. M., & Kairys, D. The emotional impact of ward rounds. *Journal of Mt. Sinai Hospital* **23**: 782–803 (1956).
7. Romano, J. Patient attitudes and behaviour in ward round teaching. *Journal of the American Medical Association* **117**:664–667 (1941).
8. Linn, L., Kahn, R., Coles, P., Cohen, J., Marshall, D., & Weinstein, E. A. Patterns of behavior disturbance following cataract extraction. *American Journal of Psychiatry* **110**:281–289 (1953).
9. Holland, J., Harris, S., Plumb, M., Tuttolomondo, A., & Yates, J. Psychological aspects of physical barrier isolation. Observation of acute leukemia patients in germ-free units. *Proceedings of the International Congress of Hematology* (1970).
10. McKegney, F. P. The intensive care syndrome. *Connecticut Medicine* **30**:633–636 (1966).
11. Sgroi, S., Holland, J., & Marwit, S. Psychological reactions to catastrophic illness. A comparison of patients treated in an intensive care unit and a medical ward (abstract). *Psychosomatic Medicine* **30**:551–552 (1968).
12. Egerton, N., & Kay, J. H. Psychological disturbances associated with open heart surgery. *British Journal of Psychiatry* **110**:433–439 (1964).
13. Blachly, P. H., & Starr, A. Post-cardiotomy delirium. *American Journal of Psychiatry* **121**:371–375 (1964).
14. Kornfeld, D. S., Zimberg, S., & Malm, J. R. Psychiatric complications of open-heart surgery. *New England Journal of Medicine* **273**:287–282 (1965).
15. Lazarus, H. R., & Hagens, J. H. Prevention of psychosis following open-heart surgery. *American Journal of Psychiatry* **124**:1190–1195 (1968).
16. Heller, S., Frank, K. A., Malm, J. R. et al. Psychiatric complications of open-heart surgery. A re-examination. *New England Journal of Medicine* **283**:1015–1019 (1970).

17. Cheek, D. S. Unconscious perception of meaningful sounds during surgical anesthesia as revealed under hypnosis. *American Journal of Clinical Hypnosis* **1**:101 (1959).

18. Levinson, B. W. States of awareness during general anesthesia. *British Journal of Anaesthesia* **37**:544 (1965).

19. Winkelstein, C., Blacher, R., & Meyer, B. Psychiatric observations on surgical patients in recovery room. *New York State Journal of Medicine* **65**:865–870 (1965).

17

Cancer, Emotions, and Nurses

SAMUEL C. KLAGSBRUN

The small cancer research unit in a major East Coast university hospital was unique in many ways. It was tucked away in a corner off a main corridor and was screened in by a glass partition that architecturally demonstrated its separateness. It was the only service to which no house staff was assigned. It was funded in a different way from all the other services. And it was the only service in the hospital that had little hope for success in its struggle to ward off death.

The patient population was selected for research purposes. If a patient experienced a remission, he was discharged to the outpatient clinic and followed by the same medical and nursing staff that worked on the inpatient unit. The entire staff got to know the patients, their families, and their friends on an intimate basis.

The psychiatric consultation service of the hospital had been called in from time to time by the cancer research unit to help in the management of difficult patients. We became aware of the tremendous strain the patients placed on the medical and nursing staff. To a great extent the staff saw these patients as walking dead; and since "one should not speak ill of the dead," the staff felt constrained to keep their feelings about the patients to themselves.

But the angry feelings—and guilt at having those feelings—did

SAMUEL KLAGSBRUN, M.D. • Assistant Clinical Professor, College of Physicians and Surgeons, Columbia University; Attending Psychiatrist, St. Luke's Hospital, New York, New York.

Reprinted from *American Journal of Psychiatry,* 1970, **126,** 1237–1244. Copyright 1970, the American Psychiatric Association.

exist and were very evident in the approach of the staff toward the patients. There was covert rejection of the patients' emotional needs, especially in the face of terminal illness. Numerous struggles between patients and staff took place over such medical issues as the side effects of some of the experimental drugs being used. The patients complained of being used as guinea pigs. "Uncaring doctors" and "unavailable nurses" were phrases that were often repeated to anyone who would listen.

This was the setting, then, in which the following pilot project was attempted.

The psychiatric consultation service assigned me to work as the cancer unit's own psychiatrist in an attempt to analyze and develop a workable approach to the problem of patient management on a cancer unit. I decided that the best approach was to try to alter the ward culture as a whole rather than to deal separately with each patient management problem. The assumption was that the patients' morale and behavior could be improved greatly if they could continue to see themselves as functioning and productive human beings. Meeting these goals would require the creation of an antiregressive atmosphere. And the creation of such an atmosphere would depend largely on the nursing staff. The nurses spent much more time with the patients than anyone else; therefore, their impact was likely to be more pervasive than anyone else's influence on the patients.

Meetings with the Nurses

My first job was to make the nurses aware of the importance of their role. After receiving clearance from the medical staff, I began to hold weekly meetings with the nursing staff. The initial object of the one-hour-a-week meeting was to discuss patient management problems. No hint or suggestion was made to indicate that the ultimate object was to deal with the ward culture or with the nursing staff's feelings toward the patients. The reaction of the staff to the appearance of a psychiatrist in their midst was a mixed one. They were gratified to have this effort made on their behalf by a medical service of the hospital, but they also felt self-conscious and somewhat threatened. An initiation phase began. Problems of an emotional nature were not brought up at all. Instead, matters pertaining to drug dosage, organic illness, or the care of weeping sores on the buttocks of patients sent in from other units rose to the surface. My medical competence was thoroughly tested during this period, and only when it became obvious that I was comfortable as well as interested in these aspects of a patient's care were the nurses willing to accept me as a member of the staff.

The head nurse, an extremely competent and perceptive person, broke the ice one day by saying, "Now look, ladies, this is a psychiatrist. Why don't we tell him things he's supposed to know about?"

With that, a flood of feelings began to come out. Many of these were directed not toward the patients, as might have been expected, but toward the medical staff in charge of the unit. What the nurses complained about most bitterly was the lack of emotional backing by the medical staff, rather than the demands of the patients or the depressing nature of their work.

The following incident exemplified their feelings: A middle-aged woman, well known to the staff, had died a few days prior to our weekly meeting, and the mood of the unit was still low. The nurses spoke of their sense of despair and frustration. At one point, a member of the staff turned toward a large, bulky brown bag sitting on the floor in the corner of our room. "Those are her clothes," she said. "I haven't called the family to pick them up."

"This patient was different," another nurse said. "She tried so hard. She was always cheerful, and when she was sent home last time to continue her treatment in the clinic she was so happy."

"And yet other patients have gone through the same thing." I commented. "There must be something different about her."

"It's the way we feel about what the doctors did on the night she died. We saw she was going, and we called the family in to be with her. We also notified the doctor on call, who knew there was nothing he could do. We had earlier decided not to use any heroic measures since there was no way for her to continue her life. The doctor said that we should help the family accept the inevitable and to let him know when she had died. That was it. I was so angry at his coldness I could have cried. But what can you do? I had to control myself because the family was there and there were other patients to take care of."

"What happened when she died?" I asked.

"The family kept asking, 'Is the doctor coming?' It was terrible. I told them that he had left all the necessary orders, but they kept on asking when he would be coming. Finally, they left after she died. We all cried and they thanked us for what we had done. We felt terrible."

"And the clothes?"

"I guess we just don't want to face them. . . . The doctors never come in when there's a situation like this. It's as though the research drug is the most important thing. If it can't be used anymore, they just lose interest. Oh, I guess that's not true, but it's not fair for them to leave this stuff to us to handle."

The meeting continued and cooled down as the nurses spoke up, with less and less anger being directed at the doctors. Finally, at the end, one of the nurses volunteered to call the family to pick up the brown bag of clothes.

The following week the nurses seemed more guarded and distant, as though they had revealed too much in the previous session. In order to let them deal with their feelings about their doctors with some degree of safety and distance, I decided to use another hospital setting as an example of the problem they had raised. I described a meeting the psychiatric consultation service had held with the surgical, medical, social service, and psychiatric staff of a major hospital devoted exclusively to cancer research. We were interested in exploring the emotional effects of some of their radical work on cancer patients. The medical staff had been placing patients in "life islands" for the purpose of keeping them in a sterile atmosphere during periods of low white counts while they were under antimetabolite treatment. They hoped thereby to prevent infections. These patients lived for weeks in a plastic bubble with ultraviolet light shining constantly. The hospital had also been doing hemicorporectomies on patients in the hope of eliminating extension of the disease. In response to some of our questions, one surgeon had summed up his feelings very clearly when he said, "If I thought about what I was doing to a person, I couldn't do it. But I don't think that that is my job."

I asked the nurses for their reaction. After talking about how gruesome they thought these research procedures were, they moved on to discuss the purpose of the procedures. Finally they came around to appreciating the truth and honesty of the surgeon's remarks. As one nurse put it, "If our doctors had to worry about all the nausea and vomiting a drug caused, they probably would feel terrible about prescribing it. I guess that puts us right in the middle. We'll have to handle the patients."

"They give the drug and we stand there with the emesis basin," another added.

Recognition of Doctors' Feelings

What emerged from that meeting was a much clearer recognition and understanding of the doctors' need for distance as well as the nurses' own central role in the care of the patient. The exciting part of the meeting was that for the first time the nurses seemed able to accept the emotional burden of the patients without expecting to be supported by the doctors. What was left unsaid was that, given the backing of a psychiatrist, they were able to free their doctors from answering their needs and thereby allow the doctors to spend more time in the labs.

Once the nurses' role was clarified, they began to look at their patients in a more critical way. They became less frightened of being put upon and therefore more open to learning. The methods patients used to express their needs were recognized more quickly. Management problems were analyzed from the point of view of "What is the patient really asking for?" The nurses became sophisticated in recognizing subterfuges for the expression of anxiety. The number of complaints—calling for nurses, turning of nighttime into daytime, repeated questions about what is really in the I.V. bottle—all these were now understood as expressions of fear, and the nurses became quite free in calling the shots as they saw them.

"Let's talk, Mrs. Jones. You really don't need the bedpan again, do you?"

"I know you didn't call, Mr. Brown, but you look sad. Anything I can do?"

The nurses were encouraged to seek out contact before the patients created a crisis situation that required their presence. They now understood that symptoms were often communications on a nonverbal level. In addition, my willingness to use more tranquilizers and antidepressants gave them a sense of confidence. They knew that methods of control were readily available in case of severe agitation and depression

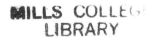

that they felt unable to handle. They experienced a marvelous new sense of freedom and openness. "When I told Mr. Smith that if I were in his shoes, I'd be asking many more questions than he was asking," reported one nurse, "I could actually see the tension coming out of his face."

This free and easy approach, however, soon led to complications. Patients were now communicating their worries to the nurses, and many of them asked fairly direct questions about their prognoses. The nurses felt comfortable in talking openly to the patients about anxiety or depression, but they felt they were overstepping their boundaries when patients started asking them about diagnoses, prognoses, and medications. The most frequent question raised was what to tell the patient in response to the question, "Am I going to die?"

The experienced nurses, who really understood their patients and the patients' families, could judge what answer was expected of them.

One example was that of a husband who had refused to bring his sick wife to the hospital because he was sure that the staff would tell her her diagnosis, and he was convinced that she would not be able to tolerate the truth. His wife, on the other hand, asked the nurses not to tell the husband that she had cancer because she was sure he needed to protect her from the truth, since that helped his manly image. But she also knew he would probably be unable to keep it to himself and would feel terrible if he blurted it out to her. She was trying to protect him. The nurses had no difficulty in refraining from talking to him about her illness while listening and talking to the patient about how she was doing.

A second example of courage coupled with wisdom was one reported by a nurse the day after a sad experience. An old woman who was failing rapidly called in one of the nurses and said simply, "I am dying. I feel it is the end, isn't it?" The nurse looked at her and said quietly, "Yes." The nurse sat down next to the old woman, took her hand and held it. "I don't want to die alone," the woman said. "I'll stay with you. You won't be alone," the nurse answered. The woman said, "That's good." And she died in ten minutes, with the nurse holding her hand.

As the nurses got to know their patients better, they realized that the patients were not dead yet and that even those who seemed to see themselves as dead could emerge from the grave in response to crises in their families or to important external events.

Experiment in Self-Care

Now everybody was ready for the next step: a radical experiment in self-care. Many of the patients who were in bed did not really need to be there for medical reasons; they simply retired to their beds as part of their withdrawal. The nurses had come to understand that. They began reorganizing the unit. They urged patients to take passes and to leave the ward. They made demands on the patients by asking them to get involved in such projects as sewing and art work. As much as they could, they pushed the patients into activity.

The patients' reaction to the new hustle-bustle varied. Those patients who saw themselves as terminally ill at first resented the expectation that they could take care of themselves. They saw it as further evidence that they were being abandoned by the world. On the other hand, those who found themselves grasping for any bit of evidence that proved they were not sick—or at least not dying—quickly latched on to the new idea that they were still responsible, functioning, and productive people. This group, in fact, began edging the nurses out of jobs and taking over some of the nursing tasks.

For example, one of the first changes made in the ward was to have the patients fix their own beds. Next they were to get their own water and ice. The nurses were a bit fearful of this revolutionary step, and they were upset when the sick patients saw it as a rejection of their needs. But the patient-activists on the ward surprised everybody. They began taking the water and ice to the patients who were too sick to care for their own needs. Then they took over the linen closet and made up beds for the very sick patients. They began eyeing the desk jobs. They wanted to answer the phone and type the admission forms. Finally, they took over the responsibility of running errands to other parts of the hospital. The "revolution" reached the point where the nurses were able to have each new admission oriented to the ward by a welcoming group of older patients.

The ward acquired a new culture. As the weeks went on, the activists took over the ward, and it was quite common to see a patient get up in the morning with an I.V. drip going into one arm, make his bed with the other, then carry trays of food to the bedridden and explain the new system to the practical nurses who were occasionally assigned to the ward.

The most important step taken, however, was the communal dining room. We decided that providing a nucleus for socialization would add to the atmosphere of liveliness and stimulate the patients further. The dieticians, who took part in all our meetings, arranged for food trays to be brought to a separate room where the patients would gather to eat. This was a major breakthrough that allowed lonely and isolated patients to talk to fellow patients. Now the patients discovered new communal strength that came from shared experience. Patients began organizing evening activities, with the inevitable showing of slides of the latest European trip. Afternoon snacks were delivered to the dining area, and an accumulation of puzzles, cards, and books found its way there. Life was suddenly being lived.

As the experience continued, some of the patients who had had remissions and had gone home began coming back when their illnesses progressed. A common reaction was a sense of relief at returning to a culture that treated them as though something was still expected of them. Some patients had visibly regressed at home, but under the competitive spirit of the ward they too returned to greater activity. Their demands for nursing attention diminished, and they appeared happier.

The self-care atmosphere periodically broke down in the face of actual death and the overwhelming illness of patients, and the nurses learned that in order to maintain this culture they had to nourish and support it. A change in the patient population had to be countered with a renewed nursing effort to teach the new admissions about the ward culture. If the old-time patients of the ward outnumbered the new ones, the culture was protected. Otherwise the authority of the nurses had to be brought into play to back self-care until the new patients could be acculturated.

Effect on Medical Staff

The impact on the medical staff of the changing culture was interesting. In the beginning they continued to maintain their distance from the patients. But as the ward atmosphere changed more and more, they began asking about the new regulations being instituted. The influence of the ward upon the medical staff was felt to be complete when one of the nurses reported the newest order she had received. The doctor had written, "Patient must each lunch in communal dining room." The doctor explained that he had noticed that the patient was slipping into a depression and was beginning to regress. He felt that a medical order pushing her into the ward atmosphere would be helpful. This gave us a clue to something we had not been aware of before— namely, that the medical staff had not necessarily ignored the emotional aspects of patient care; they had simply felt they had little to offer. Once it became obvious that there was something that could be done, they turned to it as much as everyone else did.

The increased level of activity of the patients as well as the high level of psychological sophistication of the nursing staff were proven beyond a shadow of a doubt in one incident. A 39-year-old man with cancer had been admitted, and his sexy young wife was a constant visitor. He caught on to the spirit of self-care to such an extent that he decided that he was going to live as normally as possible while he had to be on the unit. The nurse who barged in and found him in bed one day with his wife walked out without another word. At our next meeting, after the giggling died down, the nurses discussed the man's need for denial. They had some serious doubts about whether to forbid this unusual activity on the unit. The final consensus was that it was too much of a radical departure for the ward to handle, and they should not allow it to continue. The fact that they saw it first in terms of patient need and second in terms of ward management showed that the conversion had been accomplished.

In a summary session that was taped, the staff reviewed the history of the experiment after 18 months. The unanimous conclusion was that the changes in the ward were of major importance to the patients. The nurses spoke of the increased will to live that they had noted. They pointed out that patient care was more efficient. And most of all, from an administrative point of view they realized that the turnover rate of nurses, which had been very high, had decreased markedly. Now nurses wanted to work on the unit.

What are the psychological implications of this experience? Certainly the work of some of the investigators reported[1,3-6] shows some correlation between the onset of cancer and the experience of an emotional loss. The implication that such a connection exists in the onset of illness suggests that its remission, or at least its management, may be equally influenced by emotional factors of a positive nature. The effect of a positive ward culture must therefore be considered worthy of research.

Aside from considering the course of the illness, we can think about the quality of life that the patient lives. Palliation need not only be thought of in terms of physical pain; it can also be seen as a legitimate goal to achieve on an emotional level. The response of the patients to the idea that they were expected to function on an adult level decreased their anxiety, dependency, and feelings of being a burden and thereby added to their well-being. The quality of their remaining life was improved.

One of the reactions we frequently see in sick patients is that of shrinking horizons over a period of time. The patient loses interest in the world outside the hospital, then in the life affairs of friends and family, and finally in the ward. At the end, he becomes focused on his own life functions. Maintaining his interest in the surrounding world as long as possible and making him feel responsible for it retards this process and keeps him feeling fulfilled for a longer time.

Conclusion

This clinical report suggests an approach quite different from that implied by Kurt Eissler in his famous book.[2] Eissler encouraged the patient's defense mechanism of denial by allowing the patient to imbue his therapist with magical qualities. The therapist enhanced this image by showing concern, bringing gifts, and behaving in a protective way toward the patient. The method implied was "I will take care of you." In contrast, the experience of our cancer unit led us to feel that we could successfully support a patient's denial by using an antiregressive approach.

It might be valuable to test these different approaches in a research project. We certainly do not have the complete answer yet. Our experience indicated that many of our patients did well clinically in the atmosphere we had created. However, I am not convinced that this approach works well during the period just before death. This period is still an unknown entity from a psychological point of view.

There were two main "make-or-break" points in our pilot project when things could have gone very differently from the way they did. The first took place at the initial meeting with the nurses. By focusing the goals of this meeting on patient management rather than anything more radical, I made the road easier for myself. The nurses were able to get to know me without feeling threatened. I could then suggest more significant changes, knowing that I had a comfortable relationship with the staff.

The second point occurred when the nurses decided that they were ready to take a chance and run the ward differently. Without making a major issue of it, I spoke to the medical staff individually and encouraged them to show interest in and appreciation for the project. I pointed out that the more responsible the nurses were made to feel in their involvement with the ward, the less they would burden the medical staff with minor problems. As it turned out, the medical staff became fascinated with the project and invited us to report on it at one of their scientific research conferences.

In any attempt to change a ward culture, as we did, a good deal of groundwork with key people on an informal level becomes necessary. We prepared the medical staff and made sure to discuss all changes with the head nurse, the nursing supervisor, the dietician, and the hospital administration.

Finally, I would like to offer one more observation—the importance of sharing. We all realized that our ability to talk about death and cancer with the patients and to bear their needs without closing ourselves off from them grew in direct proportion to our ability to share our own anxieties at our group meetings. The more we talked together, the more easily we could listen to our patients. As a side note, I was able to serve as a sounding board for the patients and the nurses because I was able to unburden myself at psychiatric consultation service rounds. It seems that if the system works, it does so on all levels.

The implications of this project apply to the hospital as a whole. From a financial point of view the program offers the possibility of reducing costs in that patients may need fewer aides. From a personal point of view it suggests greater stability of staff by decreasing turnover rate. And from a humane point of view, if offers dignity.

References

1. Greene, W. A. The psycho-social setting of the development of leukemia and lymphoria. *Annals of the New York Academy of Sciences* **125**:794–801, 1966.
2. Eissler, K. *The psychiatrist and the dying patient.* New York: International Universities Press, 1955.
3. LeShan, L. An emotional life-history pattern associated with neoplastic disease. *Annals of the New York Academy of Sciences* **125**:780–793, 1966.

4.   Muslimm, H. L., Gyarfas, K., & Pieper, W. J. Separation experience and cancer of the breast. *Annals of the New York Academy of Sciences* **125**:802–806, 1966.
5.   Paloucek, F. P., & Graham, J. B. The influence of psycho-social factors on the prognosis of cancer of the cervix. *Annals of the New York Academy of Sciences* **125**:814–816, 1966.
6.   Schmale, A., & Iker, H. The psychological setting of uterine cervical cancer. *Annals of the New York Academy of Sciences* **125**:807–813, 1966.

Discussion

This interesting paper focuses upon a small cancer unit tucked away in a general hospital where patients with cancer were sent for treatment under conditions that for many of them inevitably meant death—either upon their first admission to the unit or a subsequent return to the ward. The author is to be commended for his description of a technique that involves an hour of work on the ward each week by the visiting psychiatrist, with techniques aimed at improving the staff morale so that there is more efficient management of patients and with the patients assuming more responsibility for their physical and emotional care while in this unit.

There are several major areas of discussion that arise from this paper. The first concerns the attitudes of the nurses and focuses also upon the nurse–doctor relationship. It was noted that there was originally high turnover of nurses in this unit and that patients did not seem to receive the best type of care because of the turnover and because of the lowered morale of the nursing staff. The type of specialty ward described in this paper seems to be developing in a number of hospitals in this country: there is a movement away from general wards in which patients with different kinds of diseases are cared for together toward a small unit oriented to a specific disease, such as the unit described in this paper. It is evident that concentrating one kind of patient with serious illness and a high mortality rate on one ward can provoke a major emotional stress in the nurse, for she has no patients with recoverable illness and a more positive prognosis with which to counterbalance the emotional strain occasioned by the gravely ill patient. Often, because of the frustration engendered in this situation, the nurse expects more of the physician than he is able to provide, with resultant discord and frustration occurring in the nurse–doctor relationship.

Problems in the nurse–doctor relationship in this kind of unit have two major elements. In a treatment situation where there is a rotation of house staff to the unit, the long-stay nurse often has more direct experience with the type of care needed on the unit than does the rotating intern. A second frustration can occur because of the increasing preoccupation in some teaching hospitals with care aimed at the molecular or cellular level and not at the level of human experience. The nurse is caught up in a twofold bind by the physician's preoccupation with the discrete rather than the general and by her own inability to motivate the physician to recognize the importance of the patient's more human needs. This is not necessarily the fault of the physician but rather is a reflection on the way in which we reward the house staff with prestige for work at this level. However, this does not help the nurse, who has to spend more time than the physician involved in the daily lives of the patients. Also, the physician's avoidance and withdrawal from the patient care situation can only intensify the nurse's feeling of frustration and isolation.

Another question concerns the way in which we treat our patients. One wonders whether or not patient treatment practices are structured for the convenience of the physician and the nursing staff or rather reflect the most appropriate way in which to care for the patients. We know that patients can respond to what they see as inelegant care by the physician or a noncaring attitude on the part of the hospital staff by assuming a demanding and complaining role in regard to the ward structure. In fact, patients "needle" us to get attention and we often needle them in reprisal. It is always easier to prescribe medication than to give of our time and empathy. With these diverse frustrations and experiences on the unit, Dr. Klagsbrun is to be commended for his techniques of recognizing and then restructuring the ward milieu of these gravely ill patients.

His use of small group techniques in which professionals are invited to discuss how to better manage their patients and the tensions involved both in the intrafamily structure and also their own intrapsychic structure reflects the techniques described in the early 1950s by Balint of London[1] and Watters of New Orleans.[2,3] These techniques can be considered helpful not only in terms of the diminished nurse turnover within the unit but also in the improvement in direct patient care. An additional use of the group technique is as a teaching device to help the staff become more knowledgeable in recognizing and managing emotional illness.

The use of the self-care system by the patients reflects a trend started in geriatric practice and in the self-care system wards of some general hospitals but is different in that these patients were in a unit where many of them were gravely ill.

The techniques described here lend themselves as models to many of the specialized units springing up around the country and offer a way in which the limited psychiatric manpower problem can be eased.

JOHN RECKLESS, M.B., CH.B.
Durham, North Carolina

References

1. Balint, M. *The doctor, his patient and the illness.* New York: International Universities Press, 1957.
2. Watters, T. A. The general practitioner and the third dimension. *Journal of the Medical Association, Georgia* **51:**567–572, 1962.
3. Watters, T. A. Continuing education programs in psychiatry and their evaluation. Boulder, Colorado: Western Interstate Commission for Higher Education, 1964.

18

Coping with Waiting: Psychiatric Intervention and Study in the Waiting Room of a Pediatric Oncology Clinic

IRWIN HOFFMAN and EDWARD H. FUTTERMAN

Medical advances have prolonged the lives and decreased the morbidity of children with fatal malignancies and have made it possible to treat these illnesses primarily on an outpatient basis. For example, children with acute leukemia, who commonly survive 2 or more years from the time of diagnosis under current medical regimens, are likely to visit the outpatient clinic about once a month during remissions and once a week when in relapse or when suffering other complications. Periods of hospitalization lasting from a few days to a few weeks are usually only necessary at the time of diagnosis, in the terminal phase, and a few additional times during the course of the illness. When in remission, a child is often symptom-free and able to carry on normal activities.

Various aspects of the family crisis precipitated by the diagnosis of fatal illness in a child have been studied in recent years.[1-9] Our own

IRWIN HOFFMAN, Ph.D. • Assistant Professor of Psychology, Department of Psychiatry, Abraham Lincoln School of Medicine, University of Illinois, Chicago, Illinois. EDWARD H. FUTTERMAN, M.D. • Associate Professor of Psychiatry, Department of Psychiatry, University of Illnois College of Medicine, Chicago, Illinois.

Reprinted in abridged form from *Comprehensive Psychiatry*, 1971, **12**(1), 67–81, by permission.

investigation, in progress at the University of Illinois Medical Center since 1964, has involved consideration of a number of adaptational issues.[10-13] Data-gathering procedures of this project have included extended interviews with parents and healthy siblings of approximately 23 families with leukemic children. The interviews have been conducted at various points during the child's illness as well as following the child's death. In addition, we have had contact with more than 100 families on an informal basis. We have found that most families mobilize their resources to meet this crisis without signs of gross psychiatric disturbance or family breakdown. On the other hand, adaptational difficulties and emotional disequilibrium and strain have been apparent at one time or another in all of the families we have encountered. In the course of our work, we have attempted to develop modes of crisis intervention[14-16] to help families cope with the adaptational tasks posed by the child's fatal illness. Effective programs for psychological care of the inpatient fatally ill child and his family have been reported.[4-7] The hospital clinic waiting room offers unique opportunities for the development of complementary outpatient programs.

In addition to being a place where regular and consistent contact with families can easily be established, the outpatient waiting room also brings a number of psychological issues to the fore. Many aspects of the adaptational crisis precipitated by the diagnosis of fatal illness in a child are encapsulated in the experience of waiting for medical care. Because of the prognosis of death, the visit to the clinic, in addition to being an assertion of mastery and hope, also activates painful feelings such as grief, anger, guilt, helplessness, fear, and despair. The physician, due to limitations of time as well as certain peculiarities of his professional role, is hampered in his ability to help family members deal with many of their emotional reactions to the child's illness. In this connection, mental health workers have an important contribution to make to the comprehensive care of the patient and his family.

In the summer of 1968, a waiting room intervention program was initiated at the University of Illinois Medical Center under the joint sponsorship of the Departments of Pediatrics, Psychiatry, Occupational Therapy, and Medical Social Work. The program was designed to help families deal with adaptational tasks as they arose in the waiting room by creating a milieu conducive to active and expressive coping. The purpose of this paper is to describe this program and some of its practical and theoretical implications.

The Intervention: Setting and Approach

The Setting

The Pediatric Oncology Outpatient Clinic at the University of Illinois Medical Center is conducted one morning each week from 9:00 a.m. to 12:00 p.m. There is a sign on the wall off the waiting room reading "Tumor Clinic." The patients are children under the age of 16 who have various types of malignancies. Although some of the children have arrested tumors and normal life expectancies, most are afflicted with illnesses likely to lead to death during childhood. Leukemia, which is the main focus of our work, is the predominant diagnosis. One or both parents, and occasionally siblings, other relatives, or friends, accompany the children to the clinic. About 10–15 children are treated each week. The population, consisting predominantly of white, lower-middle class, Catholic, suburban residents, changes considerably from one week to the next because of varying appointment schedules, terminations, and new patients. All patients are asked to arrive by 9:30 a.m. for weighing and laboratory tests. The period of waiting to see the physician and for the results of tests and procedures ranges from ½ hour to 2 hours.

The clinic generally carries a load of about 40–50 cases shared by four or five physicians, usually Fellows in Hematology. While the Department of Pediatrics attempts to provide continuity of patient care, there is usually a turnover whenever a Fellow completes his post-residency 2-year training program.

The Preintervention Milieu

At the invitation of the Department of Pediatrics, the waiting room and clinic were observed by one of the authors for a period of 6 months prior to the introduction of the intervention program. During this time, a number of behavior patterns became apparent and certain general impressions emerged. People in the waiting room were usually silent and immobile, and the atmosphere often seemed tense and depressed. There was little or no activity or play on the part of the children, who often cried and screamed during the medical procedures, but appeared sullen and tight-lipped before and after their appointments. Parents and children rarely separated, and there was little interaction either among the children or among the parents. Occasionally, parents alluded to the strain caused by the long waiting time, the traveling, the buildup of tension within the child during the week preceding the appointment, resistive or uncooperative behavior on the part of the child with respect to clinic attendance and other unpleasant factors surrounding the clinic visit. Exploratory individual play sessions with the children were characterized by the same sense of tension and constraint that permeated the waiting room. On the whole, the atmosphere was similar to the description by Bozeman et al.[2] of a comparable setting. Among their many observations, these authors noted that "clinic days were disliked by the children as well as by the mothers," and that "there was a conspicuous absence of play or interaction among the children, [who] remained close to their mothers in this feared and disliked situation."

The Intervention Approach

We viewed the preintervention milieu of the waiting room as one in which active coping with adaptational tasks was inhibited. Parents and children seemed locked into patterns of passivity, noncommunication, and social isolation. Feelings were being handled internally, without social support, without avenues for release of tension, and without opportunities for exercising control over the situation. We sought to develop a milieu conducive to more expressive, varied, and integrated coping behavior. The intervention was designed to facilitate coping with the clinic experience itself. However, the representatives of issues raised in the clinic waiting room along with the opportunity for regular and consistent contact with the families gave reason to hope that the program would have a more general therapeutic influence upon family coping.

Specifically, the objectives of the waiting room intervention were oriented around the adaptational tasks described earlier. Briefly summarized, the goals of the program were: (1) to facilitate the work of mourning the prospective loss of the child, i.e., anticipatory mourning; (2) to help family members to maintain a sense of mastery and to deal with the emotional constellation of helplessness, guilt, and anger; (3) to help the child cope with injuries to his self-image, sense of worth, and sense of trust and to reinforce the continuity and integrity of his identity; (4) to reinforce the integrity and cohesiveness of the family and the openness of interaction among family members.

To achieve these goals, one of the authors (I.H., previously the observer) along with an occupational therapist entered the situation on an active basis. Around a central focus of a play program for the children, these therapists defined their roles in terms of active availability to both children and parents. Other than a brief introductory letter and a questionnaire providing identifying information on the families, there were no formalities. While respecting the wish for privacy or solitude, an attempt was made to be accessible for communication with all family members. In addition, the therapists worked to facilitate interaction among families in the waiting room in order to develop a supportive and communicative group atmosphere.*

Coping in the Postintervention Milieu

In contrast to the oppressive rigidity observed in the waiting room prior to the intervention program, the new milieu came alive with activity, and a wide range of coping patterns emerged. Behavior in the postintervention milieu seems to vary as a function of a number of variables including the sick child's age, the child's physical condition, passage of time since diagnosis, and personality characteristics of family members. The main purpose of this paper, however, is to survey the range of coping responses to adaptational tasks in the postintervention milieu rather than to establish the underlying sources of variation.

The Task of Anticipatory Mourning

As stated earlier, family members have the task of mourning the prospective loss of the sick child while continuing to care for his physical and emotional needs. One way in which this dilemma often becomes manifest is in increased conflict and anxiety about day-to-day separations between parents and children.[10] In the new waiting room milieu, children and their parents are encouraged to deal more openly with their feelings about separation. Families respond in a wide variety of ways to the option of separation with which they are confronted by the play group. Often, children participate in the group while their parents

* Since this paper was submitted, a parent group program has been initiated in the outpatient clinic which affords parents the option of still more intensive sharing and exploring of concerns.

take the opportunity to "get away" and talk privately with other parents or with a therapist about concerns they conceal in the presence of the child. Given this opportunity, parents have verbalized many feelings associated with the work of anticipatory mourning, ranging from mixed shock, grief, and disbelief near the time of diagnosis to resignation near the terminal phase. We have found that even parents who initially seem withdrawn and inaccessible often respond to mild encouragement from the therapists by sharing openly their anticipatory mourning reactions. Meanwhile, the child is helped to assert his individuality and to deal with feelings that he suppresses in his parents' presence.

On the other hand, avoidance of separation between parents and children is also an aspect of anticipatory mourning. Clinging can have meaning as part of the magical struggle against death and death wishes at the same time that it represents a phase in the process of coming to terms with anticipated loss. Clinging to the image of the lost object is generally regarded as normal in the early stages of mourning if it gradually gives way to object decathexis.[17-24] Similarily, in the context of anticipatory mourning, temporary regressive, mutual clinging may be part of an overall successful adaptation.[10] In the waiting room, such clinging is the norm whenever there is a deterioration in the child's medical status, whether or not this setback is clinically manifest. At these times, children typically do not participate in the play program and parents are less socially responsive than usual. Nevertheless, even in this situation, the therapists have been able to help family members articulate the feelings motivating their behavior and their choice of coping strategy. This often helps to facilitate a flexible and realistic response to changing circumstances. Thus, as the child's physical condition improves, clinging can be gradually relinquished and behavior patterns fostering the continued growth and individuation of the child can be reestablished.

Another form of anticipatory mourning facilitated in the new milieu is that of participation and involvement on part of parents in the distress of other families. Parents interact much more with each other and with each other's children than they did prior to the waiting room program. It is common for parents to become attached to other parents' children, to psychologically "adopt" them, and subsequently to mourn their deaths. In some instances we have heard quite intense grief reactions to the news that a child, even when known only at a distance, has died. By mourning the loss of another child, a parent may further the work of mourning his own, indirectly, and at a level he can more easily endure.

Parents also involve themselves in the distress of other families by giving each other social and emotional support. One mother remarked, "I think Mrs. A looks tearful. She must have had some bad news today. I remember when I had bad news that I cried and everyone left me alone. I'm going over and talk with her." In supporting another mother, this parent takes a step toward coming to terms with the anticipated death of her own child. Assisting others can also help parents compensate for their feelings of inefficacy in relation to the fatal illness itself.

Greene[25] has termed processes by which the bereaved become concerned with the pain of other mourners "proxy mechanisms." He notes that while these mechanisms can assume pathological dimensions, they may also have a place in the normal work of mourning:

> That the mechanisms seen in melancholia or hypochondriasis or the proxy mechanisms described here are pathologic is evident when they assume exclusive proportions in time and quality. I consider the possibility that all three of these kinds of mechanisms may be included in successful grief work.[25]

Proxy mechanisms can be particularly adaptive in *anticipatory* mourning when the sense of helplessness arising out of inability to rescue the dying child can be so acute and the need to do "something useful" so great.

Anticipatory mourning has also been evident in the waiting room in the attempt by parents to persuade others to invest in and to appreciate their own children. In this way parents forge "anticipatory mourning alliances" with other parents or with the therapist. For example, one woman often spoke with pride of her daughter's abilities and achievements and on a number of occasions brought in samples of art work that the child had produced in school. It seemed important to her to have the therapists share her own affection for her child and, perhaps, her rage that so young a person with so much worth and potential should have to die. While on one level this mother may have been pleading the case for a reprieve for her child, on another level she seemed to be asking the therapists to share her experience of loss, including the burdens of guilt and rage that it entailed.

The processes of psychological adoption and of building alliances can complement or reinforce each other. This is the case whenever a parent seeks to "adopt" a child whose own parent is in the process of reaching out to have someone share the burden of her parental role.

While we have focused upon adaptive responses to the task of anticipatory mourning, in rare instances the mechanisms described have appeared to take on a rigid, exclusive, or inappropriate quality. For example, anxious clinging between a sick child and his parent has occasionally persisted during long periods of symptom-free medical remissions. Even more rarely, parents have ventilated anticipatory mourning reactions, including feelings of disgust or despair regarding the child's illness, with apparent insensitivity to the feelings of children or of the other parents in the area. The diagnostic and prognostic import of behaviors observed in the waiting room in regard to the success of a family's overall adaptation to the child's fatal illness requires further investigation.

The Task of Maintaining a Sense of Mastery

The child's illness is a severe challenge to a parent's sense of mastery and worth. Unlike some serious illnesses such as hemophilia[26] or diabetes,[27] leukemia requires little active participation by parents either in day-to-day preventive strategies or in the actual performance of treatment procedures. Instead, responsibility for medical management is delegated almost entirely to the physician. In this connection one mother commented bitterly, "There is nothing for us to do but wait," and a father, expressing a common reaction, remarked, "The worst thing about this is feeling so useless." In the new milieu parents have been encouraged to share with each other or with the therapists the feelings of helplessness, guilt, and anger that the child's illness inevitably provokes.

Complaints about inconveniences associated with clinic visits, lack of parking space, the long wait, brusque treatment from clerical personnel, and the like, while they may be common in public clinics, function in this particular setting to help parents to dissipate some of their indignation at being unjustly victimized and afflicted. To the extent that immediate conditions are real and correctable, the therapists have acted as practical advisers and consultants. To the extent that these conditions have been representative of deeper frustration and rage about the child's fatal condition, the therapists have supported parents in their attempt to come to grips with these underlying feelings.

Negative or critical reactions to the physician or to medical care are particularly difficult for parents to express because of their extraordinary dependency upon the doctor. Sometimes, however, the doctor has become the focus of angry feelings. One woman, for example, threatened, "If he doesn't tell me what these headaches my son is having are from, and doesn't do anything about them, I'm gonna find me another doctor." In this case, the therapist arranged a three-way conference in which a social worker, who had been working with this mother, served as a mediator, helping to bridge the communication gap that had developed in the parent–doctor relationship. The mother's confidence that the doctor knew what he was doing and that both he and she were indeed doing everything possible was restored. On another occasion, a mother reported angrily that she and her husband felt that her son was being kept alive as a "research guinea pig" and that her husband "was gonna call and give the doctor hell." After the death of the child, the pediatrician reported that the father was calling her every night to harangue her for the hospital's alleged medical mismanagement of the case and liability for the child's death. A meeting of parents, physician, and therapist was then arranged. The pediatrician and therapist were able to acknowledge legitimate complaints while providing reassurance that the child could not, in fact, have been saved. As the session progressed, the parents' anger subsided, and they began to share their intense grief reactions to the loss itself.

Another means by which parents restore some sense of mastery over the situation is through active information-seeking regarding the illnesses of other children and the ways in which other parents are coping.[2,5] In the waiting room, parents sometimes talk among themselves about the medical condition of their children and the treatment that is being received. The exchange of such information is often threatening. It can arouse anxiety about the future course of the illness, as well as uncomfortable competition among the parents. On the other hand, knowledge can also be reassuring, particularly when reality is less frightening than a parent's fantasies of what the future will bring. More common, however, than discussion of medical issues per se is conversation about problems of child rearing. Parents consult with each other and with the therapists about such matters as the tendency to indulge the sick child, ways of dealing with his anxieties, and the problem of ensuring proper care of healthy siblings. All of these efforts at intellectual mastery help parents combat their sense of helplessness to control the course of the illness and to save the child.

The Child's Task of Maintaining the Continuity and Integrity of His Identity

The play group offers the child a means of counteracting the assault of the fatal illness upon the integrity of his self-image. The dangers are immediate and intense in the waiting room, where there is an increased focus upon the child's illness, and where separation anxiety (in particular, in relation to the prospect of hospitalization) and mutilation anxiety (in response to medical procedures) are high. In this situation, the child is prone to withdraw into passivity and to be overcome with a sense of sickness and vulnerability. Play activity, in itself, can help the child to reaffirm his identity as a living and functioning person, with many varied feelings and capacities. This not only helps to restore the child's self-image, but also reminds the significant adults in his life that he is still very much alive.

The child must affirm his identity in the face of the continual life interruptions and painful experiences that accompany his illness. Through play as well as by direct communication, children have been helped to express and master specific anxieties associated with their illness and treatment. The focus of these anxieties has been shown to vary in accord with the developmental level of the child, with separation anxiety predominating in preschool children, mutilation anxiety in latency-age children, and death anxiety in adolescents.[3] How each of these has been manifested in the waiting room is briefly illustrated and discussed below.

Separation Anxiety. The therapists have provided direct support to children coping with brief separations from their parents in the waiting room. They have also been able to reduce some of the anxiety associated with hospitalization by making follow-up visits to children on the wards.

Themes of separation, estrangement, and loss are common in the children's play. One boy with leukemia who had become quite bloated as a result of medication told a story about a kitten who left home and wandered about lost for years. When his parents finally encountered him, they did not recognize him because he had become so enormous. Sometimes conflicts about separation are acted out among the children. For example, while one child imitated his mother's protectiveness of him by adamantly insisting that a sick rabbit puppet stay home, other children argued that the rabbit was better and could go outside. In general, feelings of loss and loneliness are commonly projected onto dolls and puppets who have been "put in the hospital" or otherwise separated from parents or home.

Mutilation Anxiety. Doctor play is frequently utilized by children as an effort to master anxiety associated with treatment procedures. What may start as a gentle needling with a toy syringe often develops into a violent series of injections. The needle changes from a mechanism for healing to a weapon with which to mutilate or destroy. Often the child who has been most quiet and reserved becomes the most ferocious shot-giver, betraying his underlying fear and rage. Such "identification with the aggressor" mechanisms help the child release anger that he might otherwise turn against himself. Another route to mastery involves playing the patient role bravely as the dreaded procedure is reenacted. Alternatively, the role of doctor as healer may be played out. In each case the play functions to help heal the psychological wounds associated with the feeling of being forced into a position of helpless victim subjected to painful procedures for reasons often unknown or unclear to the child.

Death Anxiety. While themes of separation, estrangement, and mutilation have been quite common in the children's play, explicit themes of death and dying have been less prevalent. Occasionally they have arisen in the course of doctor or puppet play. However, when a doll or puppet "dies" the children are usually quick to change the subject. Even older children who could be expected to have developed a concept of death differentiated from separation and mutilation[28] rarely directly communicate fears or concerns about their own deaths. In fact, explicit expressions about death are more frequent in hospitalized children than in the waiting room. Whether this is related to the immediacy of the threat during hospitalization or to the inhibition of the child's communication in the presence of his parents is not clear. From other aspects of our study, including interviews with siblings of the sick child conducted prior to our involvement in the waiting room, we have reason to believe that the children have greater awareness of the nature of their illness than what is ascribed to them by their parents. In this connection, we have beem impressed by the readiness of some parents to talk about various aspects of the illness, including indirect references to its gloomy prognosis, while apparently denying that children in hearing range can understand anything that is being said.[13] We suspect that the failure of the child to communicate concerns about death and dying is more related to taboos upon this subject, in the culture and in the family, than to lack of awareness on the part of the children.[29,30] We are continuing to explore this issue in the waiting room as well as in separate groups where the children are given an opportunity to express themselves in their parents' absence.

The Task of Maintaining Family Integrity

The intervention program has often had direct or indirect impact upon the quality of interaction among family members in the waiting room. For example, instead of silent tension in the interaction of parents and children preceding and following medical procedures, family members have been encouraged to actively play out their feelings. Children, supplied with a variety of toy medical equipment, can demonstrate "what happened in the doctor's office." Parents welcome the opportunity to play patient. This is consistent with a feeling many parents have expressed to the therapists that they often wish they could take their children's places. In addition to its guilt-relieving function, the interaction allows the parents to release some angry feelings toward the child by mimicking his whining and crying while the child does to his parents what was done to him. In effect, depressed clinging, with its underlying guilt and mutual hostility, is transformed into overt, expressive interaction. Often, the acute sense of depression is relieved as the anger of both children and parents is externalized.

The following vignette consolidates a number of adaptational tasks and coping processes we have described. It concerns observations, in the waiting room, of a healthy 13-year-old sibling of a terminally ill child, but it has general implications for family adaptation to fatal illness:

> Norma sits at the table and begins drawing, tight-lipped and intense. Her brother lies on a cart-bed a short distance away along the wall. The father stands silently by the cart, appearing to be depressed. Norma draws a horse and rider. She tells the therapist of her interest in horseback riding, and then complains bitterly that she can never go anymore because there is no one to take her now that her brother is so ill. She speaks resentfully about how her life has changed and about how her own needs and interests are now secondary or neglected. She continues drawing, demonstrating much artistic talent. Later she is seen propping her work up on her brother's bed, in his line of sight. She returns to the table and remarks, "I gave it to him; a present." She resumes drawing, cutting and pasting with much skill. . . .

Norma utilizes the activity first as a means of escape and relief of the tension of waiting by the side of her dying brother. She then ventilates feelings of resentment which she may not be able to express readily to members of her family. Finally, having indulged her own needs and interests, she expresses the other side of her ambivalence by offering her brother a gift of her own creation, thereby also expiating her guilt.

In the postintervention milieu, escape and relief mechanisms, ventilation of feelings of resentment of the burdens of the illness, and attention to personal needs have all been encouraged in family members in order to help them cope with their ambivalence toward the dying child. Incubation of "selfish" needs and wishes can cause a build-up of guilt and resentment in family members, which, in turn, can result in a greater need for systems of projection and displacement that threaten the cohesiveness of the family as a whole. In the microcosm of the waiting room the therapists have facilitated more open expression, sharing, and acceptance of such inhibited or taboo feelings than had been possible in the preintervention milieu.

Acknowledgments

The authors would like to express special appreciation to Dr. Sabshin, Department of Psychiatry; Dr. Schulman and Dr. Honig, Department of Pediatrics; Miss Wade, O.T.R., and Miss Madigan, O.T.R., Department of Occupational Therapy; Miss Preucil, M.A., and Miss Klein, M.S.W., Department of Medical Social Work, University of Illinois College of Medicine, for their cooperation and assistance in the instrumentation of this project and the preparation of this manuscript.

References

1. Richmond, J. B., & Waisman, H. A. Psychologic aspects of management of children with malignant diseases. *American Journal of Diseases of Children* **89**:42–47, 1955.
2. Bozeman, M. F., Orbach, C. E., & Sutherland, A. M. Psychological impact of cancer and its treatment—Adaptation of mothers to the threatened loss of their children through leukemia. I. *Cancer* **8**:1–19, 1955.
3. Natterson, J. M., & Knudson, A. G. Jr. Observations concerning fear of death in fatally ill children and their mothers. *Psychosomatic Medicine* **22**:456–465, 1960.
4. Knudson, A. G. Jr., & Natterson, J. M. Participation of parents in the hospital care of fatally ill children. *Pediatrics* **26**:482–490, 1960.
5. Friedman, S. B., Chodoff, P., Mason, J. W., & Hamburg, D. A. Behavioral

observations on parents anticipating the death of a child. *Pediatrics* **32**:610–625, 1963.

6. Hamovitch, M. B. *The parent and the fatally ill child.* Los Angeles: Delmar, 1964.

7. Karon, M., & Vernick, J.: An approach to the emotional support of fatally ill children. *Clinical Pediatrics* **7**:274–280, 1968.

8. Oakley, G. P. Jr., & Patterson, R. B. The psychologic management of leukemic children and their families. *Medical Journal of North Carolina* **27**:186–193, 1966.

9. Binger, C. M., Ablin, A. R., Feuerstein, R. C., Kushner, J. H., Zoger, S., & Mikkelsen, C. Childhood leukemia: Emotional impact on patient and family. *New England Journal of Medicine* **280**:414–418, 1969.

10. Futterman, E. H., & Hoffman, I. Transient school phobia in a leukemic child. *Journal of the American Academy of Child Psychiatry* **9**:477–494, 1970.

11. Sabshin, M., Futterman, E. H., & Hoffman, I. Empirical studies of healthy adaptations. Unpublished.

12. Futterman, E. H., Hoffman, I., & Sabshin, M. Parental anticipatory mourning. Unpublished.

13. Futterman, E. H., & Hoffman, I. Shielding from awareness: An aspect of family adaptation to fatal illness in children. *Archives of Thanatology* **2**:23–24, 1970.

14. Lindemann, E. Symptomatology and management of acute grief. *American Journal of Psychiatry* **101**:141–148, 1944.

15. Caplan, G. *Principles of preventive psychiatry.* New York: Grune & Stratton, 1964.

16. Klein, D. C., & Lindemann, E. Preventive intervention in individual and family crisis situations. *In* G. Caplan (Ed.), *Prevention of mental disorders in children: Initial explorations.* New York: Basic Books, 1961.

17. Pollock, G. H. Mourning and adaptation. *International Journal of Psychoanalysis* **42**:341–361, 1961.

18. Gorer, G. *Death, grief, and mourning.* Garden City: Doubleday, 1965.

19. Bakan, D. *Disease, pain and sacrifice.* Chicago: University of Chicago Press, 1968.

20. Rheingold, J. C. *The mother, anxiety, and death: The catastrophic death complex.* Boston: Little Brown, 1967.

21. Freud, A. The role of bodily illness in the mental life of children. *In: Psychoanalytic Study of the Child,* Vol. VI. New York: International Universities Press, 1952. Pp. 69–81.

22. Bergmann, T. *Children in the hospital.* New York: International Universities Press, 1966.

23. Morrissey, J. R. Children's adaptation to fatal illness. *Social Work* **8**:81–88, 1963.

24. Bowlby, J. Processes of mourning. *International Journal of Psychoanalysis* **42**:317–340, 1961.

25. Greene, W. A., Jr. Role of a vicarious object in the adaptation to object loss: 1: Use of a vicarious object as a means of adjustment to separation from a significant person. *Psychosomatic Medicine* **20**:344–350, 1968.

26. Browne, W. J., Mally, M. A., & Kane, R. P. Psychosocial aspects of hemophilia:

A study of twenty-eight hemophilic children and their families. *American Journal of Orthopsychiatry* **30:**730–740, 1960.

27. Geist, H. *The psychologic aspects of diabetes.* Springfield, Illinois: Charles C. Thomas, 1964.

28. Nagy, M. H. The child's view of death. *Journal of General Psychology* **73:**3–27, 1948.

29. Glaser, B., & Strauss, A. L. *Awareness of dying: A study of social interaction.* Chicago: Aldine, 1965.

30. Kübler-Ross, E. *On death and dying.* New York: Macmillan, 1969.

VIII

The Crisis of Treatment: Survival by Machine

In the last two or three decades medical progress has involved more and more reliance on technology and machinery. As with the complex specialized hospital environments discussed in part VII, this progress has created new psychological stresses for patients and their families. In an intensive care unit, for example, a patient must live with an array of machines and accept the fact that his life may depend on them, but he also knows his stay in the ICU will be of short duration. In this section we focus on those who must accept the use of an artificial organ or mechanical device in order to survive, on their adaptation to the loss of a normal bodily function, and on their permanent dependence on a machine as a substitute. With the pace of developments in biomedical engineering and in human transplant methodology (see part IX) the concept of replacing worn-out or diseased human organs is an everyday reality. The emotional, psychological, and social effects of these procedures must be fully understood if patients are to benefit maximally from their use.

One of the earlier developments, and one which immediately created psychological problems, was the colostomy, the creation of an artificial opening in the abdominal wall for the discharge of intestinal material after cancer or ulcerative colitis has necessitated the surgical removal of some or all of the colon or rectum. Given the distaste with which bodily waste products are viewed in our culture and the emphasis on personal hygiene, the loss of bowel control and the possibility of escaping gas, unpleasant odors, or occasional leakage present serious threats to the colostomy (or, similarly, the ileostomy) patient. In addition to anxiety about social embarrassment and even rejection, the patient must deal with a sense of mutilation and an altered and impaired body image.

Druss and his colleagues[3] describe several approaches which patients may take in handling these issues. Some develop obsessive rituals of colostomy care to bolster their sense of control. Other strategies include restriction of activities, reluctance to leave the home, and avoidance of interaction with other people; these help control anxiety but are usually less satisfactory in terms of overall adjustment. A patient's insistence on self-sufficiency in colostomy care is a more positive way in which he can avoid the risk of rejection. Members of local colostomy or ileostomy mutual aid clubs can be a valuable source of encouragement and of practical information, and can also serve as models of successful adjustment with whom patients can identify.[3]

In the years since the first cardiac pacemakers were implanted in 1957 the procedure has become almost routine for medical staff, but for patients it still has a dramatic psychological as well as physiological effect. Unlike the colostomy, the pacemaker actually controls the deficient organ rather than being under the patient's control. Blacher and Basch[1] describe three stages in the adaptation of people to pacemaker implantation. In the preoperative and immediate postoperative period the patient's main concern is death due to the cardiac surgery and fear about having his life depend on a fallible machine. Learning more about how the pacemaker works and denying the risks of serious mishaps are the common ways in which patients handle this initial anxiety. During their convalescence when they are no longer in acute danger of dying, patients tend to become more aware of the pacemaker itself: its effect on physical appearance and its implications for an altered body image. Over the long term most patients resume their activities, master their fears, and integrate the pacemaker into an acceptable self-image.

Our first article is an example of just such a successful adaptive process. Clarissa Williams, a nurse in a coronary care unit, briefly recounts her own experience with a pacemaker and her work with other pacemaker patients. Initially she resisted the idea of a pacemaker implant. She was disturbed by the thought of a mechanical device controlling her heart, especially a device which her own experience as a CCU nurse had shown her was not fail-proof. Although she resumed her usual activities she did not feel she had really accepted the pacemaker; she decided to meet her problem head on by specializing in helping pacemaker patients. To facilitate effective coping she allows patients to ventilate their feelings and fears, she gives them information about how the pacemaker works and about what to expect physically and emotionally, she shares her own experiences with them, and she encourages them to identify with her as an example of the return to full productivity which awaits them.

In the early 1960s the introduction of a permanent arteriovenous shunt made regular hemodialysis possible for patients with chronic renal failure. Unlike a colostomy, which requires a few extra hours for care and maintenance, or a pacemaker, which can almost be ignored between battery changes, chronic hemodialysis necessitates significant changes in life-style and involves major psychological conflicts for many people. The stresses which accompany this life-saving procedure are so numerous that they tax people's coping abilities to the utmost, causing some patients to ask if such a life is worth living.

The problems associated with chronic hemodialysis are of several types. There are practical matters like the financial strain caused by medical bills and reduced income, or the need to change residence to be near a dialysis center. Specific aspects of the treatment often prove troublesome, such as the strict dietary and fluid restrictions or the length of time (20–30 hours a week) needed for dialysis, time which often must be taken away from work or from family activities. The care of the arteriovenous shunt itself is another source of concern for patients because of the ever-present threat of injury or infection and because of its cosmetic effect. In addition, many patients continue to experience a sense of physical deterioration and feel unwell at least some of the time.

In the second article Harry Abram discusses the problems patients have preserving a satisfactory self-image and maintaining interpersonal relationships. These difficulties are generally related to the issue of dependence. Since dialysis is usually prescribed only as a last resort for people with permanent (and terminal) renal failure, most patients have experienced a period of severe, debilitating illness and have had to accept the status of a dependent invalid. Once they are selected for dialysis, patients are expected to resume independence and self-sufficiency outside the treatment settings, and to accept their total dependence on a life-giving machine and the staff who run it, a difficult balance for most people to find. Acknowledgement that their bodies can no longer function normally and must have mechanical assistance to survive requires major adjustment in patients' self-image and can diminish their self-esteem. Abram examines the widespread use of denial to cope with these troublesome issues and the incidence of active and passive suicide among hemodialysis patients.

People respond to problems in a variety of ways, and a broad range of coping mechanisms in addition to denial have been observed among hemodialysis patients. Seeking emotional support from family members or medical staff and turning to religion[6] are two sources of help for patients. Patients and their families who feel hostile toward each other or toward the medical staff often displace these angry feelings onto less guilt-producing or less threatening targets. Similarly, concern about his overall medical condition (over which the patient has little control) is often displaced onto the shunt, which the patient then guards vigilantly.[4] Finally, a number of patients deal with the dependent situation imposed upon them with regressive behavior, giving up some of their adult status and responsibilities (for more on regression and the artificial kidney as a maternal symbol see Viederman[6]).

In the third article Franz Reichsman and Norman Levy describe the stages dialysis patients go through in the course of successful adaptation. In contrast to their initial feelings of depression and resignation about their terminal uremia, the "honeymoon" period, when the dialysis first takes effect and physical improvement becomes noticeable, is a time of euphoria as patients feel reborn and hope for a better future returns. The next stage is often a time of disenchantment and discouragement as patients come to realize that some of their expectations (for example, for a return to their preillness level of well-being or the resumption of a full work schedule) are unrealistic. In the last stage, that of long-term adaptation, patients gradually learn to accept their limitations and the unavoidable fluctuations in their sense of well-being. An important component of this adaptation is settling into a satisfactory work pattern. The medical staff can help by advising on realistic work goals for patients, by giving the support and encouragement needed to achieve them, and by making clear that their approval and assistance are not contingent on a return to full productivity.

Home dialysis has eased some of the problems of hospital or renal center treatment, but it raises some new problems for patients and their helpers. Home dialysis gives the patient a greater sense of competence and control, but it puts a tremendous responsibility on the shoulders of the helper (usually the spouse), who must help hook the patient up to the machine and stand by in case of accidents or emergencies. (See Shambaugh & Kanter[5] for other problems which spouses of dialysis patients experience.) Also, at least in the initial transition period, patients are often bothered by feelings of anxiety and inadequacy. Since home dialysis patients do not receive close or constant supervision by trained medical personnel, careful consideration must be given to the psychological adjustment of the patient and helper, as well as to their practical ability to run the machine (see Brown et al.[2]).

References

1. Blacher, R. S., & Basch, S. H. Psychological aspects of pacemaker implantation. *Archives of General Psychiatry.* 1970, **22**, 319–323.
2. Brown, T. M., Feins, A., Parke, R. C., & Paulus, D. A. Living with long-term home dialysis. *Annals of Internal Medicine,* 1974, **81**, 165–170.
3. Druss, R. G., O'Connor, J. F., & Stern, L. O. Psychologic response to colectomy: II. Adjustment to a permanent colostomy. *Archives of General Psychiatry,* 1969, **20**, 419–427.
4. Kaplan de-Nour, A., Shaltiel, J., & Czaczkes, J. W. Emotional reactions of patients on chronic hemodialysis. *Psychosomatic Medicine,* 1968, **30**, 521–533.
5. Shambaugh, P. W., & Kanter, S. S. Spouses under stress: Group meetings with spouses of patients on hemodialysis. *American Journal of Psychiatry,* 1969, **125**, 928–938.
6. Viederman, M. Adaptive and maladaptive regression in hemodialysis. *Psychiatry,* 1974, **37**, 68–77.

19

The CCU Nurse Has a Pacemaker

CLARISSA D. WILLIAMS

It had been a restful and uneventful week of vacation. The bothersome dizzy spells, which had plagued me off and on for three years, had been fewer. Maybe they *were* due to tension and tiredness as the doctor had told me. Then, what were all these people doing standing around my bed staring at me? What were the frightening and strange sounds that kept coming and going? I was having a nightmare, from which I would soon awaken.

The familiar sound of my doctor's voice came through the confusion. What was he doing in this dream? Whatever the reason, he was there and I felt a real need to cling to his presence. The words *convulsions* and *heart block* came through my consciousness, but meant nothing to me in my fight to try to regain my stability.

Then the words *Move to coronary care* drifted into my mind and I felt relief. I was going to a familiar area, an area where my friends and co-workers were. I would be taken care of. I would wake up to find myself getting ready for work. But it did not happen that way. I was a patient.

CLARISSA D. WILLIAMS, R.N., B.S.N. ● Instructor, Critical Care Nursing, Portland Community College, Portland, Oregon.

Reprinted from *American Journal of Nursing,* May 1972, **72**(5), 900–902.

I had no fear or comprehension of the seriousness of my illness, only the knowledge that I was very ill and in need of understanding and comforting care.

An I.V. was started; the oxygen tent was on; the monitor leads were applied. A feeling of remoteness remained. This was not really happening to me. To be a patient in your own coronary care unit where you know the treatment and procedure and implications so thoroughly is beyond description.

Professionally, I knew most of the implications of Stokes-Adams syndrome; but as a patient, I neither accepted nor acknowledged my diagnosis. I continued to mentally and verbally plan to go back to work in a week or two.

Then one afternoon I was forced into the position of facing reality. The doctor walked into my room and said, "What are your feelings about having a pacemaker?" A pacemaker! Never! The medicines would work! I would not need a pacemaker—I would not have a pacemaker! I insisted on a thorough trial of medications.

I couldn't stay in the CCU forever and trying to control my heart block with medications would take time. After a week in the CCU, I was moved to the medical floor, but I was kept on the monitor so that the doctors could see the action of the medications.

I was very apprehensive about moving out of the cloistered coronary area, as are so many coronary patients. My apprehension increased considerably, however, when the alarm of my monitor went off one evening. A registered nurse came in to investigate: "I don't know a thing about these machines or what the blips mean, but since you do, you can ring the buzzer if you need help." The vision went through my mind of being in cardiac arrest, the monitor arrest bell ringing, and this nurse waiting for me to "ring my buzzer." I knew that the majority of the nurses could read the basic rhythms on the oscilloscope and would know what to do for me, but the comment of this one nurse masked the qualifications of the other nurses on the floor.

The monitor became my master. It controlled my thinking, my actions, even my breathing. When I went into any length of heart block, I would find myself hyperventilating. At times, the oscilloscope was turned away from me but the beeping noise to my trained ear was enough to dominate me. I despised that monitor.

I became very depressed. But was it really depression? I believe that sorrow—not depression—was my problem: sorrow over what I had left to do in life but felt I would be unable to do, sorrow that I might not see my children grown or see grandchildren. I was, in reality, grieving that this had happened to me.

After two months on medications with no improvement, my cardiologist said, "When do we put in the pacemaker?" The time had come.

A pacemaker implant is so-called minor surgery. So is a tonsillectomy, but both are painful and require physical and emotional support. In looking back on my reaction to having a pacemaker and observing those of my patients, I can see the similarity: the terrifying thought of a mechanical device regulating and controlling as vital an organ as the heart, the wonder of how one's life will be changed, and the concern about the cosmetic effect (which concerned me more than I would admit).

In addition to these reactions, I had the "professional knowledge" reaction. I thought of the mechanical problems that I had seen and heard about during or after a pacemaker implant. These and such thoughts as coming back every three years for replacement of the pack were going through my mind and still do.

In the end, this coronary care nurse had a Medtronic permanent demand pacemaker inserted, and went back to work in the CCU and open-heart recovery room. I defibrillated patients and worked with all types of electronic equipment without having any ill effects or apprehensive feelings.

Life picked up and became almost normal again, except for this "Thing." I cannot truthfully say I accepted the pacemaker. It made my breast sore when I pulled or lifted patients. When I reached up to get something off a shelf or to count intravenous drops, or did cleaning, my shoulder and breast area ached. I hated the "Thing."

I finally decided that I was going to have to force myself to accept it. But how? The answer came very naturally because of the area I worked in. I began to counsel prospective pacemaker patients. I read everything I could find about pacemakers. I asked the doctors questions. I wrote a pamphlet for pacemaker patients and their families.

As you learn to live each day with a prosthesis, you also learn to let it become a part of you. It is always there and it will always be.

I have learned many things about pacemakers from experience— my own and those of other pacemaker patients. When I counsel pacemaker patients, I share these experiences with them.

Counseling Others

Prospective pacemaker patients are admitted to the CCU where I work. I talk with them, ask them what their feelings are about having a pacemaker, let them ventilate their apprehensions, and then tell them I have a pacemaker. I also tell them a little about my family and my own feelings about having a pacemaker. I describe the lapses of memory and discontinuity of thought I suffered prior to my pacemaker. The majority of the patients have experienced the same bothersome problem, but most had thought it was advancing age. They are often relieved to know that it was due to heart and circulatory problems. I encourage them to ask me any questions that come to mind at that time or later. I make a point of letting them know that I work full time as a nurse and let them observe me working.

I was given a used pacemaker pack and electrode that I let the patient examine and keep at the bedside to show his family. It is surprising how carefully and absorbingly patients handle and scrutinize the pack. Some handle it almost as though it were alive. Is it because they have already associated it with life and have incorporated it into themselves to the extent that they are unable to distinguish between that which is alive, the heart, and that which is life supporting, the pacemaker? It gives me a real feeling of fulfillment when they look up at me and say, "Is this what you and I have?"

When I explain the surgery itself, I tell a female patient that the surgeon will place the pacemaker pack under her breast tissue so that there will be no cosmetic effect that cannot be taken care of with a little larger bra. This is a great relief to women of all ages. I explain to the men to be certain to let the surgeon know if they hunt so that the pacer pack can be placed in an area that will not be affected by the gun stock. This impresses them with the fact that they will not have to change their activities, but can lead a normal life. I explain to all patients that they will have a drain attached to a Hemovac for a day or two after surgery. I have had a few patients wake up from surgery thinking the Hemovac was the pacemaker unit.

One of the important things I tell patients is that they will have pain. This surgery is quite painful and the patient will have difficulty moving his arm, shoulder, and chest. It hurts to turn on the surgical side; it hurts to brush your teeth; and it is impossible to brush your hair for several days.

Most pacemaker patients are in the geriatric age group, so it is very important not to allow the shoulder joint to get stiff. Therefore, I explain to the patient and to the nurses that it is important for a pacemaker patient to receive an analgesic whenever ordered and especially a half hour before starting arm and shoulder exercises. These exercises ought to be started on the second postoperative day, but cannot be too strenuous at first because the pressure dressings and drain are binding and painful. I emphasize to the patient that the more active he becomes, the better the pacemaker can be observed to be functioning satisfactorily, and the faster he will recover.

I also give Medic-Alert information to the patients and encourage them to obtain an identification necklace or bracelet from this company. This is particularly important for women, for it is almost impossible to observe a woman's pacemaker.

My Own Discoveries

I have had quite a few interesting and amusing experiences with my pacemaker. One day, for example, I had out-of-town visitors, who decided they would like to visit one of the big paper mills in our area. While we were waiting for the conducted tour to start, a faint recollection crossed my mind of something I had read about electromagnetic fields and generators in relationship to pacemakers. I casually asked a man who passed me wearing a tin hat with "electrician" on it if they had any electromagnetic areas in the plant. "Why of course," he said. "All the buildings have generators that radiate these fields." "Oh, I was just wondering because I have a pacemaker." "On your car?" questioned the electrician. "No," I laughed, "In me."

I explained to him what I could remember reading about how electromagnetic fields would literally "turn me off." The pacemaker sensitizing device cannot tell the difference between external electric stimuli and physiologic stimuli. After consultation with his superiors, the man advised me not to go on the tour. So I spent the two hours sitting in the infirmary and visiting with the industrial nurse on duty there.

After having my pacemaker for 20 months, I decided to get a new implant. One of the reasons was that the recommended battery life of my model pacemaker had been found to be approximately 20 months. The second reason was that I was planning a trip to the Scandinavian countries. The new pacemaker I would receive, a Medtronic 5842 demand, had been perfected so that an electromagnetic field would put the pacemaker into a fixed rate unit rather than inhibit it. I would not have to be concerned about where I went in my travels. So I had a pacemaker pack or, as so many people say, a battery change. This involves changing the whole pacemaker and another surgery.

With my new pacemaker I was given a round, heavy, doughnut-shaped magnet. When I hold the magnet over the pacemaker pack, it puts the pacer into a fixed rate. It is an easy way to check the rate of the pacemaker, but the magnet should be given only to those patients who know and understand how to use it. If a magnet is used incorrectly, it can cause a serious arrhythmia, such as ventricular fibrillation due to competitive pacing.

I did not really take my doctor seriously when, as I was preparing for my trip, he informed me that my magnet was probably stronger than the weapon-detecting magnet at the airport and might cause problems. You can imagine my dismay when I approached the boarding ramp to my plane to see the guards begin to scrutinize the crowd closely. The closer I got to the entrance the more excited the men became. Suddenly, I grabbed my husband's arm and told him that we should go back to the dispatcher and tell him that I have a pacemaker and explain about my magnet. As soon as we walked away from the ramp, the men appeared to calm down.

After explaining to the dispatcher about the magnet and its possible effect on the detector, he went with us toward the boarding ramp. Again it was apparent that something was causing the guards concern. It was my magnet! Within 10 feet before reaching the detecting device and 10 feet after going through the device, my magnet sent the detector needle to its highest limit. Now I always warn the dispatcher of the plane about the magnet so he can notify the guards.

From such experiences, I continue to learn and discover new things about pacemakers which help me in counseling others. I now warn pacemaker patients to be careful of such things as microwave ovens and airport radar, as these two devices will inhibit the sensitizing components of a demand pacemaker. Radar at the airport may inhibit a pacemaker up to a mile away.

Even after they are discharged, pacemaker patients often call me concerning personal problems that they don't want to "bother" their doctors with. Actually, I have found the families to be more difficult to teach and help adjust to the pacemaker than the patients themselves. The families are inclined to treat the person as a coronary cripple which, as I know, we definitely are not!

A pacemaker patient has a slightly lower fatigue level than does a person with a healthy heart; like anyone with a heart condition, he has a lower cardiac reserve. This limits the level of activity, but not the scope. I swim, dance, mow my lawn, paint my house, work in nursing, and do almost everything else that I want to do. In fact, walking and jogging every day is a must. We who are pacemaker patients can live normal productive lives if we follow the few rules and regulations— exercise, daily pulse taking, and periodic checkups—and take care of ourselves.

20

Survival by Machine: The Psychological Stress of Chronic Hemodialysis

HARRY S. ABRAM

Chronic hemodialysis for terminal renal failure is an example of medical progress in which the patient faces new, and at times overwhelming, psychological stresses. Dependence upon machines for survival is a recurrent theme of man's response to artificial organs. In cardiac surgical patients, the patient experiences this dependence in the Intensive Care Unit with its mechanical respirators, electrocardiograms, and computerized monitoring devices. In postcardiotomy deliria, patients often project their feelings upon these devices and have illusory experiences in which they perceive the machines as menacing. Usually the ICU stay and this type of dependence on machines is of short duration. However, with dialysis it is chronic and lifelong in nature. Put in one form or another the patient must learn to "live with the machine." Through patients' thoughts and fantasies we can learn a great deal about this relationship with an inanimate object which becomes an essential part of the patient's life.

The clinical use of dialysis began in the early 1960s after innova-

HARRY S. ABRAM, M.D. • Professor of Psychiatry, Vanderbilt University Medical Center, Nashville, Tennessee.

Reprinted in abridged form from *Psychiatry in Medicine*, 1970, **1**, 37–51. Copyright 1970, Baywood Publishing Company, Inc.

tions in heart surgery already foretold some of the problems and conflicts to be expected. In dialysis, however, the environment shifts from the intensive care to the renal or dialysis unit, and the patient's concern with acute threat of death shifts to concern with the prolonging of life by artificial means.

The Prolongation of Life

If one regards operating on the heart as the paradigm of the acute threat of death, chronic hemodialysis represents a related but contrasting situation—the meaning of prolonging life by artificial means. The patient dying of irreversible renal failure does face death and is in or near the terminal stage of uremia when he begins dialysis. He usually reacts with euphoria after a few "runs" on the dialyzer. His sensorium and mental confusion clear, and his extreme lethargy and apathy dramatically diminish. Symbolically and realistically he has "returned from the dead." When he is mentally alert the dialysis may initially create anxiety, particularly when he is "hooked" to the machine and witnesses his own blood running through the clear plastic cannulae into and out of the dialyzer. Usually this anxiety is transient, particularly if someone explains the procedure beforehand and as the routine is established. However, one patient, with whom I worked, had an episode of depersonalization during an initial dialysis in which he hallucinated himself on the ceiling watching himself being dialyzed. He reacted with panic, screaming, "Oh, my God, I've got to get out of here! Let me out of here!"

However, once the patient becomes accustomed to the dialysis regimen, concern with living overrides fear of dying. This latter fear does return in later stages of dialysis and especially with the death of a fellow dialysis patient. But for the remainder of the patient's life (unless he receives a successful renal transplant) he wrestles at both conscious and unconscious levels recurrently with the question which he asks himself in one form or another, "Is a life on dialysis worth living?" Wright[29] outlined well the stresses, the losses, and the restrictions with which the patient (and his family) must contend. Particularly bothersome are the dietary and fluid constrictions, the care of the shunt and fears of its becoming infected or clotting, and a sense of bodily deterioration. Bone demineralization, pruritis, insomnia, and sexual impotence are concomitant problems. And above all the patient must learn to live with the dialyzer, the machine which sustains his life.

Chronic dialysis thus creates unique psychological situations which require further elucidation, namely: (1) dependency versus independency needs in the patient; (2) a relationship with an inanimate object (the dialyzer); (3) ambivalence over life and death; (4) the role of denial as a major defense mechanism; and (5) interpersonal conflicts related to the dialysis unit personnel and the dialysand's spouse.

Dependency–Independency Conflicts

Dependency upon the treatment regimen is a relatively constant finding among dialysis patients. Being "hooked" to the dialyzer has meaning not only in the sense of the patient being attached to it via his cannulae but in the sense of his being "addicted" to it. In reality he is dependent upon it for his life and upon the dialysis unit nurses and physicians. Keeping his shunt clean and staying on a constricted diet also impose dependency, as well as limitations being placed on his life by having to keep a certain proximity to a renal unit. The patient, however, receives conflicting messages. He must "cooperate" with the program (that is, be able to accept his dependency upon it), and at the same time be independent (lead a "normal" life by keeping up his work and family relations). He must attach himself or be attached to the dialyzer for approximately 30 hours a week. During the remainder of the week he must keep up a semblance of a "healthy" life, in spite of physical complications and symptoms. "Postdialysis lethargy" is a particular problem when the patient must return to work after a "run" on the dialyzer when he is apt to feel weak and "washed out" (as a patient phrased it). This dual message ("be dependent and independent") gives rise to conflicts, which the patient handles in a variety of ways.

The patient may react through accepting the dependency and independency requirements. He follows the treatment program and is able to return to society as an active citizen. If, however, he is threatened by the dialysis situation and has unresolved dependency needs, he reacts either by becoming excessively dependent and unable to give up the "sick role" or rebels against the problem and refuses to accept the regimen. With excessive dependency the patient becomes demanding during dialysis and has difficulties outside of the unit with his work and family. It usually requires three to six months for the patient to resolve this conflict and return to his premorbid pattern of living. For the patient who does not resolve it, he may have continued difficulties giving up his role as patient to return to the workaday world. On the other hand, the patient who is too threatened by dependency cannot accept the program. He refuses to stay on his diet, takes poor care of his shunt, is grouchy with the nurses, and comes late to the dialysis unit for his treatments.

De-Nour[13] discusses dependency in chronic dialysis in a somewhat similar vein but with more emphasis upon repressed aggression resulting from the enforced dependency.

Relationship with the Dialyzer—Disturbances in Body Image

A patient[1] wrote of his experience with dialysis and feelings about the dialyzer: "Though my contact with the machine is for only thirty hours a week, it is seldom, if ever, completely out of my mind. It maintains a powerful, almost frightening hold on my life. Were it not for the kidney I wouldn't be here to write this and yet I find it impossible to make friends with the monster."

Cooper[11] describes a thirty-five year-old woman who developed a hypomanic psychosis associated with chronic dialysis. Much of her delusional system centered around the dialyzer: ". . . she became wildly excited and irritable and threw a bottle of saline at the window. . . . She expressed considerable hatred of the machine, endowing it with human motives. She expressed the view that the machine somehow knew of her dependence for her life on it and enjoyed, patronizingly and sometimes contemptuously because of her weakness, a feeling of total power." He then interprets her reaction as follows: "The patient's attitude to the machine was exteriorized during the psychosis. She clearly resented her dependency upon it but also feared the pain it could bring her. She referred to it vehemently, almost as if it had human attributes, as 'that hateful thing,' 'I despise it,' and 'I sometimes feel like destroying it.' In fact, the patient threw a bottle of saline, intended for infusion, through a window; this can be seen as a symbolic act of destruction directed at the machine."

Although such psychoses are now rare among dialysis patients, the above description of a dialysand's primary processes does give us insight into the unconscious meanings of this relationship between patient and machine. Another source is that of the dialysis patient's fantasies about himself and the dialyzer. Shea[27] describes an adolescent patient who incorporated the dialyzer into his body image as shown in his "mechanical appearing (figure) drawings," and Wright[29] notes the "umbilical" symbolism in which the dialyzer represents the placenta and the cannulae the umbilical vessels. (Glud and Blane,[16] describe the tank respirator or "iron lung" in similar terms as "a source of security, a womblike structure which the patient fears to leave.") From a psychoanalytic viewpoint this fusion between patient and machine complicates the process of separation and individuation seen in the extreme symbiosis of the early infant–mother relationship as discussed by Mahler,[20] even though the relation is not truly a symbiotic one (as the machine receives no gratification from the patient).

It is of interest that Prugh and Tagiuri,[23] in their observations on the emotional aspects of respiratory care involving the "iron lung" in children with poliomyelitis, also note an incorporation of an artificial lung similar to Shea's adolescent. "Bill, a seven year old boy, was able to incorporate his chest respirator as part of his body image, using the acceptable and somewhat humorous fantasy that he resembled a 'man from Mars.'" The science fiction theme (that is, the "man from Mars" in the above quotation) also occurs with dialysis patients. Such fantasies as "zombies" (having arisen from the dead) or "androids" (science fiction robots who appear human) are not uncommon. A minister being dialyzed gave his first sermon after returning to the pulpit on "the rather simple story of Jesus raising someone from the dead" and described himself as a present-day Lazarus saved by "the miracle . . . of . . . advanced medical science." Another patient[10] spoke of his complexion as a "half olive color" and described himself as looking "like a candidate for a downtown morgue." He also fantasied conversations between himself and the dialyzer, and spoke of himself as a machine ("After all, I was kind of an experimental machine in a frontier world.").

Borgenicht, Younger, and Zinn[7] in an unpublished thesis on the psychological aspects of home dialysis give the following striking examples of "dehumanization and loss of identity to the dialysis machine."

> Mr. X said he thought the machine was "very funny" and that "the whole idea is very amusing to me. When I am on dialysis I am half-robot, half-machine." What he meant to say was "half-man, half-machine" or "half-robot, half-man", but the words he used are very revealing. The word "man" is omitted and he thinks of himself as all machine.

> Mrs. Y, a patient, noted with annoyance that a doctor had once told her, "If you learn to run the machine, you'll get closer to it." "I don't want to be buddy-buddy with the machine," she said angrily, "It's a machine—if it does its job, I'll do mine."

Kemph[18] also describes a dialysis patient who "depicted himself quite graphically as 'a broken man, a disjointed man,' jerked about and completely controlled by the strings to his arms, a sick puppet. At this time he had a blood pressure apparatus on one arm and the dialysis tubes on the other."

A dialysis patient with whom I have worked intensively in psychoanalytic therapy free-associated during one session.

> We're sort of zombies . . . sort of close to death. . . . I guess we're like the living dead . . . somebody who should be dead but who isn't. . . . We're sort of just marking time. In essence we're dead anyway. I'll never have the feeling of being a whole human being. Even if I have a [kidney] transplant one of these days, I'll never get over the feeling I'm already dead.[4]

He also wondered if he would be held responsible for murder if he committed one, as he was kept alive by artificial means and actually died when he was accepted for dialysis. In his words he was "already dead" and his "death warrant . . . signed and sealed a year and a half ago" (when he began dialysis). Litin[19] also speaks of dialysis patients as having "Frankenstein fantasies" associating the cannulae or shunts with the tubes protruding from the monster's neck. As I note in an earlier paper,[3] "These associations (of zombies, etc.) were of special interest to me, as they corroborated some of my fantasies in working with some of these patients. At times while watching some of them being dialyzed, I had fantasies that they were in many aspects 'the living dead' who had to be 'revitalized' twice weekly by machines or that they were machines themselves (science fiction 'androids') in the shape of humans and dependent on other machines for their existence."

The patient thus *incorporates* the dialyzer and *projects* his feelings onto it. (We noted a similar but fleeting projection in ICU patients after open-heart surgery.) In addition to the mechanical aspects the dialysis patient's concept of his body has a defective, deathlike quality to it. My analytic patient condensed many of these feelings one day by exclaiming. "What a piece of junk I've become!" Searles[25] comments extensively on the schizophrenic's view of inanimate objects. He describes patients "who react to various *parts* of themselves as being nonhuman. It is as if such patients have particularly abundant reason for their anxiety lest they become wholly nonhuman, for parts of themselves have

already, in their subjective experience of themselves, become so." With
the dialysis patient there is also objective experience that a vital part of
their existence is in fact nonhuman.

Ambivalence over Life and Death

In this section I shall deal directly with the prolongation of life, the
patient's ability to adapt to the chronic stress of dialysis, and the problem of suicide among dialysis patients. In its most simplified and yet in
its most complex form the question the patient asks himself is, "Is it
worth living?" (under the restrictions and hardships of a dialysis
program). For as Camus[9] most succinctly put it in his opening sentence
of *The Myth of Sisyphus,* "There is but one truly serious problem and
that is suicide. Judging whether life is or is not worth living amounts to
answering the fundamental question of philosophy." Most patients on
dialysis programs speak of suicide at one point or another. Most do not
commit suicide, yet there are a certain number who do through various
means either actively or passively kill themselves. The "passive" forms
consist of withdrawing from dialysis programs and an inability or
refusal to follow the medical regimen (e.g., adhere to the dietary and
fluid restrictions, take proper care of the shunt), and the "active" form
includes suicidal attempts through such means as cutting the shunt
(thereby bringing about death through exsanguination), overdosage, use
of firearms, etc.

How often does the active and passive suicidal behavior occur? In a
recent study[5] I report on the results of a questionnaire study which
contains data on 3,478 dialysis patients in the United States. The
following summarizes our findings: 29 patients withdrew from programs, 117 died from an inability or a refusal to follow the medical
regimen, and 20 successfully committed suicide (another 17 attempted
suicide but were not successful). There were also 9 "accidental" deaths
from shunts falling apart, 37 "unexplained deaths," and 107
"accidents" (such as shunts falling apart) without death. Therefore,
excluding "unexplained" and "accidental" deaths, 166 patients or
approximately one out of every twenty ended their lives through active
and passive suicidal behavior.

Here are some examples of these forms of suicide:

Death through Dietary Indiscretion. Rubini notes:

> ... We have had one suicide. He was a chap who, as a child, didn't like his
> teachers or his parents. As an adult he didn't like his bosses; they all told him
> what to do. After he was dialyzed two years, he didn't like dialysis either, as we

tried to tell him what to do also. He picked the Easter weekend. He went on a tremendous feed, almost a Roman orgy. He started off in the San Francisco docks, where he purchased a number of kinds of shell fish and a jug of chianti. He went home, put a suckling pig on the spit; he partook of all these goodies and more. When admonished by his visiting mother, he retorted he knew better than his doctors how to take care of himself. He returned to the hospital with severe hyperkalemia, suffered a cardiac arrest and he died.[24]

Withdrawal from Program. An answer from our questionnaire and a newspaper clipping:

> . . . two people requested to be taken off dialysis. In both cases, the patients were in extremely poor physical health and were unable to be successfully rehabilitated; one because of eighth nerve damage secondary to Kanomycin which resulted in permanent vertigo and complete deafness and in the other case that of a physician with personality problems prior to dialysis—simply a failure to thrive on dialysis despite the best possible management. Both patients' requests to be withdrawn from dialysis were acceded to by the staff with some degree of relief on our part.

"'It's Time to Die', Ailing Man Decides" read the headlines of an Associated Press release about a thirty-three year old dialysis patient. It describes his "wasting body and his demoralized mind." The article quotes his saying, "I'm taking myself off the machine. . . . I'm ready to die," and comments that "a day later, he signed a waiver removing himself from further treatment." He remarked, "When I signed the waiver I knew what kind of symbol that was, like signing your own certificate. . . ."

Active Suicide. Three terse responses from the questionnaire: "One patient, a fifty-four year old man unhappy with maintenance dialysis in his second year of therapy began playing with his shunt. He had two 'accidental' falls fracturing his hip. Later, his shunt 'opened' when he was alone at home and he exsanguinated."

"Sixty-four year-old male—walked into the cellar at 3:00–4:00 a.m., placed his arm in a bucket, and cut his shunt with a scissor. The patient exsanguinated."

"Patient with severe renal osteodystrophy, osteomalacic pain and multiple pathological fractures. Shot himself in head with a shotgun after three years of center dialysis."

Another response to the questionnaire brought up requesting a transplant as a suicidal maneuver, "There is also a group of patients who *request* high-risk (poorly matched) cadaver transplant. The usual statement is 'I'll try anything rather than this' (dialysis)."

Beard speaks of the dilemma of the dialysis patient as "fear of death and fear of life": "The fear of dying and the fear of living were an integral part of the whole problem of renal failure and its treatment. To these patients, their major concerns were involved with this dilemma. To them, working out some solution to this dilemma was their primary task. To these patients, the whole matter of chronic renal failure, hemodialysis, and kidney transplantation meant dealing with this dilemma."[6]

Thus the dialysis patient struggles with his life and ambivalent feelings about it. Psychotherapy is often crucial, especially to allow the patient to become aware of and work through the ambivalence. Depressions often are concurrent with physical complications, both in the patient and in a fellow patient. One of the major defenses for coping with these conflictual feelings about life and death is denial, and it is to this mechanism that we now turn our attention.

Denial

As with the dependency conflicts associated with dialysis, denial is a universal finding in psychological studies of chronic hemodialysis. Nemiah[21] defines denial as "a mechanism of defense in which the facts or logical implications of external reality are refused recognition in favor of internally defined, wish-fulfilling fantasies." With this definition "external reality" represents the dialysis regimen and its implications and the "wish-fulfilling fantasies" the wish not to be ill. Such denial not only involves the patient but his caretaking personnel as well. In one form or another they ask, "Why should dialysis be upsetting? It doesn't really affect you. It's a little inconvenient but that's all."

Short and Wilson[28] describe in detail the roles of denial in chronic hemodialysis. They note:

> The capacity for denial in these patients is phenomenal, but what are they denying? Previously, it was pointed out that these patients accept their condition and the inevitability of their outcome. What is denied is that it is happening now. When their bones become bowed from osteomalacia, and they go from a cane to a walker, and then to a wheelchair, they continue to expect and to hope that this process will be reversed. When clotting, bleeding, or infections occur at the cannula site, they accept this as a singular occurrence, only to have it happen again . . .
>
> In view of the foregoing, it would appear that increasing denial would be an inevitable consequence of chronic hemodialysis. However, in actuality, it may be

necessary that these patients be allowed to maintain their capacity to repress in order to cope with their life situation.

Hackett[17] makes a similar point (i.e., the necessity and actual beneficial aspects of denial) in his work with coronary care patients. Denial is so commonly found among dialysis patients that psychotherapeutic intervention is often extremely difficult or impossible. And indeed if denial is so strong it is best left alone. Denial becomes dangerous, however, when the patient refuses to accept dialysis, that is, when the wish not to be ill leads to a massive psychotic denial and a break with reality. Such denial occurred in four patients whom I studied. Two had "religious conversions" in which they became convinced their kidney failure was cured by God and that dialysis was no longer necessary, and a third after using massive denial since the beginning of his dialysis became transiently psychotic, developed a hysterical dysphonia (in which he could not "speak" of his troubles) and gradually declined to a state of invalidism and death. This patient shortly before his psychotic break was interviewed by a local newspaper reporter. In the newspaper article he states, "I could go on indefinitely (with dialysis) . . . the 'machine' hasn't changed my life much at all. People don't look at me as an invalid. I'm simply a whole man who needs treatment. I still work and raise a family. I guess I'm pretty normal. . . . I've learned to live with it and appreciate it" (speaking of the dialyzer). The fourth, a woman from a primitive background, refused dialysis from the onset, as she did not want to uproot her family to move to our dialysis center.

Short and Wilson also stress that denial occurs in the families of dialysis patients, the community, and the caretaking personnel. In particular the dialysis physician affirms there is "nothing wrong" with his patient, thereby compounding the patient's denial. For example, Norton[22] writes of dialysis, "When a vital biological organ fails and is adequately replaced by a workable and relatively convenient socially devised and maintained organ, the person tends on the whole to go on living in much the same manner as he did before his loss. Having been given a social reprieve from a biological death he acts like a living person rather than one dying." In response to the suicide questionnaire discussed earlier, one physician answered, "The problems appear little different than in a nondialyzed population." Another stated, "You will be making an error if you equate inability to stay on the diet with a 'death wish' or suicide. Patients have problems with the diet and other facets of dialysis because it represents a limitation of their freedom or because they cannot comprehend the necessity of close cooperation." I believe such examples of blanket denial on the physician's part are related to his emotional investment in the success of his dialysis program which prevents his stepping back and viewing objectively what is happening to his patients.

Interpersonal Relations

It is of interest that few studies deal directly with the spouse of the dialysis patient, especially as the spouse is so intimately involved and in home dialysis is responsible for the patient's treatment (i.e., attaching him to the dialyzer, etc.). As impotence and infertility in male dialysis patients and infertility in women patients are frequent complications, the lack of work in this area is all the more surprising. Aside from Shambaugh's[26] reports of his group work with the spouses of dialysis patients, there is little available material in the area. The unpublished thesis of Borgenicht[7] and his colleagues comments extensively on the marital interactions of home dialysis patients, and it is indeed unfortunate that this work is not available to a larger audience.

Shambaugh paints a rather dim picture of the spouse's response to the dialyzed partner. In his group therapy sessions with spouses (some of whom operated their partner's dialysis machines themselves) over an eight-month period, denial and guilt were common findings.

Hostility and murderous impulses toward the sick partner were quite prevalent in the group (for example, "A husband fantasied taking an axe to the kidney machine"). And although the group worked through some of these intense feelings, denial ("reluctance to face the horrible facts") and a number of deaths among the sick partners eventually resulted in the group's disbanding. Indeed, the intensity of the group's reaction and the dialysis physicians' response to Shambaugh's report (requesting he discontinue his group meetings) may account for there being so few studies in this area. However, Borgenicht's paper corroborates his work, as do isolated reports of dialysis deaths brought about by "carelessness" on the part of the spouse responsible for setting up the dialysis equipment for his partner. Borgenicht describes a death in a patient with rather serious marital discord as occurring after her husband "used the wrong dialysate in the dialysis machine." In reply to the suicide questionnaire mentioned earlier a physician remarked in an item dealing with "accidental" deaths, "The 'accidental' death may have been deliberately done by the patient's wife."

Many of the same reactions exhibited by the spouses occur with the dialysis team. As the reader is by now aware, denial is present among patient, spouse and personnel. With the latter I have already noted some physicians' responses to the suicide questionnaire, the reaction to Shambaugh's findings, and remarks such as Norton's. In spite of the multiple and independent reports of the psychological and physical hardships of dialysis, some dialysis physicians tenaciously hold on to the idea there is nothing traumatic about dialysis, that it is "a way of life" or no different from adaptation to any chronic illness. One dialysis physician refused to let a psychiatrist talk with his patients as he feared "it would upset them." Such physicians look upon the expression of any feelings, especially negative ones, as harmful and to be avoided. And indeed the conspiracy of denial in the patient, family, and physician can make psychiatric intervention or exploration extremely difficult or impossible. "Cooperativeness" is also stressed by dialysis physicians. Often "cooperative" describes the uncomplaining patient who passively accepts all that comes his way and even "thanks" nurses and physicians for procedures which are painful and unpleasant. As noted earlier Brown[8] discontinued therapy in "uncooperative" patients, and apparently patients have been taken off of dialysis in other centers for similar reasons. Therefore complaints are discouraged, and the patient quickly perceives that negative attitudes are not tolerated. Some dialysis patients fear rejection by the unit and believe (perhaps correctly in some instances) that if they are not "good" patients their dialysis will be terminated.

Although interaction between doctor and patient is important, the dialysis nurse actually spends more time with the patient and the intensity of this relationship may create more of a problem (Abram,[1] Fellows[15]). With the patient coming to the dialysis unit twice weekly for 15 hours the remainder of his life, intense transference and countertransference reactions develop. De-Nour[13] and Cramond et al.[12] both discuss this area and the problems of possessiveness and withdrawal which occur in nurses and patients. Nurses are frequently frustrated by the patient who will not let them take care of him, the patient who becomes demanding, or the negativistic patient. Sexual advances by a patient are also threatening, and in some units nurses report male patients becoming exhibitionistic or openly masturbating. I have found group therapy helpful with the renal unit nurses to help them understand their patients' reactions and not be threatened by them. For example, understanding the demanding patient as one with excessive dependency needs, or sexual advances as a symptom of the patient's fear of impotency and a regressive phenomenon in which he is looking for "mothering" from the nurse can be reassuring and prevent her rejecting the patient entirely. Nurses often identify with their patients and have dreams of themselves being dialyzed. The following is an example:

> I had a dream just today about cannulae and the kidney. I didn't ever think I would this soon after starting to work with them. Anyway, I barged in unexpectedly on a class at a college and started talking about the artificial kidney. I told the teacher that I "just had to tell these people all about the kidney." So I did—I had cannulae in my leg by the way. I woke up just after leaving the classroom, but the teacher was running after me and yelling, "You forgot to show them your cannulae."

In summary, chronic dialysis serves as a paradigm not only of man's response to a chronic illness but to a treatment which requires dependence upon an artificial device for survival. As such, it has some similarities to use of the "iron lung" in patients with respiratory poliomyelitis and also serves as an example of how patients may react to artificial organs. With chronic dialysis certain psychological conflicts are highlighted, and we are given an unusual opportunity to look at such aspects as the patient's relationship to a machine, the role of dependency and independency in chronic illness, the use of denial as a major defense mechanism and interpersonal relations involving patient, family, nurse, and physician. An editorial in the *Journal of the American Medical Association*[14] speaks of the problems in chronic dialysis which may prove pertinent to other transplanted and artificial organs.

> An unknown number of people are today alive and working under biweekly hemodialysis who would otherwise be dead. Even committed to their slavery to a machine, it is understandable that life may be sweet, in its limited way. The submission, with the reaper smiling grimly behind every movement, knowing that his turn will come, does not lead to a placid temperament and easy acceptance. To the contrary, the person who lives successfully with hemodialysis lives in a state of suppressed inner turmoil from which there can never be an escape except in death. The history of those who have lived with and at the mercy of hemodialysis confirmed the difficulty of the position. . . .
>
> The man who lives on borrowed time lives uneasily, and the latest medicosurgical creations of borrowed time must eventually be questioned in terms of

the moral result, as well as their physical result. They may be creating nothing, except something of that which philosopher Unamuno called the "too long" life.

References

1. Abram, H. S. The nurse and the chronic dialysis patient. *A Dialysis Symposium for Nurses.* Philadelphia, April, 1968. (a)
2. Abram, H. S. The psychiatrist, the treatment of chronic renal failure, and the prolongation of life: I. *American Journal of Psychiatry* **124**, 1351–8, 1968. (b)
3. Abram, H. S. The psychiatrist, the treatment of chronic renal failure, and the prolongation of life: II. *American Journal of Psychiatry* **126**, 157–67, 1969. (a)
4. Abram, H. S. Psychotherapy in renal failure. *Current Psychiatric Therapies,* **10**, 86–92, 1969. (b)
5. Abram, H. S., Moore, G. L., & Westervelt, F. B. Suicidal behavior in chronic dialysis patients. *American Journal of Psychiatry* **127**, 1199–1204, 1971.
6. Beard, B. H. Fear of death and fear of life. The dilemma in chronic renal failure, hemodialysis, and kidney transplantation. *Archives of General Psychiatry* **21**, 373–80, 1969.
7. Borgenicht, L., Younger, S., & Zinn, S. Psychological aspects of home dialysis. Unpublished, 1969.
8. Brown, H. W., Maher, J. F., Lapierre, L., Bledsoe, F. H., & Schreiner, G. E. Clinical problems related to the prolonged artificial maintenance of life by hemodialysis in chronic renal failure. *Transactions of the American Society for Artificial Organs* **8**, 281–91, 1962.
9. Camus, A. *The myth of sisyphus.* London: Hamish Hamilton, 1960.
10. Chadd, K., & Estlack, M. Transplant . . . A layman's account of a kidney transplant. Unpublished.
11. Cooper, A. J. Hypomanic psychosis precipitated by hemodialysis. *Comparative Psychiatry* **8**, 168–74, 1967.
12. Cramond, W. A., Knight, P. R., Lawrence, J. R., Higgins, B. A., Court, J. H., MacNamara, F. M., Clarkson, A. R., & Miller, C. D. J. Psychological aspects of the management of chronic renal failure. *British Medical Journal* **1**, 539–43, 1968.
13. De-Nour, A. K. Emotional problems and reactions of the medical team in a chronic hemodialysis unit. *Lancet* **2**, 987–91, 1968.
14. Editorial. On borrowed time. *J.A.M.A.* **195**, 13, 168, 1966.
15. Fellows, B. J. The role of the nurse in a chronic dialysis unit. *Nursing Clinics of North America* **1**, 577–86, 1966.
16. Glud, E., & Blane, H. T. Body-image changes in patients with respiratory poliomyelitis. *The Nervous Child,* **11**, 25–39, 1956.
17. Hackett, T. P., Cassem, N. G., & Wishnie, H. A. The coronary-care unit: An appraisal of the psychological hazards. *New England Journal of Medicine* **279**, 1365–70, 1968.

18. Kemph, J. P. Renal failure, artificial kidney and kidney transplant. *American Journal of Psychiatry* **122,** 1270–4, 1966.
19. Litin, E. M. Discussion of three papers on Man and the Artificial Organ. Read at the 123rd Meeting of the Amer. Psychiat. Assn., Detroit, Mich., May, 1967.
20. Mahler, M. On human symbiosis and the vicissitudes of individuation. *Journal of the American Psychoanalytic Association* **15,** 740–63, 1967.
21. Nemiah, J., *Foundations of psychopathology.* New York: Oxford University Press, 1960.
22. Norton, C. E. Attitudes toward living and dying in patients on chronic hemodialysis. Abstract, New York Academy of Sciences Symposium "Care of Patients with Fatal Illnesses", February, 1966.
23. Prugh, D. G., & Tagiuri, C. K. Emotional aspects of the respirator care of patients with poliomyelitis. *Psychosomatic Medicine* **16,** 104–28, 1954.
24. Rubini, M. I. Proceedings, the conference on dialysis as a practical workshop. New York: National Dialysis Committee, 1966.
25. Searles, H. F. *The non-human environment.* New York: International Universities Press, 1960.
26. Shambaugh, P. W., & Kanter, S. S. Spouses under stress: Group meetings with spouses of patients on hemodialysis. *American Journal of Psychiatry* **125,** 928–36, 1969.
27. Shea, E. J., Bogdan, D. F., Freeman, R. G., & Schreiner, G. F. Hemodialysis for chronic renal failure: IV. Psychological considerations. *Annals of Internal Medicine* **62,** 558–63, 1965.
28. Short, M. J., & Wilson, W. P. Roles of denial in chronic hemodialysis. *Archives of General Psychiatry* **20,** 433–7, 1969.
29. Wright, R. G., Sand, P., & Livingston, G. Psychological stress during hemodialysis for chronic renal failure. *Annals of Internal Medicine* **64,** 611–21, 1966.

21

Problems in Adaptation to Maintenance Hemodialysis

FRANZ REICHSMAN and NORMAN B. LEVY

After the introduction of the permanent arteriovenous shunt in 1960 by Scribner and his associates,[1] maintenance hemodialysis became a practical possibility for the long-term care of patients with terminal renal disease. Since then, many investigators have reported behavioral and psychologic observations in such patients[2-12] and have formed hypotheses based on their observations.

Our review of this literature will focus on patients' adaptation to terminal renal disease and to dialysis, on the reported mechanisms of defense, and on the patients' problems relating to dependency.

Shea et al.[2] reported that their nine patients "never quite accepted the shunt as an integral part of themselves," apparently because they found in it "constant reminders of their condition and their dependence on the dialyzers." Furthermore, they interpreted the patients' difficulty in verbalizing their reactions to the machine as strongly suggesting that "their most obvious dependency is too threatening [to them]. . . ." Wright and his associates[3,4] described a variety of major life stresses

FRANZ REICHSMAN, M.D. • Professor of Medicine (assigned from Psychiatry), State University of New York, Downstate Medical Center, College of Medicine, Brooklyn, New York. This study was supported in part by Public Health Service training grants MH 08990 and MH 06317, as well as by Career Teacher Grant MH 10403 (recipient: Dr. Levy) and Foundation's Fund for Research in Psychiatry (fellowship: Dr. Reichsman).

Reprinted from *Archives of Internal Medicine*, December 1972, **130**, 859–865. Copyright 1972, American Medical Association.

during dialysis, as well as the patients' adaptations to them. They found that denial was a defense mechanism used extensively in reacting to these stresses; failure of this defense frequently seemed to lead to depression. They also observed that the treatment process placed the patients "in a position of greatly increased dependency." DeNour et al.[5] in a one-year study of six women and three men, found the patients' main defenses to be denial, displacement, isolation, projection, and reaction formation. They hypothesized that the main stress of maintenance hemodialysis stemmed from the patients struggle *against* dependency. Other writers[6-8] have observed the ubiquitousness of the defense mechanism of denial. Depressive feelings were emphasized particularly by Cramond et al,[6] who attributed these feelings to the patients' reaction to terminal renal disease. Kemph[9] and Abram[10] similarly attributed their patients' "depression" either to chronic renal disease or to maladaptation to hemodialysis. Abram[11] also outlined phases of adaptation in patients undergoing long-term hemodialysis. In order of progression, starting with the uremic state, his patients manifested apathy, euphoria, anxiety, convalescence, and "the struggle for normalcy."

The present report will deal with the origin of the depressive phenomena, their interrelationships with chronic renal disease and maintenance hemodialysis, and their possible connections with shunt complications. It will also describe certain periods of adaptation to hemodialysis and will attempt to correlate them with events in the patients' lives and their affects. Finally, it will describe what we consider a central stress in our group of patients.

The Unit and the Patient Population

Observations were made over a four-year period, beginning late in 1964 with the inception of the hemodialysis unit, until the end of 1968. The patients underwent hemodialysis twice or three times weekly in overnight "runs," each lasting 12 to 16 hours. Each patient was attached to an individual bedside-modified Kiil dialyzer and dialysis fluid was circulated by a central pump.

This report deals with 25 of the 28 patients accepted into the program between late 1964 and early 1968. It excludes two patients who had only short-term dialysis and one patient in whom hemodialysis had been started at another institution. Of the 25 patients, 17 were referred from the wards of the Kings County Hospital, while eight were referred by physicians at other institutions or in private practice. The ages of the 7 women and 18 men ranged from 15 to 56 years; the median age was 31 years. Six patients were black and 19 white, including two of Puerto Rican descent. Two were college graduates, ten were high school graduates, 5 had completed elementary school, and five had less than an eighth-grade education. Three were students while undergoing dialysis, one at high school and two at college. Of the remaining 22 patients, there were two salesmen, one pizza parlor owner, three clerks, three in professions, five in skilled trades, and two had been unemployed; six patients were housewives.

Collection of Data

Candidates for the program were interviewed by one of the authors in two or three sessions of about one hour's duration, most of which were tape-recorded and then transcribed. After acceptance into the program, each patient was seen by the initial interviewer frequently in brief sessions throughout the period of the study. Longer interviews took place at more irregular intervals. Frequency of interviews was determined by the emergence of medical complications, of other stressful life events, or of distressing affects. The patients were usually interviewed at the bedside during hemodialysis or, at times, in offices.

Additional data were obtained at weekly conferences with the staff of the hemodialysis unit, frequent conferences with the unit's social worker, and occasional conferences with the nurses. During the four years of the study, the authors visited the unit most mornings following hemodialysis to learn from nurses and other professional personnel their observations—physical and psychological—about the patients.

While the interviews with patients, relatives, and unit personnel were conducted in an open-ended manner, we focused on collecting data about the following: the patients' affects and defenses; the relationships between life events (including complications of hemodialysis), affects, and physical illness; the patients' character structures; and the patients' overall adaptive patterns.

After conclusion of the period of observation, each investigator analyzed all the material recorded in his own patients. This included not only study of the initial transcribed interviews, but often also relistening to the tape records. Each investigator's findings were then scrutinized by both investigators together in many meetings.

Selection of Patients

Patients were selected by a committee consisting of the director of the unit, its clinical director, and the two senior urologists in the program. Their decisions took into account the data obtained in our initial interviews that we presented to the group without recommendations. The general criteria for acceptance into the program were the following: (1) presence of terminal, irreversible kidney failure in which conservative management would not support life; (2) the absence of other life-threatening, chronic disease; (3) the patient's age; because of the serious medical problems associated with hemodialysis in the adolescent and in the aged, there was a preference for patients between the ages of 18 and 50 years; exceptions were made on four occasions, when patients who were 15, 51, 54, and 56 years of age were accepted; and (4) an assessment of psychosocial factors. This included the following: an evaluation of the patient's ability to cope with stress and to tolerate frustration to a degree that would enable him to engage in the program; the absence of psychosis or of a severe character disorder (one paranoid schizophrenic man was accepted into the program because his psychosis, in a quiescent period, was not detected); and the presence of a responsible family member willing to help in the care of the patient.

During the study, 23 patients were not accepted into the program. Eight were rejected because of marked emotional instability in which addiction to alcohol or narcotics played an important role, and nine others because of severe character disorder without addiction; in some of these there was also no supporting adult at home. Four were rejected primarily because of their age, and 1 because of severe psychosis long antedating his renal disease. The high rejection rate because of psychosocial factors is attributable to the candidates having been screened before referral to us in regard to the other criteria for acceptance.

Affective State before Acceptance into Program

At the time of the initial interviews, the 25 patients were significantly depressed. Depressive feelings had clearly preceded the symptoms of uremia in nine patients and were associated in time with the experience of a meaningful loss that occurred a few weeks to three months before the onset of physical symptoms. Such losses occurred shortly preceding the uremic state in nine additional patients but without the patients giving a history of associated depressive feelings. In the remaining seven patients, there was no history of meaningful object loss or depressive feelings before the onset of uremic symptoms; their depressive feelings seemed to be a response to the progressive uremic state that also deepened the depression in all other patients.

Of the depressive affects, those of sadness and helplessness were present in all patients. The intensity of the feelings of helplessness, at the time of the interviews, as well as during the preceding period (ranging from a few months to two years), was particularly impressive. We use the term *helplessness* here in the specific sense defined by Schmale[13] as feeling let down, abandoned by one's objects, and a feeling of being unable to cope by oneself; the patient ascribes this situation to failure of the *environment*. However, in hopelessness, according to Schmale's definition, the patient holds *himself* responsible for the dire situation or for the need to give up. This was observed in only two patients, interestingly both of them women.

At the same time, the great majority of the patients had felt hopeless (in the colloquial sense of the word), i.e., that they had little or no hope in the future. By the time of the interviews, this feeling had been attenuated by their realization that they were candiates for the life-saving program of maintenance hemodialysis.

As to other affects, expressions of overt anger—according to data obtained from patients, relatives, and hospital personnel—were conspicuous by their absence, in contrast to their prominence later on during hemodialysis therapy. Even in disguised form, anger was expressed in only four patients. The other patients felt so helpless and so dependent upon family members and medical personnel that they did not express anger in order to avoid the danger of losing their help.

Feelings of anxiety concerning their present life situation and the future were experienced and expressed much less than depressive feelings. Furthermore, anxiety was limited mainly to two specific areas: the possibility of being rejected for the program and the future care of the patients' children. The latter played a greater role in the women who voiced great concern and distress over the fate of their children if they themselves were to die. To some extent, this represented the displacement of the affect to a vicarious object, as described by Greene.[14] As to the degree of anxiety deriving from the possibility of rejection for the program, there was wide variation among the patients depending on their basic feelings of self-confidence or lack thereof, and also on their usually realistic perceptions of the feedback received from medical personnel concerning the likelihood of acceptance or rejection.

The Stages of Adaptation to Maintenance Hemodialysis

In most patients, we could distinguish three distinct stages during the course of maintenance hemodialysis. We have named these (1) the "honeymoon" period, (2) the period of disenchantment and discouragement, and (3) the period of long-term adaptation.

The "Honeymoon" Period

We defined this as a period of marked improvement, physical and emotional, of which the patient had clear and conscious awareness. It was accompanied by a marked emergence of joie de vivre, confidence, and hope.

For example, a 21-year-old college student stated five months after the initiation of dialysis: "I'm no longer sick, my self-image is not being sick . . . I have no symptoms, no nausea, no throwing up, no diarrhea . . . ." He made this statement despite the fact that his "honeymoon" was marred by experiencing intense free-floating anxiety and severe headaches during many hemodialyses.

Another patient, a 44-year-old cutter in the clothing industry, said: "I'm feeling now like before. . . . It's a difference like day and night . . . . I am a mensch again. . . ."

A 44-year-old housewife stated that she did not feel sick anymore, saying: "I feel like living . . . now I have hope again." A few months later she stated: "It's like being born again."

The onset of the "honeymoon" occurred one to three weeks after the patient's first hemodialysis. Its duration ranged from about six weeks to six months except for one patient in whom it lasted for 2½ years.

A clear-cut "honeymoon" occurred in 16 (11 men and five women) of the 25 patients. In three additional patients (two men and one woman) the sense of well-being and the emergence of hope was not as clearly expressed as in the other 16, although they obviously showed significant improvement physically and emotionally. Five patients (four men and one woman) did not have a "honeymoon": four of these had serious medical complications, particularly repeated clottings at the shunt site, from the very beginning of dialysis. In the one remaining patient, a paranoid schizophrenic man, sufficient data were not available.

During this stage most patients accepted their intense dependency upon the "machine," the procedure, and the professional staff very readily and gratefully, with few if any expressions of displeasure.

The "honeymoon" was not an unclouded one for most patients. They all, more or less, experienced repetitive, intense episodes of anxiety in relation to their hemodialyses. For example, the 21-year-old college student showed all behavioral signs of anxiety and expressed the feeling that undergoing hemodialysis was "like watching a Dracula movie." He attempted to diminish his anxiety by having in operation his radio and television set and by writing letters, all at the same time. A great majority of the patients had serious difficulties sleeping while undergoing hemodialysis, for periods ranging from two months to about a year. These patients were aware that their insomnia was related to fear and anxiety that some kind of mechanical failure might occur either at the shunt site, in the artificial kidney, or in the central unit that they called, not unaffectionately, "the monster."

Another manifestation of anxiety, a reaction to the stress of dialysis, was the occurrence of unconcealed masturbation in many of the male patients during the early months of dialysis. At a time when there was a total of 11 male patients in the program, seven were observed to masturbate frequently during runs. Masturbation seemed to be primarily related to the patients' anxiety: they stated that it helped them to "forget" about the danger of the procedure.

During the "honeymoon," distressing affects were experienced also in relation to stresses other than those of dialysis. In contrast to the predialysis period, apprehension was experienced and verbalized about the patient's life expectancy, his ability to return to work, and a variety of other factors in each patient's life situation. We regard the patients' resurgence of anxiety feelings as an indication that they reverted from the predialysis adaptive stage of conservation–withdrawal, as manifested by primarily giving up and depressive affects, to the fight–flight pattern.[15] The emergence and verbalization of periods of irritation and anger in many patients during the "honeymoon" also point to the same phenomenon.

Despite the periodic external stresses and the unpleasurable affects experienced, the "honeymoon" period was, nonetheless, clearly dominated by feelings of contentment, confidence, and hope.

The Period of Disenchantment and Discouragement

In all 16 patients who experienced a clear-cut "honeymoon," a distinct change in affective state was observed, occurring in some patients quite abruptly and in others more gradually. The feelings of contentment, confidence, and hope decreased markedly or disappeared. Instead, the patients began to feel sad and helpless, an affective state that lasted from about 3 to 12 months.

Of the 16 patients, 12 (nine men and three woman) showed a definite chronologic relationship between the onset of this period and a specific preceding stressful event, namely the planning or the actual resumption of an active and productive role at work or in the household. In the setting of the depressive affects associated with this life change, repeated physical complications related to dialysis and to the shunt site in particular were noted. The most common complication was clotting of the arteriovenous shunt. Other complications were infections of or bleeding from the cannula, and marked venous or arterial spasms of the shunt vessels during hemodialysis. In all 12 patients, the sequence of life stress, affective change, and complications at the shunt site was clearly established. This sequence will be illustrated by two case vignettes.

A 54-year-old former salesman felt considerably stronger, more contented, and hopeful during his "honeymoon" period, which lasted about two months. Shortly after the social worker discussed job opportunities with him, he began to develop increasing weakness that could not be explained on a physical or biochemical basis. He felt "lonely and gloomy," expressing anxiety and diffidence about getting and holding a job. The patient was troubled by "violent dreams" that sometimes involved authority figures who reproached and punished him for tasks he had not performed. Shortly after a physician discussed job plans with him, the patient carelessly fell out of bed at home and felt pain in his shunt arm. Disregarding instructions, he did not call the hemodialysis unit, nor did he inspect the shunt properly. Following revision of the irreversibly clotted shunt, he continued to be severely depressed and had a series of disabling accidents culminating in his death at home, by exsanguination from his disconnected shunt.

A 30-year-old carpenter's period of disenchantment and discouragement began abruptly on the day when, for the first time since starting hemodialysis therapy, he was to subcontract for a major carpentry job. A few hours before his appointment, his shunt clotted irreversibly. Asked how he had felt about the job, he said: "I didn't know whether I could do it. . . . I felt down in the dumps. . . . I was willing to try . . . you never know until you try. . . . I'll have to try again." He also felt that the physicians at the hemodialysis unit would strongly disapprove of him if he did not reestablish himself as a carpenter. The patient continued to be discouraged and depressed and to have major shunt difficulties for several months. In the three years since then, he has never returned to carpentry and has worked only intermittently as a bartender.

Helplessness and sadness, the dominant affects observed during this period, are illustrated in the second patient. In the first patient, in addition to these affects, there was also intense hopelessness (in the colloquial sense of the word), an affect observed in four other patients also. Guilt of varying degree was noted in nearly all patients in relation to dietary indiscretions, which increased during this period. Shame concerning the nature of the illness and its complications, and concerning the appearance of the shunt site was relatively frequent and intense. The affects of annoyance and anger occurred frequently and, in some patients, very intensely, particularly in relation to the personnel at the hemodialysis unit.

During this period, five patients died. These deaths included three of the four patients accepted into the program who were outside the usual age range, being 15, 54, and 56 years old when entering the program. Also, four of these patients were among the five who had not had a "honeymoon," while the fifth had a "probable honeymoon" only.

The Period of Long-Term Adaptation

This stage was characterized by the patient's arriving at some degree of acceptance of his own limitation and of the shortcomings and complications of maintenance hemodialysis. The transition to this period was gradual in all patients. This stage was marked by fluctuations in the patient's sense of emotional and physical well-being. The intensity of the fluctuations varied greatly from patient to patient and also in the same patient from time to time. All patients experienced prolonged states of contentment alternating with episodes of depression of varying duration. During both these states the patients' primary and most commonly used mechanism of defense was that of denial. We have not seen denial used as massively as by this group of patients, as a whole, in any other patient population with physical illness. The patients' denial seemed to serve an effective adaptive function in many instances: during periods of depression it protected the patients from experiencing even more intense helplessness, and during periods of contentment it helped to preserve the patient's sense of well-being.

Complications at the shunt site, most commonly clotting, continued to occur during the period of long-term adaptation, although less often than during the preceding period. Frequently, the chronologic relationship of life stress, depressive giving-up affects, and clotting were evident. During this period the life stress was, at times, related to the patients' work situation, but more often to a wide variety of losses—real, threatened, or fantasied. For example, a 35-year-old housewife experienced intense grief on learning of the death of her mother with whom she had had a very ambivalent relationship. Within half an hour she noticed that her shunt was clotted. After the shunt was declotted, she decided not to go to the funeral in order not to get "too upset." While she sat at home grieving during the funeral, her shunt clotted again. As she continued to grieve over the next few weeks, the shunt clotted repeatedly; she stated toward the end of this grief period: "Since my mother died, my shunt has never stopped clotting."

While the close chronologic relationships between object loss, depressive affect, and clotting occurred in many patients, the incidence of this phenomenon was not determined because some patients were not seen by us soon after the clotting episodes. However, not only we, but also the personnel of the unit—physicians, nurses, and social worker alike—were impressed by the frequency of the dramatic association of object loss, distressing affect, and clotting.

During this period, the patients became keenly aware of their abject dependence upon "the machine," the procedure, and the staff of the hemodialysis unit. They repeatedly expressed anger that they attributed to the inconveniences and hardships of life while undergoing dialysis. As during the period of disenchantment and discouragement, their anger and aggression was often directed more or less openly toward the personnel of the hemodialysis unit. They verbalized their displeasure at not being cared for with sufficient expertise and understanding. Their statements made it clear that they wanted more help and support from the unit, be it in relation to job opportunities, to finding apartments, to getting financial support, or in the relationship to the spouse and to other family members. They were not striving for greater independence but rather for more support. This seeking or demanding help and support was more evident in the men than in the women. The manifestations of aggressive feelings were limited to verbal expressions in most patients, but some of them acted out by repeatedly coming in late for hemodialysis therapy, by disregarding instructions concerning shunt care, or by openly flaunting dietary indiscretions. Their anger and aggression diminished when they perceived the unit as more giving and as more supportive of their needs. The staff of the hemodialysis unit, on the other hand, was clearly aware of the patients' attitude and found it at times difficult and even annoying to deal with what they regarded as excessive demands and as the patients' attempts to "cling" to the professional person.

Despite these difficulties, most patients were able to adapt to life while undergoing dialysis on a long-term basis. This adaptation was attributable in part either to their beginning some meaningful work and continuing in it much of the time, or to their settling down to doing little or no work at all. In the latter situation, the patient's adaptation was made easier when he became aware that the unit personnel were willing to accept him despite his failure to become productive. This recognition tended to dilute the patient's apprehension about being rejected by the unit and by the physician in particular.

Each patient's school or work record (for women, this included housework) was assessed throughout this period. On the basis of our interview data, we estimated the percentage of "available time" devoted to work or school activities. (The term "available time" is defined as time available to the patient for work or school activities, excluding such periods as hospitalizations and time spent in actual hemodialysis.)

Ten men and one woman were active 0 to 25% of the "available time," whereas eight men and six women were active 75% to 100% of the time (Table I). While the difference between the sexes in the two

Table I. Percentage of "Available Time"
Spent on Work

	0–25%	25%–75%	75%–100%
Men	10	0	8
Women	1	0	6
Total	11	0	14

groups is impressive, the *P* value was just less than .05. Not one patient fell into the intermediate group of 25% to 75% work activity. It is noteworthy that the assessments of these patients' work activity by Chaundhry et al.[16] made independently from us and in a somewhat different manner, revealed almost identical results.

Comment

It has been emphasized[5] that patients on maintenance hemodialysis are abjectly dependent upon a machine, a procedure, and a professional staff. The willingness or relative willingness of the patients to accept this dependence came at first as a surprise to us. Later, it became understandable in terms of the patients' predialysis experiences and the corresponding intrapsychic processes. While some of the patients seemed at times to resent the dependent role and acted out against it, the conflictual situation arose from the fact that the patients' dependency needs could not be gratified sufficiently even by a very conscientious, care-taking staff.

Patients undergoing maintenance hemodialysis experience a variety of frequent and intense life stresses; some of these have been described in the literature[2,3,5] and were apparent in the present study as well. Beyond these, we noted one stress that was central for our patient population; it was related to the patients' experience before and during hemodialysis.

Before being considered for maintenance hemodialysis, the patients were severely ill with uremia, usually for many months, and had gradually reached a stage where they were at death's door. At some level of the spectrum of consciousness–unconsciousness they were aware of being near death, with attendant varying degrees of giving up and of giving-up affects.[17] They had reached a point where striving or competing had become a matter of the past. While many patients used the mechanisms of denial and repression, these defenses seemed to be successful only in part in helping the patient to cope with the situation. Whatever the success of the individual's ego defenses, it is clear that a great amount of "grief work"—perhaps better called in this context "death work"—was done in this giving-up process. These processes and this work were going on largely at an unconscious level.

Then, often suddenly, the possibility of hemodialysis arose. As the patient was evaluated as a candidate for the program, he realized how thoroughly he was being scrutinized from every angle: physical, biochemical, social, and psychological. When finally accepted, after weeks of clinical and laboratory evaluation, the patient knew that he was joining the chosen few, the "chosen people." Then, through dialysis therapy, he was returned to life, he was "resurrected." The patient's resurgence of hope was at first accompanied by denial of the expectations placed upon him because of his renewed well-being. However, he soon had to face the reality of paying a price for having been rescued, namely having to strive and to compete again, to produce. This objective was always the implicitly, and usually the explicitly, stated expectation of the dialysis unit. It was also the usual expectation of the patient's family.

To become productive again presented a major conflict for most patients. The patient's preconscious or unconscious wish was to continue in the dependent role, to be taken care of in the manner in which it occurred during the uremic state and during the early stage of maintenance dialysis. At the same time, the expectations of important figures around him, the dialysis personnel in particular, were that he become independent, active, and productive.

In this setting the main affect experienced by the patients was that of helplessness: They felt trapped between the wish to be passive and dependent on one hand, and the expectation of the unit of their being active and independent on the other. The patients felt that their relationships with the staff, particularly with the physicians, would be seriously disturbed if they did not fulfill the high expectations of the unit's personnel for productivity. They thought that their failure to live up to these expectations would result in their being rejected or abandoned by the hemodialysis unit.

The data concerning patients' character structures, particularly of the men, may also help to explain the intensity of the conflict in the area of dependency and the intense feelings of helplessness. Except for three of the men, all had been very passive with strong dependency needs. From the data obtained in the initial interviews, this character structure had been present for many years, long antedating the appearance of the symptoms of uremia; their character style strongly resembled that described by Schmale[18] in patients with "high helplessness predisposition." These men had lacked drive; many of them had been underachievers at school and at work. A good many were wanderers and drifters, not in an independent manner, but in someone's tow, often until they got married. Those who married chose wives who were stronger and more aggressive than they. Frequently, the wife was the more stable, better-functioning partner in the relationship and, invariably, the dominant figure in the household. Before the onset of uremic symptoms, many of the men had preserved a semblance of playing the masculine role in the family, a role relinquished during the uremic stage. Then, after dialysis had restored their physical and emotional well-being to a considerable extent, they had major difficulty in reestablishing even a semblance of their masculine role in the household and at work. Their awareness of this difficulty reinforced the feeling of threatening abandonment, particularly by the personnel of the dialysis unit, if remaining unproductive when they were expected to resume masculine activities. At the same time, the threat of failing gave rise to feelings of shame in only one man, because in most of the others the goals were set for them from the outside, not from within themselves.

The seven women patients had been more active, as well as less dependent and less passive than the men. Their greater productivity as compared with the men may reflect differences between the sexes in their social roles and also, perhaps, a difference in character structure between them and the men.

Additional evidence for the presence of unusually intense dependency needs was obtained by using tests of cognitive style (field dependence–independence) in our patient population. Witkin et al.[19] have shown that a significant correlation exists between field dependence (as assessed by tests of cognitive style) and emotional dependence, and that a subject's field dependence remains rather constant over many years of observation. Preliminary screening of the data on the hemodialysis patients, as compared to three "control" groups, shows that many patients undergoing dialysis are markedly field-dependent, although there are also a few field-independent patients in this group.

Our observations lead us to agree with De-Nour et al[5] that the main problem of patients maintained with hemodialysis is in the area of dependency. However, we disagree with their hypothesis that the problem stemmed from the patients' struggle against dependency. Even their own observations seem to show that the patients did not struggle against dependency, but rather that dependency needs were not sufficiently gratified when the patients had to function independently. While their data as well as our own observations indicate that the patients had very intense dependency needs and that their show of independence was an expression of compliance with the unit's expectations, the differences in social status, culture, and in sex distribution between their group and our group of patients may have resulted also in an actual difference in data.

As to the onset of the present illness in our patients, in 18 of the 25 there was a history of meaningful losses and separations preceding the onset of uremic symptoms by a period of weeks to three months, at most. Of these 18 patients, nine reported feelings of helplessness in response to these life events. It is likely that stressful life events and the emergency of feelings of helplessness preceded the onset of uremic symptoms more often than elicited. While most patients spoke freely of their helplessness and sadness as responses to the uremic state, many seemed to deny or to withhold the occurrence of such feelings preceding their physical symptoms. These patients emphasized having been "strong," "normal," and "not nervous" because they feared that acknowledging the existence of depressive affects prior to the onset of physical symptoms would stamp them as "weak" persons and hence would jeopardize their acceptance into the program.

While there was a wide variety of object losses prior to the onset of the uremic syndrome, at the end of the "honeymoon" the threatening loss was usually related to the expectation of the unit and of the family that the patient become productive again. Feeling unable to fulfill this expectation, they anticipated loss of support, esteem, and affection from key persons at the hospital and at home. The chronologic relationship of stressful life event, depressive affect, and clotting of the shunt at the end of a clearly experienced "honeymoon," was observed in 12 of 16 patients. We are conceptualizing these relationships along the lines postulated by Engel[17] (to whom we refer the reader for an explicit elaboration of these concepts), i.e., biological change being associated with the giving-up affects of helplessness or hopelessness that may contribute to the onset and exacerbation of physical illness through biological interactions.

We shall limit considerations about the management of patients undergoing maintenance hemodialysis to the transition from the "honeymoon" to the period of disenchantment and discouragement, a time of great psychologic stress for most patients. In order to reduce this stress, careful consideration should be given to how the patient's return to work activity is to be dealt with. To accomplish this, the dialysis physician should be thoroughly acquainted with the patient's work history prior to the onset of the uremic phase of the illness. He should then appraise the possible effect of the patient's continuing illness and its demands upon the potential productivity of this patient. His realization of the patient's need to comply with the physician's wishes will enable him to set goals that are realistic for the patient and, later, to give him appropriate support and encouragement. In those patients for whom return to work presents a particularly intense threat, it may be indicated to delay this event or to introduce work activities only very gradually. Furthermore, the physician needs to realize that in some patients return to work is not a realistic goal at all and that no attempt should be made to induce the patient forcefully to become productive. At the same time he should make it clear that continuing acceptance by the dialysis unit will not be dependent upon the patient's future productivity. It will also be well for the dialysis physician to have some understanding of his own character style and of its potential impact on his patients. Many of these physicians are men of high productivity who are highly motivated and intensely dedicated to what we consider one of the most demanding tasks in medicine. They are viewed by many others, including their patients, as having high expectations of themselves and of others. It is important that the physician know himself and modify his attitude, in the direction of permissiveness, toward patients vulnerable in the area of productivity.

On the basis of all these considerations the physician now may guide the patient and his family to realistic expectations for work, school, or household activity. With the groundwork carefully laid as outlined above, the adaptation of the patient to his illness, to maintenance hemodialysis therapy, and to his new life would be greatly enhanced.

Acknowledgment

Eli A. Friedman, M.D., Gerald E. Thomson, M.D., and Norma J. Goodwin, M.D., provided assistance in this study. Lily Chaundhry, the unit's social worker, provided particular help in making and recording her observations of patients.

References

1. Scribner, B. H., et al. The treatment of chronic uremia by means of intermittent haemodialysis: A preliminary report. *Transactions of the American Society for Artificial Internal Organs* **6:**114–121, 1960.
2. Shea, E. J., et al. Hemodialysis for chronic renal failure: IV. Psychological considerations. *Annals of Internal Medicine* **62:**558–563, 1965.
3. Wright, R. G., Sand, P., & Livingston, G. Psychological stress during hemodialysis for chronic renal failure. *Annals of Internal Medicine* **64:**611–621, 1966.
4. Sand, P., Livingston, G., & Wright, R. G. Psychological assessment of candidates for a hemodialysis program. *Annals of Internal Medicine* **64:**602–610, 1966.
5. De-Nour, A. K., Shaltiel, J., & Czaczkes, J. W. Emotional reactions of patients on chronic hemodialysis. *Psychosomatic Medicine* **30:**521–533, 1968.
6. Cramond, W. A., Knight, P. R., & Lawrence, J. R. The psychiatric contribution to a renal unit undertaking chronic haemodialysis and renal homotransplantation. *British Journal of Psychiatry* **113:**1201–1212, 1967.
7. Short, M. J., & Wilson, W. P. Roles of denial in chronic hemodialysis. *Archives of General Psychiatry* **20:**433–437, 1969.
8. Glassman, B. M., & Siegel, A. Personality correlates of survival in long-term hemodialysis program. *Archives of General Psychiatry* **22:**566–574, 1970.
9. Kemph, J. P. Renal failure, artificial kidney and kidney transplant. *American Journal of Psychiatry* **122:**1270–1274, 1966.
10. Abram, H. S. The psychiatrist, the treatment of chronic renal failure, and the prolongation of life. *American Journal of Psychiatry* **124:**1351–1358, 1968.
11. Abram, H. S. The psychiatrist, the treatment of chronic renal failure, and the prolongation of life. *American Journal of Psychiatry* **126:**157–167, 1969.
12. Abram, H. S., Moore, G. I., & Westervelt F. B., Jr. Suicidal behavior in chronic dialysis patients. *American Journal of Psychiatry* **127:**1199–1204, 1971.
13. Schmale, A. H., Jr. Relationship of separation and depression to disease. 1. A

report on a hospitalized medical population. *Psychosomatic Medicine* **20**:259–277, 1958.

14. Greene, W. A. Role of a vicarious object in the adaptation to loss. 1. Use of a vicarious object as a means of adjustment to separation from a significant person. *Psychosomatic Medicine* **20**:438–447, 1958.

15. Engel, G. L. Anxiety and depression-withdrawal: The primary affects of unpleasure. *International Journal of Psychoanalysis* **43**:89–97, 1962.

16. Chaundhry, L., Goodwin, N. J., & Friedman, E. A. Long-term employment performance in center hemodialysis patients. Read before the Fourth Annual Meeting, American Society of Nephrology, Washington, DC, 1970.

17. Engel, G. L. A life setting conducive to illness: The giving-up–given-up complex. *Annals of Internal Medicine* **69**:293–300, 1968.

18. Schmale, A. H. Depression as affect, character style and symptom formation. In L. Goldberger (Ed), *Psychoanalysis and contemporary science.* New York, Macmillan Co, 1972.

19. Witkin, H. A., et al. Psychological individuality, in *Psychological Differentiation.* New York, John Wiley & Sons, 1962. Pp 381–389.

The Crisis of Treatment: Organ Transplants

Recent developments in the field of immunology, combined with improved surgical techniques and the advances in long-term hemodialysis treatment discussed in part VIII, led to the emergence of organ transplantation as a significant method of treatment for patients with certain life-threatening illnesses. The majority of the current work is confined to kidney and, to a lesser degree, heart transplants, but it seems likely that the next decade will bring a substantial increase in the use of transplantation. In addition to the general problems patients encounter in the period of serious illness which generally precedes an organ transplant, there are specific emotional and psychological difficulties associated with transplantation itself. These include the side effects of immunosuppressive drugs, the patient's relationship with the organ donor, the uncertainty of rejection episodes, the alteration of the recipient's body image, and the effort to resume self-reliance after a period of chronic illness and dependence.

In our first selection Viki Vaughn relates her personal experience with chronic kidney failure, hemodialysis, and transplantation. She is typical of the majority of renal transplant patients in her long period of chronic illness and in the temporary use of maintenance hemodialysis to keep her alive while the best possible donor match was arranged. Her method of dealing with unpleasant or upsetting medical procedures was to seek full explanations of what was happening and what to expect. She took comfort in the constant support offered by her family and made an effort to enlist the understanding and support of the medical personnel who treated her. Of particular help were the explanations and encouragement offered her by another young transplant recipient. She mentions her concern with the side effects (the puffy cushingoid face, for example) of the immunosuppressive medication; younger children sometimes experience retarded growth, including delayed sexual maturation, as well. Viki deals with it by focusing on the importance of the drugs in saving her life and on the possibility of eventually reducing the dosage. She maintains her general optimism, apparently by denying the likelihood of future rejection episodes (she glosses over one such crisis), and by mobilizing hope that her condition as a hepatitis carrier (which prevents her from baby-sitting, kissing anyone, or visiting friends for meals or overnight) will eventually clear up, allowing her to enjoy a normal life once again.

In our second article Michael Adler focuses on the issues of altered body image, the patient's relationship with the donor, and the reliability of the transplant. His careful study of one woman's way of handling these issues offers insight into the major adaptive tasks associated with organ transplants. In addition to the problems of loss of normal function due to the original illness and the sense of mutilation when the diseased organ is removed, transplant patients must learn to adjust their established body image and accept the donor's organ as their own. Extreme overprotectiveness or vigilance toward the organ or references to it as "the baby" are indications that the incorporation process is not yet completed. One heart transplant recipient learned to think of the new heart simply as a mechanical pump, thereby isolating from it the symbolism and emotional significance which would make it more difficult to accept a replacement organ as her own.[7]

The patients' relationship with the donor can have a significant impact on their acceptance of the new organ and their general readjustment. Because only one kidney is necessary to maintain good health, one encounters the situation in which a healthy person may volunteer to give up a kidney to save someone else. This sacrifice may lead to feelings of guilt and overwhelming obligation, identity confusion, or other complications in the donor–recipient relationship. In the case of Dr. Adler's patient, her feelings of closeness to her brother (the donor) made the process of psychological incorporation of the new kidney easier for her.

Her efforts to make the gift the basis of a stronger tie between them (efforts which her brother successfully resisted) serve as an example of the adjustments which are required when a live donor is used. The medical advantages of securing a genetically closer tissue match and of avoiding the delay of waiting for a cadaver match are said to outweigh the psychological difficulties mentioned and the medical risk to the donor. In recent years more attention has been directed at the donor, the role of the family in selecting a donor, the motivations of the volunteer, the psychological rewards of the act, and the posttransplant changes in the donor–recipient and donor–family relationships.[4,5]

With a cadaver donor the question of obligation is not raised, but the patient may face months of waiting for an appropriate match and must also deal with the fact that his survival depends on someone else's untimely death.[7] Transplant teams often try to keep the actual identity of the cadaver secret from the patient in order to minimize the natural tendency to fantasize about, and perhaps identify with, the deceased donor (for example, see Mowbray,[8] p. 260). With kidney transplants where two patients receive organs from the same donor, the "surgical siblings" have additional identification problems to resolve.[3]

Although the possibility of a transplant represents the patient's best hope of survival and cure, it also entails a massive threat both from the surgery itself and from the continuing possibility of rejection episodes. Recipients must come to terms with the uncertainty and anxiety of their situation and find a workable balance between necessary concern and precautions and a disabling fear of losing the transplant. Miss R, Adler's patient, had several methods of managing her anxiety during her illness, methods which were characteristic of her approach to nonmedical problems as well. By attributing power and responsibility for her condition to her surgeon, she could deny her considerable fears for herself and depend on his skill and confidence to reassure her. After her surgery Miss R focused her attention on minor medical complaints, like constipation, and on other patients and their problems, thereby displacing her fears about her new kidney onto areas which she found less threatening and more manageable. Beard[1] describes several renal transplant patients who, after several months of demonstrated improvement, were able to rely on their newfound physical competence to ease their fears and begin to plan for the future.

Chronically ill people such as those accepted for transplants have of necessity reached some acceptance of the dependent position in which their illness places them. When a successful transplant removes the need for such dependency, these patients or their families may have difficulty giving up the dependent patterns.[2,6] Betty Johnson, who received a heart transplant, described her family's continued caretaking attempts after her recovery and her need to resume full responsibility for herself.[7]

In our third article Lois Christopherson and Donald Lunde examine some of the key factors in the adjustment which cardiac transplant recipients make. Heart transplants differ from kidney transplants primarily in the fact that for the heart there is no mechanical substitute for long-term use, like a dialysis machine, which can keep the patient alive and permit a second attempt if the first transplant fails. The Stanford transplant team found that most patients and their families were well aware of the nearness of death. The team supported the open acknowledgment and discussion of the possibility of death in order to discourage the development of elaborate coping strategies based on denial and pretense and to foster an atmosphere of frankness and realism in which mutual support could be provided and necessary anticipatory grief work begun.

The quality of emotional support available to a transplant recipient can be a critical factor in his ability to withstand the stresses of his situation. Christopherson and Lunde suggest that open communication patterns help prevent the isolation of the patient and allow the patient and his family to help each other. The vital importance of the family's support is evident in the case of a young lung transplant recipient.[9] For the first seven months postoperatively he did very well, taking pride in his participation in a major medical experiment and maintaining his confidence and high hopes by denying his doubts and by keeping busy with light handiwork. His wife remained very supportive throughout, but when he began to have difficulties with his parents-in-law and one quarrel led to a serious fall and rehospitalization, he became depressed and uncooperative. He died shortly afterwards in an acute rejection episode with massive infection.

So far heart transplants offer only a very limited reprieve, albeit one during which patients can function once again at a normal level. Christopherson and Lunde maintain that those who had specific reasons for wanting the transplant adjusted better to their new condition and found greater satisfaction in the extra time the transplant bought them. With kidney transplants, which potentially offer a long-term cure, the concept of living on borrowed time with certain specific goals to achieve may not represent a good adjustment. For those patients who have survived uremia, dialysis, and one or more transplants, the ultimate goal is to be able to accept the new kidney as their own and to live as normal and full a life as possible.

References

1. Beard, B. H. The quality of life before and after renal transplantation. *Diseases of the Nervous System,* 1971, **32,** 24–31.
2. Bernstein, D. M. After transplantation—the child's emotional reactions. *American Journal of Psychiatry,* 1971, **127,** 1189–1193.
3. Christopherson, L. K., & Gonda, T. A. Patterns of grief: End-stage renal failure and kidney transplantation. *Journal of Thanatology,* 1975, **3,** 49–57.
4. Cramond, W. A. Renal transplantations—Experiences with recipients and donors. *Seminars in Psychiatry,* 1971, **3,** 116–132.
5. Fellner, C. H., & Marshall, J. R. Twelve kidney donors. *Journal of the American Medical Association,* 1968, **206,** 2703–2707.
6. Hickey, K. M. Impact of kidney disease on patient, family, and society. *Social Casework,* 1972, **53,** 391–398.
7. Johnson, B., & Collier, C. *Change of heart.* Logan, Utah: Sayre Press, 1973.
8. Mowbray, A. Q. *The transplant.* New York: David McKay, 1974.
9. Versieck, H., Barbier, F., & Derom, F. A case of lung transplant: Clinical note. *Seminars in Psychiatry,* 1971, **3,** 159–160.

22

The Vicissitudes and
Vivification of Viki Vaughn

VIKI VAUGHN

I am fifteen years old, five feet two and one-half inches, weigh 110 pounds, and live in Wilton, Connecticut, 50 miles northeast of New York City, near Long Island Sound, where we go sailing. I have two cats, a Great Dane, and two older brothers—David, who is twenty-five, living in Tennessee, and Randy, who is nineteen and living at home. I am in the tenth grade at Wilton High School, holding my own, with some tutoring, because I missed two years of school.

My recognized kidney failure began about eleven years ago, when I was four. Because I was drinking so many fluids, including mud puddles, dew off of bicycle seats, and water in the toilet bowl because I couldn't reach the faucet, my mother took me to my doctor in Westport. He told her it was lack of discipline and to lock the kitchen and bathrooms so I couldn't get any water except what she gave me. Because of my constant drinking and throwing up, my mother changed doctors. One said it could be diabetes insipidus; another doctor put me into Norwalk Hospital. The doctors there knew it was a kidney problem and I was put through all the tests that this hospital had for my problem; my doctor there sent me to Babies' Hospital in New York, where I had six more weeks of tests. The doctors then said that I had a chronic kidney disease; the only medication for the next seven years was sodium bicar-

Reprinted from *Transplantation Proceedings*, 1973, **5**, 1087–1090, by permission of Grune & Stratton, Inc. and the author.

bonate. Things started to get worse when I was 13. I had to go in for blood tests every six weeks, and my medication was increased, with calcium, Vitamin D, sodium chloride, and sodium bicarbonate. Then, in December 1970, I had convulsions and went into coma for three days. In April 1971, I had a stroke, began dialysis, and was transplanted in January 1972. After nine months I am doing very well. I have had one relapse, which was successfully treated as a rejection crisis. In reviewing this entire period, three main experiences have remained foremost in my mind: my stroke, the period of dialysis, and the kidney transplantation.

The Stroke

One day, my mother and I were going out for lunch, and I complained of a headache and shaky hands. So I went into the car without any lunch, and fell asleep. I don't remember anything from then until I awoke in the middle of the night to go to the bathroom. When I stood up, I fell. I tried to stand up and I fell again! Then I screamed for Mom; Dad came and helped me up. Mom called an ambulance and I was off to the emergency room at Norwalk Hospital; the next day, I was taken to Babies' Hospital in New York.

While in the emergency room, I was wondering what would come next, what they would do to me, and why they were doing it. At Babies' Hospital, I had to get to know the nurses, because at first I didn't like any of them. They didn't understand what they should do or what I asked of them, and I would be miserable and difficult all the time. When they finally understood what I wanted and needed, they kept me happy. This makes me think that if the doctors and nurses had just understood better at first what I needed and wanted them to do, we could all have been a lot happier.

Mom came in every day from Connecticut (100 miles round trip), and she and I played games. She would leave at 3:00, and then I would watch TV for the rest of the night. I also had a tutor, who came in to help me with some school work, to help me regain my school memory. Sometimes I would play with my roommate, and we had a contest— which one of us would get to go home first. Another game was who would receive the most get-well cards. When I got to know the nurses better, they would listen to what foods I liked best, and even got a dietician up to see what I liked to eat, and if I could have it. There was one nurse whom I really hated, however. She would take up all my stuffed animals and throw them on the floor as punishment when I wet the bed and she had to change it. While she was making my bed, she would swear to herself aloud. Yet, I had been wetting my bed all my life, because of the fluid intake that I needed to keep up.

I would sometimes burst into tears when my mom brought friends to visit; I would just turn my head to the wall, scream, and bawl my eyes out. This was probably a combination of the effects of a depressant drug and my stroke. Luckily, I recovered fully from this episode, but I still cannot help but wonder, as a human being, why no one told me what was happening to me when I couldn't move my hand and leg or even talk. Nobody took the time to tell me what they were going to do to me, or what was going to happen to me. I just had to lie there and think the worst.

Dialysis

It wasn't *what* happened to me, but how I felt about it that really affected me. Other people might enjoy sticking needles in me, but I certainly would not enjoy doing it to them. Dialysis was all so new to me that I was not sure how things would go. The thing that scared me the most at first was that I did not know that dialysis involved needles. During my stay at the hospital to have my fistula put in, a nurse showed me the dialysis room. I saw that the people on the machines were all grown-ups, sitting up, eating, and reading. For them, the machines seemed easier, as they appeared able to accept all the pain. But, when I got on the machine, it was nothing like what the others had told me—it was worse!

I was on dialysis for a total of six months, that is, I was dialyzed approximately seventy-five times. The most that I was on the machine was twice a week at first, and then three times a week. During all of this time, and later, it was possible for me to accept all that was happening to me, such as the insertion of the fistula, the dialysis, the later nephrectomy, transplantation, and medications, because I was *told* what was expected of me and exactly what was going to be done. My parents and doctors carefully explained all of this to me. The pediatrician told me about dialysis; my nurses, Nancy and Rita, told me what would be expected of me after my nephrectomy, and in the transplant unit I was also told everything that would happen. During dialysis, I would prepare myself by trying not to forget the transplant, by knowing that it would happen. The nights before dialysis, I would just get ready—I knew what was coming up—the dialysis, first, then the nephrectomy, dialysis again, and finally, the transplant, and I would just have to face it. Knowing everything exactly in advance was a great help!

The daily routine of dialysis began when I was weighed, to see how much fluid I had retained; I never gained more than two pounds. Before each dialysis, I took valium, to keep me from getting tense, and to help get the needles in easier, because I would be relaxed. Also, every day, on the way in from Wilton, I would wonder how long it would take to get those needles in, and whether I would have any problems with them during dialysis, as sometimes happened. During dialysis, Mom and I would play games that could be played with one hand. This kept my mind off the needles, and made the time go faster. If all went well with the machine, Mom would bring me a milk shake and candy (that was the only time that I could have milk products). If I was having a bad time, I could not always eat or drink.

Sometimes it was very easy to get the needles in, because the first one, where the blood came out of my vein to go into the machine, was closest to my fistula. But the *second* needle, which returned the blood back into my body, was the hardest step, because it was not close to my fistula, but half-way up my arm, where the veins got smaller the further away they were from the fistula. The most important factor in making things go right during this period was that I had my mother to keep me company while I was on dialysis. The nurses helped a lot. Marsha was the best at putting me on the machine, because she was the first one ever to put me on it. I liked her, because she would tell me exactly what was going on, what she was going to do, when, why, and how. Also, she gave me a stuffed frog, which I named Jeremiah, from the rock song "Joy to the World." I would keep him on my stomach, facing me, or on my head, on my pillow. I also had a doll with a happy face on one side and a sad face on the other. I kept this doll with me when I went up for my nephrectomy; it even went into the operating room with me. I felt best when the nurses put the needles in where I asked them to, which would be where they had been put in before. I asked them not to put the needles in a new place, because it would hurt more than putting them into old scars. The nurses said: "That would hurt more," but I said: "No, it wouldn't." I won that battle.

If I had to talk to someone going into dialysis for the first time, I would make a real effort to tell them exactly what to do and to expect:

first, to get to know the nurses, so that they will understand what you would like them to do, and what could make you most happy and comfortable. One must especially be made to understand why you are on dialysis, why they are sticking needles into you, why your blood is going through these tubes and machines. Then, maybe it will be easier to live with dialysis.

A number of things went wrong during my six months of dialysis. The main reason that I did not like dialysis was because it hurt so much to have the needles put in. I would be so tense that I could not sleep, as the nurses wanted me to. It was the actual pain of needles that I feared the most—how much it would hurt, and whether the Novocaine would ease the pain, because sometimes it would not work, or sometimes not enough Novocaine was put in to help. I was also afraid of the length of time that I had to spend on the machine. Each time, on the way from home to New York, I would think of how long it might take that day to get on the machine; then, I would wonder whether the needles would have to be taken out and readjusted, as had to be done many times. The most time it took, on one occasion, to get me on the dialysis machine was two hours; the longest time I spent on the machine was six hours. While I was being put on dialysis, Mother would have to leave the room, because she could not bear to hear me cry and scream. Sometimes, the needles would "bump"—that meant that the blood vessel was pressing against the needle, because of low blood pressure or tension, which causes the veins to contract. I would also go absolutely nutty during the last ten minutes of dialysis, I guess because I was so glad to get off and go home!

Transplantation

If I had to explain the ins and outs of transplantation to dialysis patients, I would urge them to get to know the nurses very well, and to *ask questions*. Thus, you can help others, as I was able to do. If I had to, I would rather have a transplant than dialysis, for one reason: With chronic dialysis, I would have a scarred-up arm for the rest of my life. Instead, I now just have scars on my stomach, where they hardly show. I can always wear one-piece bathing suits, but most of the time I wear a two-piece suit to the beach, because my whole life is in those scars. I don't mind taking antirejection drugs, since they keep me well. I am able to accept all of this because my parents, my doctors, and the nurses made a special effort to tell me what to expect, and when, and also what was expected of me. As a result, the thing went smoothly, and has now lapsed into a daily routine.

About two years ago, I did not even know how to swallow pills; Mom would always crush them into fruit punch, which tasted terrible! Now, I have learned how to swallow the pills.

Some side effects of the prednisone are pimples all over my face, and puffy cheeks. The less I take, however, the fewer side effects I have. I was taught *very well* how to take my new medication, and the nurses made sure that I would do it properly by standing over my shoulder.

My new kidney was given to me by my father. It was such a successful transplant that it started working even before they got me stitched up! I was very happy that it went so well, and I was even able to call Mom the same night that I got the transplant. There is only one other problem now—I have become a hepatitis carrier. How this happened, I do not know. However, I must not baby-sit, work in a hospital, or kiss my boyfriends. I also cannot go to friend's houses for dinner or overnight, unless I take special precautions, such as plastic cups, plates, etc. All I can do is hope, however, that this carrier state will leave my system soon, so that I can lead a normal life again.

Some Suggestions to Doctors, Hospitals, Other Teen-Age Patients, and Their Parents

I think that the doctors must decide what is to be done, and must make sure that the nurses and the hospital know exactly what they have planned. The doctors should particularly tell the *patient* what is going to happen, when, how, and *why*, and must make sure that the *patient understands* what the doctors are telling him. Hospitals generally try to do their best to help patients, and the nurses do what is best for the patient; however, I think it important that they do it in a way that *also makes the patient* think that this is best for him or her. Just to have the nurses listen patiently and with attention to what the patient says and feels will make him so much happier and more comfortable.

As for other teen-age patients and their parents, I would urge you all to ask the doctors all possible questions, and to make sure that you get clear-cut answers. Also, ask questions of other patients. My dialysis and transplant were made much easier because a nineteen-year-old girl who had received a transplant before I did told me what I wanted to know. She helped me, and now I have helped another nineteen-year-old to get over her own fright.

In summarizing, I think that others facing the problem that I have had should have the addresses or phone numbers of people such as myself and others, so that they can ask questions and get the help they need.

23

Kidney Transplantation and Coping Mechanisms

MICHAEL L. ADLER

Introduction

This study is an attempt to evaluate the intrapsychic mechanisms utilized by a patient to cope with the emotional impact of a kidney transplant procedure.

When a patient receives a kidney transplant, he or she faces a unique situation. He is to have a new organ put into his body, a part of someone else's body, a foreign object upon which life depends. Conflicts will arise because of the patient's having to incorporate this new organ into the body and self-image. Added to this is the emotional adjustment he must make in relying on this new part of his body's machinery to live. Another aspect to be considered is that of the donor's relationship to the recipient. If the donor is known to the recipient, which is often the case with kidney transplants, the recipient's attitude toward the gift of the kidney and to the kidney itself can be greatly affected by their previous relationship.

Studies of the coping behavior of patients with life-threatening crises, requiring long-term hospitalization, have been done by D. Hamburg[1,2] and H. Visotsky.[3] These are recommended to the reader as

MICHAEL L. ADLER, M.D. • National Health Service Corps, Dixon, California.

Reprinted from *Psychosomatics,* 1972, **13,** 337–341.

general, basic accounts of the coping behavior of such patients. This study will attempt an in-depth analysis of one patient's ways of coping with the impact of a kidney transplantation procedure and the numerous emotional adjustments which must be made.

Coping mechanisms are mental mechanisms in the service of mastering the environment, thus used as special psychological methods of adaptation to the surroundings. These adaptations ofttimes involve special role-playing and attitudes which have been used before in other relationships at other times. A variety of mental mechanisms and aspects of the personality are used in the service of adaptation, i.e., used as mechanisms for coping, especially those mechanisms which are used to maintain intrapsychic equilibrium by repressing unpalatable impulses, the so-called ego defenses of repression, reaction formation, projection, regression, displacement, etc. Thus while these defenses serve mainly to repress unpalatable impulses, intrapsychically they are also used to master the environment. The mechanism of displacement from one concern to another may temporarily relieve a patient, thus an intrapsychic defense may and does serve to assist in coping with the environment.

Premorbid Personality

To better understand and evaluate this patient's behavior while hospitalized, a review of the personality and especially normal modes of coping with adult life must be examined. I shall present a condensation of some relevant conversations with a patient concerning her childhood and adult life and then a short summary of her personality and methods of coping with life.

> Interviewer: "What kind of child were you at eight years old?"
> Miss R: "I'm surprised I accepted as much as I did . . . my parents were selfish. . . ."
> Int: "Did you have many friends?"
> Miss R: "No . . . I couldn't play with them; my mother wouldn't let me."
> Int: "Why not?"
> Miss R: "She didn't know anything about them . . . I was afraid to question her word. . . . She hung onto the old customs—I can understand that . . . I don't want to paint her as an ogre. . . . She dressed well and she liked to see us dressed well. . . . But she always got us (Miss R and her sister) the same clothes."
> Int: "How about your father?"
> Miss R: "He brought us food, big boxes of Hershey bars. . . . He hated shopping for clothes; mother did it. . . . He never bought us clothes. . . . He was

intelligent, capable, well-loved, friendly. . . . Everybody adored him. . . . I was his favorite." "I always felt rejected by my mother; she always paid more attention to my sister."

"My mother was very strict and stern with me so I would turn out right and the rest would follow her ways. . . . Once she paid a compliment to me while I was in college. . . . She said I turned out good."

> Int: "Where would you go if you ever had a problem?"
> Miss R: "I never went to my mother with a problem. . . . My father was always too busy. . . ."
> Int: "Where would you go then?"
> Miss R: "Nowhere. . . . If it was serious enough, I went to my father."

Miss R taught grammar school and lived in her parents' home until the age of 31, when she moved out and after earning a Ph.D., began teaching educational methods, which she has done ever since. Though never married, Miss R had stated: "I could have, it's not that I didn't have a chance," but when discussing a female doctor on the ward: "It's more important to be a Mrs. than a Dr."

With the above data we can extrapolate that Miss R lacked a loving mother image. Instead there was a mother of powerful authority and strictness, giving love only in return for strict obedience. Miss R's father was probably internalized as a kind man, "good, intelligent, well-liked," but in Miss R's early life, having none of the influence that the mother had. Since adolescence Miss R has identified with her father, giving her life to her work as he did, trying to be liked yet remaining at a distance.

From this relatively emotionally starved childhood, Miss R developed into a normally integrated, stable adult, but with some lack of basic trust and some unresolved conflicts from her oral (dependency) and anal (obsessional behavior) periods. In adult life Miss R thrived in dependent relationships, such as working under the heads of departments, yet she feared and distrusted those very same authoritarian figures.

> Int: "What's the status of your job now?" (Miss R had begun teaching at a Chicago school two years ago.)
> Miss R: "Don't remind me. They changed my office, [they] wanted to put me in the portables; they got cold and I have to be careful about colds. They have a tendency to do this. . . . They granted me tenure. You need security. A committee of eighteen people voted to give me tenure."
> Int: "That must have made you feel good."
> Miss R: "Yes. . . ."

She has had a lonely life: "I didn't stay in my apartment too much, I never got used to living alone . . . I usually was over at school," devoting her concerns and energies to her students. She has led a mildly obsessional life, significantly lacking in aggressive and sexual outlets. Her main methods of coping with adult life would seem to be a reliving of old relationships and modes of dealing with people which she adopted in her childhood, seeking a relationship in which she can come under an authority figure's control (fulfilling dependency needs), rationalization, identification with her father, and the displacement of concern about herself to concern over others (especially her students).

Modes of Coping Behavior

The mechanisms to be discussed are in no way to be considered pathological, or as evidence of abnormal behavior. It is my purpose to present them as the various means which Miss R employed to help her cope with fears and anxieties, to maintain an equilibrium in the face of the emotional onslaught of the operation and the attendant emotional adjustments which had to be made. The major adaptations are regression, rationalization, repression, and displacement.

Regression.   The patient was very frightened and attempted to postpone the date of her transplantation. Upon meeting her surgeon, Miss R was very impressed and in her words "all my doubts and fears vanished." Miss R came to depend more and more on her surgeon for confidence and assurance. The surgeon became an omnipotent parental figure. She could deny any fears for herself by projecting the responsibility for her medical condition onto the surgeon.

Directly after being informed of the scheduling of one of her numerous operations to repair her ureter, Miss R experienced great anxiety and depression until she had time to reinstate this defense to its previous strength and could again answer any question concerning her medical condition or her progress by replying: "That's their [the doctor's] problem."

Rationalism.   Several months after the transplant operation, in describing the things which alleviated her fears the most, Miss R mentioned the surgeon, meeting previous transplant patients and the fact which she took great pride in, that she felt she was "part of a [great] scientific experiment." Following the operation, this latter idea was used as a rationalization for involving herself in a risky procedure of which she really was very frightened and because of the surgeon's quick decision to operate, for which she felt unprepared. Miss R could not adjust to hemodialysis, thus the operation was her only alternative and her resignation to this fate was aided by her general dependency desires and by the rationalizations she could construct.

Another idea which helped the patient to accept the procedure and have faith in its beneficial outcome was her pride in obtaining the best functioning kidney ever transplanted at the hospital, a fact which she frequently mentioned. Her fears of the kidney not functioning well and the operation not being worth it, could thus be even further alleviated.

Repression. When the patient was admitted for her first dialysis session, she was severely uremic and experienced a state of altered consciousness secondary to it. Dialysis was unsuccessful at first and the patient had great difficulty adapting to it. When asked about this period, she doesn't remember anything and says that from what she's heard from the staff, she's lucky she doesn't remember. It would serve no purpose to remember and could only be detrimental to the maintenance of her equilibrium.

Displacement. When asked what it was like after the transplant operation, the patient said that she didn't have time to think about the kidney because of her bad case of constipation, which, she stated, continued for the three weeks immediately following the operation. Her chart, however, showed no indication of severe constipation and described the patient as being relatively complaint-free.

Throughout her hospitalization the patient displayed more interest in her minor medical problems, to the extent of her automatically shifting any conversation concerning the new kidney and its transplantation, to her more immediate and less significant concerns.

> Int: "How is your medical condition today?"
> Miss R: ". . . the catheter disappeared."
> Int: "It disappeared?"
> Miss R: "Yes, [I] can't see it anymore . . . it must have gone inside."
> Int: "Can you just forget about it?"
> Miss R: "Yes. . . ."
> Int: "They're [the doctors] not worried?"
> Miss R: "No, I'm on liquid restriction, it's rough on me. . . ."

On a warm summer day: "The kidney doesn't bother me, sweating so much does." Another example of this mode of handling anxiety, a personality characteristic of the patient, is the fact that she consistently displayed more concern over the other patients and their medical problems.

In these incidences Miss R was using a major defense mechanism which was called upon to help rechannel her anxiety over her new kidney to concern over conditions better understood by her. Since they could be understood, they were easier to confront and to cope.

Donor-Related Adaptations

As noted above, the donor–recipient relationship before this crisis has great bearing on the recipient's acceptance of the kidney. Therefore, we must investigate this relationship to be able to understand the dynamics of the recipient's acceptance of this gift from the donor and of incorporating it into her own body and self-image.

History

The donor is the recipient's youngest brother. The patient feels that she and the donor are very much alike. Miss R also feels that she, her youngest brother, and their father are different from their mother and sister, who Miss R feels are the same kind of people. Miss R states that she has always been in fierce competition with her sister. The sister was given the responsibility of raising the youngest brother and thus Miss R blames her for what she feels is her brother's misguided and misspent life.

After the patient had been accepted to the transplant program, her family was immediately contacted and her youngest brother volunteered his kidney. Upon learning of this, the patient attempted to talk him out of volunteering, but her brother insisted and the operation was accomplished. The donor progressed excellently and has had no complications to date.

Modes of Coping Behavior

The main dynamic in the patient's original acceptance of the kidney, and the eventual incorporation of the donor's kidney into her own body and self-image, is elucidated by the patient's attitude towards her brother and what she feels her role in his life should be. Because of the sister's raising of the donor and the patient's lifelong competition with the sister (with Miss R's resulting attitude that her brother's life has been ruined by his bad upbringing), the brother's donation of a kidney meant a final victory over her sister's lifelong influence over the brother. Thus the gift was accepted readily, with great pride and with hopes of being able to exert more control over his life in the future.

The fact that the patient felt that she and the donor were, as Miss R stated, "alike" somewhat lessened her concern about the "foreignness" of the kidney.

As with the acceptance of the procedure, the anxieties over the possible deleterious consequences of removing one of the donor's kidneys were alleviated by the assurance of her surgeon that there would be no problem.

The brother's insistence on his donation and his refusal to accept the indebtedness which the patient felt toward him and attempted to force on him after the operation made the patient accept the kidney, but she accepted it without a greater bond between herself and the donor being achieved. This fact destroyed one of the secondary gains Miss R had hoped to achieve by her acceptance of his kidney, but because of the secondary nature of the possible gain, the patient was only mildly upset and no permanent problems in their relationship developed.

General Behavior on the Ward

Miss R's general behavior on the ward displayed prominent aspects of regression and her utilization of the process of displacement. For a hospitalized patient, some regression is necessary to fit into the normally submissive role that must be played. Depending upon the individual patient, the regression and necessity of sublimating normal aggressive adult behavior may be readily accepted or be the cause of anxiety. As could be predicted, Miss R readily fit into her new role as a patient and after some time in the hospital she began to view her eventual "dismissal" with dread.

She loved all of the attention she could and did command at any hour of the day or night. She would nag at the orderlies and other service personnel, while demanding much attention from the nursing and especially the biochemical staff. Visits by interns, residents, and staff doctors were eagerly awaited, not for the information they could impart, but their presence and interest gave great comfort to her. Any variance in the schedule or amounts of her meals and snacks would greatly upset and anger her.

I frequently visited and spent much time with her and she told me she looked forward to my visits. After my leaving the ward, it was related to me that Miss R became quite anxious and that this anxiety was relieved by her developing another close relationship with another young man, thus reestablishing a relationship satisfying her need for attention.

As noted above, a certain degree of regression is normal, however, too great a regression can disrupt the ward and even retard the patient's progress.

1.   Miss R at times demanded much time from the staff and upset the staff with her nagging.

2.   Late in her hospital stay, Miss R was told that she might be able to leave the hospital in a few weeks. Several days later an "accident" occurred. The tube draining her kidney (necessitated by the nonfunctioning ureter) became detached from the catheter and hit the floor. Miss R picked it up and in her words "stuck it back in, without thinking." Being in immunosuppressive therapy, this could have resulted in a severe, even fatal infection. She did experience a high fever of undetermined origin and suffered a setback in her progress. Her desire to remain in the hospital resulted in an unconscious act, dangerous though its consequences might have been, aimed at keeping her there longer.

Transferring concern from her own problems to concern over the problems of others, considered above, was a mode of behavior observable every day on the ward. When Miss R was able to leave her room, she spent much time conversing with relatives and friends of other patients. Being able to talk about and express concern over others' problems allowed her to displace much of the anxiety she felt over her own problems to the much less threatening concern over others' problems.

Summary

This case demonstrates the value of coping mechanisms in maintaining an equilibrium during a difficult period in this patient's life. It demonstrates the value of understanding coping mechanisms so as to appreciate the stresses the patient is undergoing and also to be able to evaluate which mechanisms the patient might need to investigate and gain insight into so that she can effectively face the situation which is stimulating the defense and coping device.

In viewing Miss R's methods of handling the anxieties arising from having to accept a foreign object into her own body and self-image—an object upon which her life depends—and the donor-related conflicts of indebtedness and possible guilt, we have observed that her main methods of coping might be predicted by a knowledge of her premorbid personality and of the basic modes of coping behavior that the patient used. This seems a plausible hypothesis to set forth and only further study can test its validity.

References

1. Hamburg, D., et al. Adaptive problems and mechanisms in severely burned patients. *Psychiatry* **16:**1–20, 1953.
2. Hamburg, D., et al. Clinical importance of emotional problems in the care of patients with burns. *New England Journal of Medicine* **248:**355–359, 1953.
3. Visotsky, H., et al. Coping behavior under extreme stress. *Archives of General Psychiatry* **5:**423–448, 1961.

24

Selection of Cardiac Transplant Recipients and Their Subsequent Psychosocial Adjustment

LOIS K. CHRISTOPHERSON and DONALD T. LUNDE

The selection of recipients for organ transplantation and the relationship of selection to the patient's psychosocial adjustment after transplantation have received much attention in the past several years. No set of definitive criteria for the selection of suitable candidates for transplantation has yet been formulated. Although at many centers the criteria for selection are predominantly medical, it seems reasonable that other criteria of a psychosocial nature should enter into these selection procedures since candidates are being chosen for complicated, expensive, and somewhat experimental procedures involving long-term, intensive medical follow-up.

Abram,[1,2] in discussing selection of patients for chronic hemodialysis, suggests that psychoses (unrelated to uremia) and mental deficiency should be the "only psychiatric contraindications per se." He

LOIS K. CHRISTOPHERSON, M.S.W., A.C.S.W. • Chief Social Worker, Department of Surgery; Lecturer, Department of Family, Community, and Preventive Medicine, Stanford University School of Medicine, Stanford, California. Supported in part by NIH Grant HE 13108-01.

Reprinted from *Seminars in Psychiatry*, 1971, 3, 36–45, by permission of Grune & Stratton, Inc. and the authors.

adds that "'sociological' rejections should be rare" and questions whether any decision can be made on the basis of "social worth." Abram's beliefs are similar to the philosophy of the Stanford transplant team in selecting patients for cardiac transplantation, namely, that only mentally deficient or actively psychotic patients would likely be rejected on nonmedical grounds. At the same time, however, we have been aware both that informal screening of candidates for transplantation is constantly occurring and that there may be a future necessity for additional screening should cardiac transplantation become more successful and the demand for such surgery exceed its availability.

This paper discusses the characteristics and motivations of patients seeking transplantation and the process by which they were selected at Stanford. It suggests apparent relationships between these variables and the subsequent psychological and social adjustment of transplant survivors.

Of the 20 patients receiving transplants from January 1968 to February 1970, 11 were classified as "survivors" (patients discharged from the hospital following transplantation with no plan for readmission and with the expectation that they were medically able to return to relatively normal lives). The other 9 died following transplantation before leaving the hospital.

The Process of Recipient Selection

Medical Criteria

The primary criteria which have evolved for recipient selection are medical. Terminal heart disease, unamenable to medical and lesser surgical therapy, must be present in each case. Separate disease in other organs, which would independently limit life expectancy, should be absent, and organ dysfunction secondary to congestive heart failure should be potentially reversible.

Preliminary Screening

Approximately two-thirds of the patients evaluated for cardiac transplantation were referred by sources outside Stanford Medical Center. These patients received their initial care from family physicians who subsequently referred them for further evaluation and treatment. Whether or not it was discussed with the patient and family, most perceived this as a significant turning point in the patient's illness. Some reported, "He [the family doctor] didn't say much, but we knew that [the patient] was really in trouble." Others described a specific discussion with the physician in which they explored not only the referral to a specialist but also the likelihood that transplantation would be considered if no other mode of therapy could be recommended.

Thus, the initial process of selection for transplantation often began at this point. The family physician made his own decision about suitability for transplantation. The patient and family were in the position either of reinforcing the transplant possibility or of deciding against it. In one particularly interesting case, the patient and his family saw this referral as an opportunity to introduce the topic of transplantation to their physician, a man who was generally known to be opposed to heart transplants.

Although it is not possible to report extensively on those patients who did not reach Stanford's selection process, we are aware that physicians have ruled out patients for transplantation because of an "unsuitable personality" or "unstable family situation," even though they had previously referred other patients for evaluation. There have also been cases in which the patient himself refused to consider transplantation.

One such patient was a widow in her late 50s who responded to her physician's and family's encouragement for transplantation by indicating her own acceptance of death. "I just don't think I'd want a transplant. When your time comes, you just have to go." Another patient, a 20-year-old man with terminal myocarditis, was so overwhelmed by the mention of transplantation that he withdrew from communication with others and refused to eat. His fears appeared related both to his inability to cope with the possibility of his death and to his perception of surgery as a mutilating assault upon his person. This latter case also illustrates the problem of transplant selection when a minor is involved. Technically, the parents are responsible for surgical consent if the patient is under 21. Yet, although the mother of this 20-year-old was strongly in favor of transplantation, the patient himself made the final decision.

In contrast, the parents of a 7-year-old girl considered for transplantation were clearly responsible for the decision and monitored with the family physician and transplant team the type of information shared directly with the child. The little girl's understanding of the operation was that it would be something like the tonsillectomy she had experienced a few years earlier. She said she understood there was something wrong with her heart, and if she had an operation, she would be able to go back to school.

Screening after Referral

Patients considered likely candidates for transplantation by their private physicians were then seen at Stanford where the final decision was made. At this point, psychiatric evaluation was focused primarily on informed consent and the patient's psychiatric history in relation to prediction of the patient's response to surgery and associated stresses. Patients also were examined for evidence of severe depression, first, to identify individuals who were actively suicidal and second, because of reports that the risk of open heart surgery is greater for depressed patients.[5]

While it was relatively easy to identify the few individuals whose motives for seeking transplantation were seriously pathological or self-destructive, evaluating the degree to which others had made an informed decision was a difficult task. Fellner and Marshall[3] have raised sharp questions about the validity of claiming "informed consent" in the case of renal transplant donors. They observed that donors appeared generally to decide for or against organ donation when they were first approached. Information given them subsequently by team physicians was used only to support the decision they had already made. A similar situation was found to exist in regard to the decision about cardiac transplantation.

One man arrived at the hospital against the advice of his previous physicians, who had discouraged transplantation on the grounds that it was too new and experimental a procedure. When first interviewed, he stated, "I came to get a new ticker. My wife and I talked it over and I'm ready. I don't want to be an invalid. I'm no good to my wife or children now. I'm just a burden. I would rather take a chance on this [transplant] than go on the way I am living."

In other cases, the patient or family had already obtained much information from family physicians, friends, or the news media. They felt that transplant team members were being honest with them, but they had little interest in exploring the situation beyond what they already knew. The absence of a guarantee for survival was balanced for them by the presence of some long-term survivors and/or by the fact that there was little question of the patient's impending death.

Patients themselves were presented with as much information as was available regarding transplantation and the likely postoperative problems and expectations. Twice, however, the potential recipients were moribund because of severe cardiac failure. In one of these cases, the patient did become alert enough to participate in the discussion regarding transplantation; in the other, however, the burden of consenting to the operation fell entirely upon his wife.

Although the number of cases is too limited to permit firm conclusions, it can be hypothesized that the presence of numerous "challenging" questions about transplantation often masked a desire that it not be considered at all. One couple, for example, spoke at length of their wish to make an "informed decision."* They requested private interviews with one team member after another and produced feelings of discomfort in the physicians who were seeking to answer the apparently logical questions they posed.

When interviewed by the social worker, the patient's wife spoke sharply. "You people have to realize that we're just here to look you over. We're not making any promises and we don't know if the transplant is for us." Exploration revealed that the couple felt pushed towards transplantation by the enthusiasm of close friends and their family physician. They felt further constrained by the "rational" answers given their "logical" questions—when they were really seeking a way out of the trap in which they found themselves. Resolution of the dilemma occurred when the couple decided they could not move to the Stanford area since their children were in the midst of a school year several hundred miles away. (It has been made a requirement at Stanford that heart transplant patients either live in the area or be willing to move to the vicinity to permit adequate long-term follow-up care.)

* Interviews with this couple occurred during the middle of the transplant series. They thus had access to information about deceased transplant patients and patients who were doing well following posttransplant discharge from the hospital.

Pretransplant Interview Themes and Posttransplant Adjustment

Three subjects which were consistently explored in interviews prior to transplantation appeared to be significant when related to posttransplant adjustment. These were patterns of family communication, awareness of death, and the presence of specific, realistic reasons for wanting an extension of life through cardiac transplantation.

Family Communication Patterns

The question was routinely asked, "Have you discussed the possibility of a cardiac transplant with the rest of your family?" In the case described above, the wife became visibly upset: "We don't think that is any of their concern [referring to their children, ages 8, 10, and 13]. They could become horribly disturbed by something like this. We just told them Daddy was getting some treatment to make him better." The couple also denied any thought as to what they would tell the children should transplantation be decided upon. It was "a bridge we'll cross if we come to it."

A second kind of response was observed in cases in which patients and/or immediate family members reported they had discussed the transplant "a little bit" or had no intimate friends with whom to discuss transplantation. Following surgery, feelings of loneliness, efforts to find some meaning or significance in the transplant, or conflicting feelings about whether it should have been performed at all were sporadically observed.

Parenthetically, these feelings did not necessarily correlate with the emotional panic expressed during the transplant by a number of spouses, "Did I do the right thing?" This question surfaced frequently no matter how many family and friends participated in the decision. It disappeared in all but one case immediately following surgery.

A third type of response was quick and enthusiastic, "Yes, we've all talked it over and agreed"—usually followed by a detailed listing of calls made, relatives contacted, and the variety of responses obtained. Family members from this group were mutually supportive during and after transplantation and generally showed the least evidence of denial, either of the severity of the patient's illness or of the transplant's guarded prognosis.

Families seemed to achieve consensus by verbalizing the patient's nearness to death and by deciding that transplantation was his "only chance" for extended survival. One wife described talking to the patient's mother: "When I first told her we were considering a heart transplant, she couldn't believe it. She has read about them in the papers, but she didn't think John was that sick. . . . Now she agrees."

Awareness of Death

A second element common to interviews with most patients and families concerned their awareness of pending death. The words *death, dying,* or *survival* were often present in the everyday vocabulary of waiting recipients and their families. The phase which Glaser and Strauss[4] have described as "preparation for death" had begun on the part of both the families and the hospital staff caring for the patient.

The open discussion of death was initially encouraged and aided by team members for several reasons. It helped to release the emotional energy of key family members for use in coping with the stresses of transplantation rather than in protecting tenuous patterns of denial; it helped family members continue their grief work if a patient died relatively soon after transplantation; it helped to create an atmosphere of frankness about the transplant which included family members as well as patients; and it reflected our concern that the concept of informed consent in clinical investigation be fulfilled.

An additional reason for exploring the subject of death has been formulated more recently and is related to the posttransplant adjustment of survivors. It is illustrated by the following case. Steve X was transferred to Stanford in critical condition after a series of myocardial infarctions. Although his wife was clearly aware of his nearing death, she actively discouraged relatives and staff from mentioning death to her husband. When he appeared alert, Mrs. X assured him he would soon recover at the same time that physicians were giving him as much information as possible about cardiac transplantation. The patient signed the consent form for surgery himself, but Mrs. X also strongly emphasized her willingness to sign should her husband be unable. There was not sufficient time to help Mrs. X communicate her thoughts about dying to her husband—nor were all the possible implications of this denial recognized at the time.

Shortly after transplantation, as the patient became aware of his ease in breathing and freedom from chest pain, he remarked, "I think I almost died." His wife, in the presence of a nurse, quickly reassured him. "Oh, no, you weren't nearly that bad. They just thought this transplant would help." The nurse, caught up in the drama, supported the reassurance.

The patient did well and survives, at the time of this writing, beyond one year. His feelings about the death of a fellow survivor and friend finally served as a catalyst in helping him talk with the social worker about his own feelings regarding death. Psychologically and in terms of family dynamics, however, this patient had a relatively difficult course. His sensitivity to pain, complaints about medical procedures, and demands upon family and hospital staff exceeded those of most other patients—survivors or not. Several times he used in a veiled or direct fashion the "helpful" rather than "necessary" nature of the transplant to support his claims. He has described himself sporadically as a "guinea pig," referred to research "being done on me," and at least once told his wife he blamed her "for all this transplant stuff." In retrospect, the transplant team feels strongly that in future cases such dissonance in perception should be dealt with before transplantation whenever possible.

Reasons for Transplantation

A final recurring element in pretransplant interviews with many recipients which appeared to be a predictor of good adjustment in survivors was the presence of positive reasons for wanting "more time" through cardiac transplantation. We were struck by the frequency with which highly motivated recipients used the phrase, "I've got some things left to do." When this was explored, specific, realistic answers were usually given. "I would like to live for one more Christmas." "If I survive, I'll get to be president of Kiwanis." "I'd like to see my youngest child start school."

These answers gained further significance as it became apparent that although the same recipients would make comments such as, "I'd like to get another 20 years out of this," or "I'd like to live as long as my father," they actually planned day-to-day activities in a much more time-limited way. In contrast, two survivors who originally "didn't want to plan ahead, just to live" had difficulty planning their use of time posttransplant and reported fewer events which had special significance for them.

Hospital Discharge and Subsequent Psychosocial Adjustment

When a recipient began planning for hospital discharge, he would undertake certain tasks. Foremost was the task of deciding what to do—psychologically and socially—about the very fact that he was, irrevocably, "a heart transplant." The ease with which this was discussed with hospital personnel was about to be replaced with curiosity, "ridiculous questions" from persons he didn't know, and fear when he had no one to explain symptoms he would previously have discussed immediately with transplant team members.

Most patients began the adjustment process by trying to integrate their old identity with their new status as transplant survivors. Several wrote letters and made phone calls to relatives and old friends. The content was usually reassuring to both writer and recipient of the message: "I feel better than I have for years. I'm really the same person. These transplants are great." One man called the principals of the schools each of his children attended. "This is Jack Doe, heart transplant—Jane's father. I just wanted to catch up on how she is doing."

It was at the point of discharge also that the reasons a patient originally gave for wanting a transplant became significant (see Table I). While the two who gave no specific reasons displayed a lack of excitement or developed mild somatic complaints, the rest eagerly began negotiations for the resumption of normal activity.

One man began daily visits to the social worker to discuss the progress of his referral to Vocational Rehabilitation and his subsequent "new career." A housewife became critical of the baking she was doing in occupational therapy, pointing out how much easier it would be for her in her own home with her own equipment. A man who had always been active in civic affairs called the volunteer fire department and said, "Never fear—Bill X is here!"

Families often experienced more misgivings with discharge than the transplant survivor. Spouses who had given every evidence of

Table I. Pre- and Posttransplant Activities of Heart Transplant Survivors

Recipient	Sex	Age	Working or housewife during pre-transplant year	Working or housewife during post-transplant year	Some specific reasons for transplant	Follow-through on reasons	Moved to SUH area (others already there)	Working spouse
A	M	50s	No	Yes	Work again / Learn golf	Yes	No	No
B	F	40s	Yes (very limited)	Yes	Another Thanksgiving and Christmas	Yes	No	Yes
C	M	50s	No	No	Fish and hunt / Visit family again	Yes	Yes	Yes
D	M	40s	Yes	No	Civic leader / Have a good time	Yes	No	Yes
E	M	50s	No	No	None	—	Yes	Yes
F	M	40s	Yes	Yes	Write again / See daughter grow	Yes	Yes	Graduate student
G	M	50s	No	No	Daughter graduate	No[a]	No	No
H	F	40s	Yes (very limited)	Yes	Wife and mother again, see children graduate	Yes	Yes	Yes
I	M	40s	Yes	Yes	New career / Time with children	Yes	No	Yes
J	M	40s	No	Yes	None	—	No	Yes
K	M	30s	Yes	Yes	Work again / Have a good time	Yes	No	Single

[a] This patient died suddenly shortly following discharge.

eagerly awaiting the patient's discharge had trouble sleeping, compulsively monitored the patient's pills and diet, and in a couple of instances reported frightening fantasies of having the patient suddenly drop dead.

Delineation of the problem by team members brought about steps which minimized it for both patients and families. Physicians gave hospital passes of increasing length prior to final dicharge; nurses devised charts so that the taking of pills was routine rather than a feat of memory; the amount of attention given the patient was gradually decreased so that he was virtually caring for himself by the time he went home. Other survivors and their families discussed this period with those approaching discharge; and the social worker discussed with both patient and family the tensions which might still be expected to remain.

Publicity was initially rejected by most patients. "I just want to go home." "I wouldn't know what to say anyway." Plans were made to deal with questions of those outside his close circle of friends. There was sometimes an underlying feeling of being an "in" person. "I won't say much because they wouldn't understand anyway."

Sensitivity to publicity diminished once the survivor returned to work or became engaged in activities which had meaning for him. People whom the survivor met during his daily activities "discovered somehow" he was a cardiac transplant recipient. An entertainer who was successful in his own right decided to add to his public image by talking more often of transplantation. A man who was well known and active in his community thoroughly enjoyed the additional attention he received as a "transplant survivor."

Differentiation must be made between the eight survivors who integrated their posttransplant goals with their new self-image of "transplant survivor" and the two who had no specific goals.* While the latter two also gradually developed a desire for publicity, they appeared at times to use this to replace rather than to supplement meaningful activity of their own.

Moving to the Stanford area, as four patients did, was not of itself as significant a factor in long-term adjustment as might have been anticipated. In only one of the four cases did it pose serious problems. This family had lived all its life in one community and had neither the practice in making new friends nor the transferability of job skills needed to adjust comfortably to a new living situation. A second patient missed his rural surroundings but compensated fairly well by taking

---

* The 11th survivor died suddenly shortly after discharge.

long trips and through his wife's ability to find work and new friends immediately. The remaining two experienced no difficulty with moving or readjustment.

Personality changes in survivors were limited and consisted mostly of accentuation of characteristics present before transplantation. A recipient who had a history of developing expansive business schemes was eager to raise a great deal of money for the transplantation program and hoped to strike it rich himself. A patient whose pretransplant personality was cautious and compulsive showed extreme care in regulating his activities as a survivor. Two who had been extraverted and gregarious developed new relationships and entertained at a rapid pace.

The Prednisone requirement of 15–60 mg per day posed a number of problems for survivors. Some noted difficulties with concentration, emotional lability, and irritability. All experienced some difficulty controlling their weight, and some have had to follow restricted diets. One man suffered a spontaneous fracture of a thoracic vertebra because of decalcification secondary to steroids. Although the side effects of steroids were at times annoying and frustrating to the survivors, they did not assume major proportions in most cases. None of the survivors experienced psychotic reactions, steroid or otherwise, although these reactions were seen in four of the nine patients who died postoperatively without ever leaving the hospital. Three of these patients who became psychotic have been described in a previous paper.[6] Since then there has been one more case of paranoid psychosis and one of organic brain syndrome secondary to poor cerebral perfusion, which ultimately cleared.

The Death of a Fellow Survivor

Four of the 11 transplant survivors described in this paper had died by the time of the paper's completion. Survival following transplantation for these four patients ranged from approximately 5 to 21 months. Although two of the four families suffered severe grief reactions because of the central role the patient had played in his family, none expressed regret that transplantation had occurred. There was marked emphasis on the special quality of the "extra time" the patient had received as a result of transplantation. Members of one patient's family expressed anger that the physicians had not been able to keep the patient alive longer; the wife of a second patient openly expressed her feeling that a "less worthy" patient (who was doing very well) should have died instead of her husband.

When a fellow survivor died, remaining patients tended to avoid discussion among themselves but actively sought out members of the transplant team to talk over "the cause of death." An effort has been made to notify other patients of the death before public announcement is made, and this has provided an opportunity to help them and their families with feelings of fear and loss.

Each surviving patient typically protects himself emotionally by developing, after a few days, theories about the death which make him different from the deceased. "He smoked (or drank) a lot." "He didn't exercise enough, but I do." "He died of something not related to the transplant." Each of the reasons expressed has an element of truth, but each also serves an obvious protective function for the patient who remains.

While families of heart recipients who died before leaving the hospital generally have broken off contact with the transplant team within a matter of weeks, families of survivors have continued to keep in touch and often describe themselves as "still part of the transplant program," even if the patient dies following discharge.

Summary

Pretransplant screening and counseling of potential cardiac transplant recipients enables the transplant team to predict and to influence the subsequent psychosocial adjustment of transplant survivors. Patients who receive extended family support for the decision for transplantation, who are able to discuss their awareness of pending death, and who have specific uses for the "extra time" gained by transplantation tend to have the best psychosocial adjustment if they become transplant survivors.

References

1. Abram, H. S. The psychiatrist, the treatment of chronic renal failure, and the prolongation of life: II. *American Journal of Psychiatry* **126**:157–167, 1969.
2. Abram, H. S., and Wadlington, W. Selection of patients for artificial and transplanted organs. *Annals of Internal Medicine* **69**:615–620, 1968.

3. Fellner, C. H., & Marshall, J. R. Twelve kidney donors. *JAMA* **206**:2703–2707, 1968.

4. Glaser, B. G., & Strauss, A. L. *Awareness of dying.* Chicago: Aldine, 1965. Pp. 1–305.

5. Kimball, C. P. Psychological responses to the experience of open heart surgery. *American Journal of Psychiatry* **126**:348–359, 1969.

6. Lunde, D. T. Psychiatric complications of heart transplants. *American Journal of Psychiatry* **126**:369–373, 1969.

X

The Crisis of Treatment: Stresses on Staff

Health care professionals enjoy many rewards for their work in terms of intellectual stimulation, social status, and a sense of self-worth based on accomplishment and service to others. However, regular interaction with seriously ill people can be emotionally as well as physically taxing. In addition, certain medical situations in which the staff cannot fulfill their primary role as healers necessitate personal and professional reevaluation and adaptation. In this section we examine some of the special stresses medical staff encounter, how they cope with them, and the implications for patient care.

In the first article Susan Quinby and Norman Bernstein examine the experiences of nurses in a unit for seriously burned children, in particular, the severe challenge posed to their self-image as healers and the process of readjustment in response to this challenge. Because of the nature of burn treatment, with its painful dressing changes and debridement procedures, nurses frequently found themselves inflicting pain rather than providing comfort for their young patients. In many cases even the hope of eventually returning the child to a normal healthy life (which might justify the painful therapeutic measures) was denied them because of the likelihood of permanent disfigurement. When the children's screams of pain and anger provoked angry feelings in the nurses, they felt even more guilty.

Over several months nurses on the unit developed a combination of coping strategies to handle the emotional upset their work involved. They relinquished their idealistic and perfectionistic goals in favor of more realistic ones. They learned to use denial constructively (for example, to ignore permanent disfigurement and concentrate on a patient's assets), to derive satisfaction from having met the challenge of a difficult job, to use humor to ease the tension, to accept their own feelings (such as temporary depression or anger) as natural human reactions, and to find support in the strong group feeling which developed among the unit staff. Nurses' projection of blame for imperfect outcome onto family members or onto other medical personnel involved in the patient's care lessened their own feelings of responsibility and guilt somewhat. In general, those who found workable solutions for their internal conflicts felt new strength and integrity in their ability to appraise more realistically the inherent problems in their situation and to define their own contribution in an acceptable way.

Another environment which presents staff with special problems is the intensive care unit. As we have seen in part VII, patients are often disturbed by the high-pressure crisis atmosphere and the omnipresence of complex machinery, but there are difficulties for the staff of these units as well. In the second article Donald Hay and Donald Oken focus on the stressful aspects of ICU nursing; they look at how nurses cope with these stresses and suggest some administrative changes to facilitate healthy adaptation. The constant threat and frequent reality of death, and the need to continue full nursing care and involvement with patients who have no hope of surviving, or who are in an unconscious limbo where life is maintained only by machines—all these force nurses to confront their own feelings about death on a daily basis. The repetitive routine of close observation (e.g., taking vital signs every 15 minutes), the constant alertness required to handle complex machinery and procedures, the heavy work load, and the frequent acute emergencies make the job extremely demanding.

In the interpersonal realm nurses must act as mediators and coordinators in maintaining smooth relations among the many people who come into the unit.[4] They deal with distraught families, frightened patients, and doctors who often cope with their own distress at losing a patient by directing their anger and frustration at the nearest nurse, or by abdicating their responsibility and leaving the nurse to take charge and inform the family. All these demands are made on the nurses, but very little support is offered them. Seldom do they even have the satisfaction of seeing a patient fully recovered.

The most common defensive approaches the nurses use are to deny the disagreeable aspects of their work, and to limit their emotional involvement. Most of the nurses derive some support from the strong group ties which usually develop. Hay and Oken propose group meetings as an arena for ventilating and sharing feelings and strengthening the group as a source of emotional support. They also suggest measures to bolster nurses' self-esteem and counteract the sense of frustration and inadequacy that ICU duty generates. Having a doctor on duty full time who can carry some of the responsibility for crisis decisions and provide advice and support to the nursing staff, having a private lounge near the ICU for temporary "escape" and recovery, and providing brief rotations to non-ICU posts could all ease the pressure under which the ICU nurse must function. Gardam[1] points out the value of daily teaching rounds and other forms of continuing education in building nurses' confidence in their own knowledge and medical judgment and in their ability to handle the heavy responsibility incumbent in ICU duty.

Studies of other settings in which medical personnel deal on a regular basis with chronically or terminally ill patients raise some similar issues. On cancer units which serve patients who no longer have much hope of remission or cure doctors and nurses often feel a sense of failure and inadequacy. Doctors may deal with these feelings by retreating from the patient, limiting their visits, and focusing on their research interests where they can find intellectual rewards and some emotional immunity.[2] When doctors use distancing as their main coping strategy, they shift the responsibility for the patient's emotional health to the attending nurses. Klagsbrun (chapter 17) found that this behavior was one of the chief sources of complaints by nurses. Only after discussion revealing the essentially adaptive nature of this strategy could the nurses recognize the doctor's need for such defenses and accept their own role as mediator. Through group meetings with a psychiatrist the staff gained new insight into patient needs and learned to interpret and respond to those needs more effectively. As was the case for the ICU nurses, group meetings served as a valuable source of emotional support and an appropriate place for ventilating and resolving the nurses' feelings in response to the many demands made on them.

The hemodialysis unit is another specialized environment which presents the staff with some unusual stresses. Because of patients' total dependence on the unit, they often find it difficult to express their feelings openly for fear of alienating the staff (see part VIII). The staff in turn must deal with their own sense of responsibility and guilt for their role in deciding which patients will be accepted for this life-saving treatment.[3] When patients are not accepted, the staff quickly withdraw from further involvement. Unit personnel have a tendency to develop rather high expectations of patients in the program, pushing them to prove their worthiness and thereby justify the staff's decision to admit them.

Because a life of dependence on dialysis is fraught with difficulties, medical staff are likely to experience some of the same ambivalence the patients feel (see Abram, chapter 20). They may deal with this by denying that the patients are still seriously ill, by ignoring the fact that dialysis has not provided a real cure, or, in other cases, by overindulging the patient in his remaining sources of pleasure in an attempt to compensate for his misfortune.[3] Just as greater awareness of the patient's problems and coping strategies are essential in helping him meet the crisis of serious illness, staff must look at their own reactions and recognize the most appropriate ways of dealing with the psychological demands of their work.

References

1. Gardam, J. F. Nursing stresses in the intensive care unit (Letters to the editor). *Journal of the American Medical Association,* 1969, **208,** 2337–2338.
2. Janes, R. G., & Weisz, A. E. Psychiatric liaison with a cancer research center. *Comprehensive Psychiatry,* 1970, **11,** 336–345.
3. Kaplan de-Nour, A., & Czaczkes, J. W. Emotional problems and reactions of the medical team in a chronic hemodialysis unit. *Lancet,* 1968, **2,** 987–991.
4. Vreeland, R., & Ellis, G. L. Stresses on the nurse in an intensive-care unit. *Journal of the American Medical Association,* 1969, **208,** 332–334.

25

Identity Problems and the Adaptation of Nurses to Severely Burned Children

SUSAN QUINBY and NORMAN R. BERNSTEIN

The challenge involved medically and psychologically in caring for burned children appears to be unique. Although some of the problems are the same as those usually experienced by both the patients and staff of a general hospital, caring for burned children is quite special in that it encompasses a wide range of medical and surgical procedures and involves the psychological issues of trauma, separation, isolation, threat of death, chronic pain, repeated surgery, and protracted stressful hospitalization. Permanent individual and family changes of lifelong importance frequently ensue as a consequence of these injuries.[1] When a child is severely burned and disfigurement is inevitable, the staff wonders what kind of a life he can have.

Although the circumstances associated with the care of burned children affect any individual who is professionally or personally involved with them, we feel that these factors had particular relevance for the nurses in our study. The nurses provide most of the child's care,

SUSAN QUINBY, M.A. • Director of Psychology Training, Worcester Youth Guidance Center, Worcester, Massachusetts. NORMAN R. BERNSTEIN, M.D. • Director of Psychiatry, Shriners Burns Institute, Boston, Massachusetts.

Reprinted from *American Journal of Psychiatry,* July 1971, **128** (1), 58–63. Copyright 1971, the American Psychiatric Association.

their contact is closer and more continuous than that of any other individual, and they function as intermediaries between the child and his environment, whether it be medical or familial. We also felt that the situation presented these young women with an unusually intense and demanding challenge to their personal and professional identities.[2] Their value systems, including their images of themselves as alleviators of pain and effective mother figures, were threatened in the course of their work. They were also beset by the conflict between their personal knowledge of the importance of attractive appearance and the necessity to deny this as significant in an attempt to sustain hope for the children and optimism about their future as disfigured individuals.

We studied the adjustment of the nurses over a one-year period, from the time they first started work in a newly established hospital devoted exclusively to the treatment of burned children. The nurses were seen for semistructured, open-ended, tape-recorded interviews shortly after their orientation period and again approximately a year later (or at the time of their termination if they left sooner). Some limited testing of attitudes toward disfigurement was done initially. Meetings with psychiatric staff members were held twice a week and continued throughout the year, and on-the-ward observations were carried out on an unscheduled basis during the same period.

In focusing on the nurses' psychodynamic adaptation we did not intend to slight the presence of complex problems related to the establishment of the hospital itself. However, we felt that the most significant adaptive process was directed toward the nurses' working out a modus vivendi between the demands and gratifications of a stressful life experience and their achievement of an equilibrium between what they accepted as ego-enhancing and what they rejected as devaluative or destructive of their concepts of themselves as nurses and as individuals. The process of developing a successfully adaptive identity approximated the sequence described below.

Idealized Expectation

In initial interviews the beginning nurses expressed enthusiasm about participating in a new and truly grand endeavor that included a service to society as well as to individual patients. Their image of their role was that of "supernurse"—one with an avant-garde status as a consequence of the high level of technical competence and professional specialization required in this field. They envisioned themselves in wide-ranging roles as counselors of mothers, expert consultants to outside groups interested in care of the burned, participants in research projects of various kinds, and psychotherapists to individual patients who were suffering from emotional trauma. Although they expected to work hard and often mentioned the possibility of depressive reactions in response to the demanding aspects of the job, they clearly did not anticipate that their own feelings would become a central problem.

The nurses' pervasively positive and confident expectations contrasted with opinions and reactions they heard from numerous sources. Without exception, every nurse interviewed mentioned *dramatic* negative reactions from friends and from family when she spoke to others about her decision to work with burned children.[3] This was not confined to nonprofessionals. Several nurses reported that fellow nurses and doctors voiced the same opinion. The work was considered not only discouraging but also horrible and repulsive. Thus commitment to this kind of work involved accepting a personal challenge; the nurse was putting the strength of her convictions and value judgments to the test in the face of strong opposition.

During later interviews, after considerable bedside experience, all of the nurses still remarked on outsiders' reactions to their work. Some admiration was reported, but in the main they felt that there was no one with whom they could discuss their experiences. "They don't really understand" or "It upsets people to hear about it" were frequent comments. Several nurses indicated that, with the exception of a fiancé or husband who would listen to them almost as a therapist would, they just did not talk to anyone about their work in other than the most superficial terms. One can comment on the difference between this particular experience and that of nurses who work in other arduous situations such as on emergency wards or on terminal cancer wards.

After several months there was a striking contrast between the earliest anticipations and later evaluations of the job. Some nurses had difficulty in even responding to questions about gratifications from their work, as though it were an alien thought. There was often a long pause, followed by "Well, there must be *something* . . . !" Sadness was obvious in this reaction, as well as puzzlement and the loss involved in the dissolution of idealized hopes.

The nurses' early expectations about the mothers of the burned children need special mention. Initially, nurses often spoke of the "disadvantaged," "disorganized," or just plain "poor" families the patients were expected to come from and the difficulties in discipline and understanding this might produce. Often there was a patronizing tone to these comments and an expectation of humble gratitude from the families. The nurses anticipated that the mothers of burned children would feel guilty and abashed and that the nurses would help them with these feelings. They characterized a "bad" mother as one who showed no interest in her child, but they also often mentioned the "interfering" mother, who questioned everything and would not follow advice. However, they expected that these problems would be solved or minimized by rational explanation and educational sessions with the mothers.

In brief, the nurses began with mixed expectations. Reasonably, they expected professional approval, but they also anticipated receiving professional and nonprofessional admiration and interest, in spite of evidence to the contrary from their friends and colleagues. They expected hard work involving them in many emotion-laden situations with which they had had little experience or training, but they did not expect to be seriously upset or threatened about their personal worth and integrity. They confidently looked forward to being accepted as lovable authority figures by both the children and their parents.

Confrontation and Confusion

The hospital began functioning gradually. The first few patients were admitted for rehabilitation, plastic surgery, release of contractures, rebuilding of ears, improvements in range of motion, and revision of scars. Everyone assumed that surgery would be successful in markedly improving the patients' appearance and functioning. All of the children had been hospitalized before, and although this did not necessarily lead to any greater ease in caring for them, they were already familiar with hospital procedures and tended to be rather surprised and pleased with many aspects of the new hospital, e.g., the abundance of toys and activities, the availability of nurses to play with or read to them, and the generally optimistic atmosphere.

The arrival of the first acute patients and the aftermath of surgery with the rehabilitative patients marked a point of change. At this stage unfamiliarity with the emergency care techniques made the nurses feel additionally incompetent and anxious. Painful dressing changes and debridement became a cruel task. The children invariably screamed, and often expressed their fear and anger toward the nurse in accusations of "You're killing me" and "I hate you." The nurses vividly described the buildup of anxiety in themselves and in the children as one child after another was "done." When asked during interviews what was the one thing that was the worst about their work, by far the most common answer was "dressing changes—the screaming, it really gets me."

Although the nurses expected to cause pain in the process of treatment and anticipated occasional outbursts of anger, the situation with burned children was an intense and protracted assault. The nurses were exhausted by the repetitiveness of the stress and frustrated by their inability to successfully alter the child's reaction, but most of all they seemed ashamed and guilty about their anger at the children's hostility and uncooperativeness. They very reluctantly acknowledged that even if they had time available, they felt unwilling to spend it doing the pleasant, extra activities they had previously valued—individualized playing or talking with a child. They preferred to escape from a child with whom they had previously gone through an abrasive session of conflict, mutual hostility, and frustration.

Although the nurses brought up problems with the behavior of individual patients at this time, most of the complaints centered around deficiencies in organization and equipment. This was true even in relation to the dressing changes referred to previously. Their efforts centered on getting soundproof treatment rooms, altering the timing of dressing changes, or evolving better "teamwork" in the procedures. Some of this was certainly justified, but it was also a distancing and displacing process by which the nurses attempted to avoid closeness to the patient and to forestall recognition of their failure to live up to their high expectations of themselves as individually effective nurses.

Distancing was also apparent in instances in which a nurse was struggling to resolve her relationship with one of the children. There was a tendency to use technical terminology in describing the child and his behavior. All sorts of unpleasant or annoying actions were referred to as "regression" or "acting out." One boy's abusive and threatening language toward the nurses was termed "paranoia," and there was speculation as to whether those infants or toddlers who did not respond positively to a nurse's cuddling or playfulness might be "autistic" or "mentally retarded." Nurses regularly reacted to some children with frustrated anger and attempted to rationalize or to intellectualize the problems by using psychiatric language or blaming the family's child-rearing practices. They finally acknowledged defeat by referring the problem to the psychiatrist to "cure." Many nurses reported bad dreams during this phase.

Ambivalent Identification

During this stage the nurses were engaged in relating to disfigured children in ways that were new and difficult for them. They uneasily faced the questions about their own identity that these interactions raised.[4,5] The techniques and routines of nursing care had been mastered, although these were not accompanied by the expected gratifying feeling of accomplishment. Problems in the management of hostile impulses, feelings of rejection, and guilt over producing pain continued to be pervasive, but they were now approached in different ways. Sometimes it came up directly and with considerable anguish: "All I do is hurt him. How can he possibly like me—or trust me?" Simultaneously, many nurses began to question the extent of pain actually suffered by a child during dressing changes or immersion in the hydrotherapy tank. They needed to decide how "real" the pain was in order to respond in a way that was justifiable. If the pain was genuinely severe, short rests or breaks in the procedure were necessary; if not, one might just as well go ahead and get it over with. "Faking" or dramatizing warranted firmer measures to encourage the child to control himself and "not to act like a baby." On the rare occasions when a child did not react to pain, there was sharp concern about what was wrong with him and why he was not acting as though he were suffering. One notion that many nurses clung to hopefully was the idea that "they really know we're helping them even if they don't act that way and even if we have to hurt them." This was a tenable and supportive idea as long as it did not conflict with their feelings that despite all of the treatment, the children would still look abnormal and would never fully recover.

Several separate issues converged at this stage. "If I cause pain and if I am angry at a sick helpless child, how can I still see myself as a good nurse and a good person and a competent professional?" These young women agonized over the kinds of lives disfigured children could have.

The nurses could incorporate many conflicting feelings about themselves and about the children into the framework of an eventually constructive and benevolent outcome despite pain, anger, and disappointment. However, if the end result was a damaged product, the worth of all the effort and struggles could be undermined. The importance of appearance and of the limitations imposed upon the life of a disfigured person were underlying issues in intense, prolonged emotional exchanges. One clear-cut example was that of a two-year-old child admitted to the hospital with such severe burns that it was obvious that, if he survived, his existence could be expected to be one of lifelong agony as a consequence of a face so distorted that it was barely recognizable as human. He had no ears, a scalp open to the skull, a hole for a nose, charred eyelids and lips, and only his thumbs remaining on his hands. One nurse said: "As a person you wish they'd go fast and go quietly. I'm just glad I'm leaving, and I won't have to see him when he goes home. You can talk to me until you're blue in the face, but you can't convince me that he's going to be a happy, well-adjusted kid—but you don't really know, maybe he'll be a genius. But as a person you wish he'd go; as a nurse you have to do everything you can to save him."

Less intense variations of this ambivalence occurred with children whose disfigurement was not so overwhelming. There was considerable projection of devaluative feelings upon "outsiders," i.e., anyone the child came into contact with outside the hospital and who recoiled in horror. There was overidentification in some instances in which a nurse would, to some extent, act out the resentment, humiliation, and despair that the child presumably felt in response to his experiences outside the hospital. Nurses now showed a determined, almost compulsive, effort to recognize and praise any and all positive features in a disfigured child's appearance and behavior.

"Realistic" Resolution

After several months, it was possible to regard many of the most difficult problems as a thing of the past. Distancing by means of time and categorization seemed to be quite useful. Acute difficulties with particular children continued, but mutual reassurance could be accomplished by remarking, "Remember how awful so-and-so was? You'd hardly know he was the same boy" or "Remember the trouble we had with that child? Nothing could be that bad." There were few pessimistic discussions about a child's future, almost as if by mutual agreement to suppress such thinking. Interest and involvement narrowed, with greater concentration on technical issues and limited goals. The notions that many of the nurses had entertained about playing a significant and meaningful role in the child's long-term adjustment and life outside the hospital had largely been abandoned. This was partly due to practical considerations: They simply did not have the time to accompany a child when he returned to school, or to make home visits, or even to engage during working hours in planning or training sessions related to school and home arrangements.

However, subjective factors were also involved. Even the most optimistic rescue fantasy could not be maintained in the face of obvious reality: No matter how thoroughly explained a child's disfigurement was, strangers still reacted adversely; no matter how close and trusting a relationship a nurse might have with a child, it would not make up to him the loss of a previously attractive or unblemished appearance. The hostility the nursing staff had previously displayed toward outsiders was less evident. Instead, there seemed to be more annoyance focused on specific incidents or individuals, such as allegations that local clinics or health services had not provided follow-up care. The children's mothers were the recipients of the most intense and pervasive displaced feelings. They were blamed for lapses in physical treatment, for keeping children out of school and away from social contacts, for not changing dressings properly, and generally for not providing the ideal acceptance, guidance, and perfect home environment that the children deserved. These criticisms had some basis in reality, but they ignored the obvious fact that most of the children come from multiproblem homes with limited resources.

This was a stage of outward calm in which unresolved issues had been laid aside and internal conflicts were managed by an externalized distinction between the "good guys" and the "bad guys" surrounding the children.

Commitment and Acceptance

It was surprising to discover, after the hospital had been functioning for approximately a year, that despite the stresses and disappointments of their work and the repetitive crises related to the well-advertised departure of a few nurses, 75% of the nurses originally hired were still on the staff. Assuming that originally there was a self-selection process that determined, to some extent, the special characteristics of these nurses as a group who were perhaps more professionally ambitious, with a greater tendency toward counterphobic reactions, with a greater need to prove themselves, and with a more pervasive interest in the psychosocial implications of nursing, this was unexpected in comparison to the turnover rate in general hospitals. Extremely difficult challenges have been met and integrated as contributions to ego strength, a maturing identity, and feelings of self-esteem.

In the course of long and repeated hospitalization of these children, the nurses gained a sense of the continuity of life through tragedy and crisis to recovery and reintegration, with a growing acceptance of the unreality of idealistic and perfectionistic goals. This acceptance occurred simultaneously toward themselves and toward the children and their families. Increasing flexibility in relationships developed between the nurses and with the patients and their families. Individual professional nursing styles crystallized. Temporary states of depression became more accepted, as when a nurse had "just had it" with a patient or had blown up at an exasperating, overwrought mother. Denial was used constructively in unalterable or hopeless situations. When the nurses demonstrated pleasure at a child's improved appearance, this often involved considerable blocking out of negative stimuli: A disfigured little girl, all dressed up and beribboned for her first trip home after a long and trying hospitalization was sent off by the nurses with many exclamations of "how pretty you look," despite the distorting effect of severe scarring and contractures of her neck. A 12-year-old boy, returning to the hospital for further rehabilitative work was greeted with "Hey, you look great!" despite the fact that his entire face and part of his body were covered with a network of raised, reddened scar tissue. The sincerity of these remarks was obvious, as was the unlikelihood of their being uttered by others having a different relationship with the child. There was a pervasive group feeling of having been through great trials together. Some disillusionment and cynical appreciation of the discrepancies between promise and fulfillment were shared by the nurses who remained. They were campaign veterans who "knew the score," and could reminisce together about past experiences—both pleasant and unpleasant. They had taken their measure and had come through.

However, as greater closeness and empathy with the badly burned and emotionally distressed children became possible for them, so did the painful awareness of the future suffering the children would undergo; an increasingly subtle and selective use of denial to maintain an appropriate emotional distance was necessary. A new equilibrium came into being in which humor was frequently used. Some blame continued to be projected onto clinics, families, and professionals, always with a kernel of justification but also serving the function of relieving the nurses of some of the responsibility for imperfect results. Tolerance for *causing* pain while treating burned children was much greater, while sympathy and empathy were augmented and were less contaminated by the nurse's own frustration, guilt, or anxiety.

We do not imagine that this experience settled for these nurses all of their identification problems as nurses, young women, mother figures, or contributors to society. However, on the whole we felt that whatever was lost in terms of unfulfilled expectations and fantasies was replaced by the capacity to obtain gratification from a realistic contribution to bettering the condition of life for the children and their families and by enhancing the nurse's own sense of worth and of integrity.

References

1.   Dembo, T., Leviton, G. L., Wright, B. A. Adjustment to misfortune—a problem of social-psychological rehabilitation. *Artificial Limbs* 3 (2):4–63, 1956.
2.   Etzioni, A. (Ed.). *The semiprofessions and their organization.* New York: Free Press, 1969.
3.   Goffman, I. *Stigma.* Englewood Cliffs, New Jersey: Prentice-Hall, 1963.
4.   Hanks, J. R., & Hanks, L. M. The physically handicapped in certain nonoccidental societies. *Journal of Social Issues* 4 (4):11–20, 1948.
5.   MacGregor, F. C. Some psycho-social problems associated with facial deformities. *American Sociological Review* 16:629–638, 1951.

26

The Psychological Stresses of Intensive Care Unit Nursing

DONALD HAY and DONALD OKEN

Much has been written about the stressful psychological experience of being a patient in an Intensive Care (ICU) or other special care unit.[1-5] Less well recognized, however, are the problems posed for those who work in an ICU that provides the complex nursing care required by critically ill, often dying, patients. Notable exceptions include the contributions of Vreeland and Ellis[6] and of Gardam.[7]

The quality of a patient's care, and, hence, outcome, depends greatly upon the people providing that care, and the effectiveness of the latter is a function of their psychological state no less than of their technical expertise. This has special meaning for the ICU patient, whose very life hangs upon the care provided by the nursing staff. Yet, in this special environment, the psychological burdens imposed upon the nurse are extraordinary. Her situation resembles, in many ways, that of the soldier serving with an elite combat group.

Our understanding derives from the experience of one of us (DH) working directly as a member of the nursing staff of a 10-bed university

DONALD HAY, M.D. ● Medical and Clinical Director, Eastern Montana Regional Mental Health Center, Miles City, Montana. DONALD OKEN, M.D. ● Professor and Chairman, Department of Psychiatry, Upstate Medical Center, State University of New York, Syracuse, New York. Supported in part by Training Grant MH-06525 from the National Institute of Mental Health.

Reprinted from *Psychosomatic Medicine,* 1972, **34**(2), 109–118.

hospital ICU over a period of approximately one year, plus multiple interviews and informal contacts with ICU nurses.* From these observations, we have developed some insights into the nature of the nurses' experience and the methods they develop to handle it. These, we believe, provide useful clues for lessening the stressful nature of the experience, and hence benefit the nurses and (through them) their patients.

The ICU Environment

A stranger entering an ICU is at once bombarded with a massive array of sensory stimuli,[3] some emotionally neutral but many highly charged. Initially, the great impact comes from the intricate machinery, with its flashing lights, buzzing and beeping monitors, gurgling suction pumps, and whooshing respirators. Simultaneously, one sees many people rushing around busily performing lifesaving tasks. The atmosphere is not unlike that of the tension-charged strategic war bunker. With time, habituation occurs, but the ever-continuing stimuli decrease the overload threshold and contribute to stress at times of crisis.

As the newness and strangeness of the unit wears off, one increasingly becomes aware of a host of perceptions with specific stressful emotional significance. Desperately ill, sick, and injured human beings are hooked up to that machinery. And, in addition to mechanical stimuli, one can discern moaning, crying, screaming, and the last gasps of life. Sights of blood, vomitus and excreta, exposed genitalia, mutilated wasting bodies, and unconscious and helpless people assault the sensibilities. Unceasingly, the ICU nurse must face these affect-laden stimuli with all the distress and conflict that they engender. As part of her daily routine, the nurse must reassure and comfort the man who is dying of cancer; she must change the dressings of a decomposing, gangrenous limb; she must calm the awakening disturbed "overdose" patient; she must bathe the genitalia of the helpless and comatose; she must wipe away the

---

* While our detailed observations were made on a single ICU, superficial contact with several other such units, which have many features in common, leads us to believe that our conclusions have significant generalizability. However, there may be some significant differences from other types of specialized units such as coronary care units, neurosurgical ICUs, transplant and dialysis units, etc.

bloody stool of the gastrointestinal bleeder; she must comfort the anguished young wife who knows her husband is dying. It is hard to imagine any other situation that involves such intimacy with the frightening, repulsive, and forbidden. Stimuli are present to mobilize literally every conflictual area at every psychological developmental level.

But there is more: There is something uncanny about the-picture the patients present. Many are neither alive or dead. Most have "tubes in every orifice." Their sounds and actions (or inaction) are almost non-human. Bodily areas and organs, ordinarily unseen, are openly exposed or deformed by bandages. All of this directly challenges the definition of being human, one's most fundamental sense of ego integrity, for nurse as well as patient. Though consciously the nurse quickly learns to accept this surrealism, she is unremittingly exposed to these multiple threats to the stability of her body boundaries, her sense of self, and her feelings of humanity and reality.

To all this is added a repetitive contact with death. And, if exposure to death is merely frequent, that to dying is constant. The ICU nurse thus quickly becomes adept at identifying the signs and symptoms that foretell a downhill trend for her patient. This becomes an awesome addition to the burden of the nurse who has been caring for the patient and must *continue* to do so, knowing his outcome.

The Work Load and Its Demands

If the sense of drama and frightfulness is what most forcefully strikes the outsider, what the experienced nurse points to, para-doxically, is the incessant repetitive routine. For each patient, vital signs must be monitored, commonly at 15-minute intervals, sometimes more often. Central venous pressures must be measured, tracheas suctioned, urimeters emptied and measured, intravenous infusions changed, EKG monitor patterns interpreted, respirators checked, hypothermia blankets adjusted, etc., etc. And, every step must be charted. The nurse begins to feel like a hamster on a treadmill: She finishes the required tasks on one patient just in time to start them on another; and when these are com-pleted she is already behind in doing the same tasks all over again on the first, constantly aware of her race with the clock. A paradox soon becomes apparent. Nowhere more than in the ICU is a *good* nurse expected to make observations about her patient's condition, to interpret subtle changes and use judgment to take appropriate action. But often, the ICU nurse is so unremittingly involved in collecting and charting information that she has little time to interpret it adequately.

The work load is formidable—even in periods of relative calm. Many tasks, which elsewhere would be performed by nurse's aides, require special care in the ICU and become the lot of the ICU nurse. Changing a bed in an ICU may require moving a desperately ill, comatose patient while watching EKG leads, respirator hoses, urinary and intravenous catheters, etc. Moreover, the nurse must maintain detailed records.

Night shifts, weekends, and holidays all means less work on other floors. Only urgent or fundamental procedures are performed. But, in an ICU, emergency is routine: There is no surcease—no holidays. In fact, the regular recovery room in our hospital shuts down on weekends and holidays so that patients must be sent to the ICU after emergency surgery. It is not rare, on a weekend, to see several stretchers with these patients interposed between the fully occupied beds of the ICU, leaving the nurses with barely time enough to suction patients and keep them alive.

The quantity and variety of complex technical equipment poses tremendous demands on the knowledge and expertise of the nurse.[6,7] Because of this and the nature of her tasks, temporarily floating in nurses from elsewhere when staff is short provides little in the way of help; indeed, this may even prove a hindrance. Yet, ICU nurses are fully able to fill in elsewhere when staff shortages occur; and they are not infrequently asked to do so, leaving the ICU understaffed.

The emergency situation provides added work. Although an ICU's routine is another floor's emergency, obviously there are frequent situations of acute crisis, such as cardiac arrest. These require the nurse's full attention and prevent her from continuing her regular tasks on her other patients. A few remaining nurses must watch and calm all other patients, complete as many of their regular observations and treatments as possible, and prevent other emergencies. Meanwhile, the nurses assisting at the emergency are called upon not only to do things rapidly but to make immediate and accurate decisions that oftentimes include determining the priority of several emergencies.[6]

Habituation is both inevitable and necessary if the nurse is not to work in an exhausted state of chronic crisis. Yet, she must maintain an underlying alertness to discern and respond to cues which have special meaning. This is like the mother who hears the faint cry of her baby over the commotion of a party.

Nor is the work without its physical dangers, and the nurses know this. It is impossible to take fully adequate isolation precautions against infections because of time pressures and the bodily intimacy required to provide the needed level of care. Portable X rays are sometimes taken with inadequately shielded nurses holding immobile patients in proper positioning. Heavy comatose patients must be lifted. Sharp needles, scalpels, etc., must be handled rapidly. Electric equipment must be moved, adjusted, and attached. Physical assaults on nurses by a delirious patient, though infrequent, can and do occur.

There are occasions also when distraught relatives misinterpret a situation, feel that their loved one is getting inadequate care and become verbally—and sometimes physically—abusive. The roots of these more dramatic misunderstandings lie in more general problems about visitors. On other floors, visiting hours occur daily at specified times, but in the ICU there can be no such routinized schedule. Close relatives are allowed to see the patient at any time of the day or night. Though restricted to a brief (commonly 5-minute) period, their presence soon becomes a burden. In his constant inquiries about the patient's condition and prognosis, the relative is asking for more than information. He is seeking reassurance and support.[6,8] The nurse may wish to respond at this deeper level, but usually she cannot, because she has tasks that require more immediate attention. The relative, feeling rebuffed, begins to critically scrutinize the nurse's every action. With so much to be upset about, he is prone to jump to unwarranted conclusions. While many visitors see the nurses as "angels of mercy," others develop a projection of their worst fears. Seeing a nurse spend more time with another patient, he may feel his loved one is not getting adequate attention. Or, he may see blood, vomitus, or excreta soiling the patient's bed and misinterpret this as an indication of poor care, not appreciating the nurse's preoccupation with lifesaving activities. Moreover the nurse has little escape from hovering relatives: She has "no place to hide."

Doctors and Administrators

Visitors are not the only ones who cause problems. Some of the very people who might be expected to provide substantial support add to the stresses on the nurse. The potentially fatal outcome in the gravely ill ICU patients tends to stimulate feelings of frustration, self-doubt, and guilt in their physicians. The ways he deals with these may have major consequences for the nurse. He may, for example, use projection and behave in a surly, querulous manner. He may bolster his self-esteem by becoming imperious and demand that the nurses "wait on" him.* He may also rely on avoidance as a way of distancing himself from his feelings about his seeming failure as a lifesaver. Though the nurse must remain on the unit for almost her entire shift, the physician can make good use of his prerogatives to move about freely. Especially at the time of a patient's death, the physician seems to have a way of not being present; the full burden of breaking the news and supporting the family through the acute grief reaction is left to the nurse to handle as best she can. Conversely, compensatory overzealousness may occur, and unnecessary heroic gestures be made to save someone beyond recovery. The physician may order special treatments and an unrealistic frequency of monitoring. The not uncommon incongruity of orders is especially revealing about this. A patient on "q15 minute" vital signs will have nothing done—and correctly so—when these deteriorate. Or, the physician will recognize the inappropriateness of frequent monitoring, yet insist on fruitless *emergency* attempts at resuscitation (e.g., a pacemaker) when death supervenes. This not only increases the nurse's work load but adds to her frustration by diverting her energies from patients who could be saved.

The physician's immediate availability is essential to the nurse. He is needed not merely for emergencies but for frequently updated changes in treatment orders, for advice—and for reassurance. Thus, whether his absence arises as a consequence of defenses, competing demands for his time, or merely ignorance of the need, the nurse suffers. This is especially prone to happen in situations where medical responsibility for each patient rests with the staff of a specialty service (e.g., medicine, surgery) headquartered elsewhere.

Similarly, the nurses often feel that they do not get much support from their administrative superiors who, they believe, fail to appreciate the realities of the ICU situation. ICUs and similar special facilities

---

* Another factor in this overdemanding behavior may be his sense of inadequacy and self-doubt if he is unfamiliar with the unit and its highly organized functions.[9] This may culminate in his issuing dictatorial orders and commands that are not commensurate with the realities of the situation.

have come into their own only in the past decade, and, as Gardam has pointed out,[7] a generation gap exists between ICU staff nurses and senior nurse administrators. As a consequence, nursing administrators find it difficult to recognize the unique characteristics of the ICU, and tend to consider it merely a slightly busier and more acute service whose needs can be met simply by a numerically larger staff. Often they seem to regard the complaints of a dissatisfied or battle-weary ICU nurse as a sign of emotional unfitness rather than as a basis for changes in policy or procedure.

Some of the anger felt toward these superiors is, certainly, scapegoating. This is particularly likely in regard to the ICU head nurse or nursing supervisor-instructor. Nurses in these positions are intrinsically in a difficult bind. While they may be arguing valiantly for the ICU in the front office, on the unit they must conscientiously implement the orders of their superiors. They become enmeshed in an assignment to two simultaneous, incompatible roles: the tough top sergeant and the loving mother. These dual roles resonate, in turn, with the ambivalent attitude of staff nurses (who, as predominantly young, single, incompletely emancipated women, are prone to develop a strongly ambivalent maternal transference to female supervisors). They are, moreover, readily available and sufficiently close in age and status to temper the transference and become permissible targets for hostility.

The Psychological Experience

We will now shift from a situational frame of reference to a psychological one and take a closer look at the concerns and feelings of ICU nurses. We will also examine the adaptive devices, individual and group, which they use to cope with their situation.

The work load, so great in its sheer quantity, is unusual also in its variety and the intricacy of its tasks as well as in the rapidity with which these must be performed. Great flexibility is required (which may partly explain why ICU nurses are predominantly in their early 20s).

Mistakes are, of course, inevitable. But, when every procedure is potentially lifesaving, any error may be life-endangering. Hence the ICU nurse lives chronically under a cloud of latent anxiety. The new nurse, particularly, begins to view the never-ending life-dependent tasks as a specter of potential mistakes and their imagined dreadful sequelae.

Some, of course, cannot shake this and soon arrange a transfer. The experienced nurse achieves a more realistic perspective, but a degree of residual uncertainty always remains, given the complexity of machines and procedures. Especially at times of stress, she too may become anxious. When this anxiety exceeds minimal levels, it reduces efficiency and decision-making capacity, inviting additional mistakes—the classic vicious circle.

When the inevitable error does occur, the nurse is in a dilemma. To make it public is likely to enhance her guilt and invite criticism. Moreover, it leads to the need to fill out an incident report, a further drain on her time and a potential blot on her record. Yet to fail to do so may compound the error by blocking corrective treatment. The experienced nurse develops a subtle adaptive compromise, reporting serious mistakes but fudging over inconsequential ones. In either case, she must live with her guilt.

The ICU nurse has much in which she can take great pride. Yet her self-esteem takes an awful beating in many ways. Her awareness of her mistakes, both real and exaggerated, is one such factor. Another is her repeated "failure." The ultimate goal of the health professions is to save lives; yet, frequently, her patients die. Nor do the dying patients or mourning relatives provide much source of gratification, as do patients on other floors who go home well. (Even the ICU major successes are usually still seriously ill and are merely transferred.) On the bulletin boards of other units there are warm, sentimental cards and notes of appreciation. In the ICU, the cards are of a different and macabre quality. They say: "Thank you. You did all you could."

Further, the deaths provide a situation of repetitive object-loss, the intensity of which parallels the degree to which the nurse has cathected her patient. The intimacy afforded by the amount and frequency of direct personal contact, involving some of the most private aspects of life, promotes this attachment. This is further enhanced when the patient is conscious and verbal, since he is then so obviously human. Young patients are easily identified with friends and spouses—or with the self, stimulating anxiety about one's own vulnerability. In this country, with its cultural premium on youth, the death of a young patient tends to be regarded as inherently more tragic. Older patients may become transference objects of parental or grandparental figures.

All these warm personal attachments obviously provide great comfort for patients and family and make the job worthwhile. But they expose the nurse to a sense of loss when the patient dies. The balance is a delicate one. With comatose patients, it is easy to limit emotional involvement and subsequent grief. But here, paradoxically, one often sees the nurse project vital qualities into her patient.*

The threat of object-loss is pervasive. The nurse simply must protect herself—from grief, anxiety, guilt, rage, exhausted overcommitment, overstimulation, and all the rest. She has no physical escape. But she can avoid, or at least attenuate, the meaning and emotional impact of her work.[10] For example, she may relate more to the machines than to the patient. And, it comes as a surprise to an outsider to observe routinely some of the nurses in the ICU joking and laughing. Even whistling and singing may be observed, phenomena which are inexplicable and unforgivable to distraught relatives. Some of this ebullience arises as a natural product of the friendly behavior of young people working closely together. But a major aspect is gross denial as a defense against their stressful situation. Schizoid withdrawal or a no-nonsense, businesslike manner (isolation) also are used, but cheerful denial is more common. The defensive and, at times, brittle nature of this response is especially evident at times of crisis. At a lull in procedures after a cardiac arrest, for example, giggling and outrageous joking of near hysterical proportion suddenly may supervene. Sometimes the blowup is in the form of anger. But, there are great constraints placed upon the expression of anger by the situation and the group.

The Group

The new ICU nurse experiences the trials of her early days on the job as a *rite de passage*. Some do not make it through. Those who do, learn that they have become members of a special, tightly knit group.† Naturally, they work together on a common job, sharing common experiences. But, there is far more to it than this. Most have volunteered. They have one of the most difficult jobs in the hospital.

---

* Sometimes this mechanism backfires in an interesting way. The nurse begins to project specific attributes onto the comatose patient. When he recovers and asserts his real personality, especially if this has unpleasant characteristics, she feels a sense of disappointment and betrayal.

† We have seen similar, though usually less intense, group formation among psychiatric nursing personnel, for some of the same reasons.

Nowhere else does a nurse so often literally save lives by her own direct actions. It stands to reason that nurses who operate special machines and perform special procedures for special patients must be special too! Rightfully, they take pride in their abilities and accomplishments. The very stressfulness of the job is a further source of pride, albeit with masochistic overtones. Like commandos or Green Berets, they have the toughest, dirtiest, most dangerous assignment; and they "accomplish the impossible."

Further cementing group ties are the conditions of the work. They carry on their duties in a common area, using common equipment.[6] In emergency situations particularly, they share the responsibility for each other's patients. Even in nonemergency situations there is a general factor of enforced interdependency. Routinely, for example, one girl must ask another to cover her patients when she goes for a meal. Here an unspoken but potent group norm becomes manifest. Refusal is impossible. Cooperation is absolutely essential for unit function. When a nurse returns from an absence, she may well find that only the most minimal monitoring has been carried out on her patient. No matter how justified its basis, she is likely to be irritated. Yet, group pressures for cooperation and the very fact that there is no time for anger on the job make it imperative to suppress or repress the hostility. These same forces inhibit the expressions of anger that arise inevitably during the course of everyday work when people are in regular close contact. In the total context, this ambivalent hostility serves to bind the group ties with still more intensity.

At the end of a shift of constant work and emotional turmoil, it is near impossible for the nurse to "turn it off" and return to normal pursuits. She needs to unwind. To do so requires the understanding ear of someone who knows what she has been through. Who, then, is a more logical choice of an off-duty companion than another ICU nurse? Thus, one finds much group social activity: parties, showers and just informal off-duty get-togethers. While these might provide an opportunity to express interpersonal hostility, they more often result in "bull sessions" of shared experiences and problems. Similar discussions take place at lunch or coffee breaks, to which they go preferentially with co-workers. These shared feelings feed back to enhance group ties further.

External forces further define the group. The ICU is typically located in an area away from other nursing units. Frequently ICU nurses wear scrub gowns or other protective devices to decrease contamination and soiling; thus they have a distinctive uniform. Very significant is the attitude of other nurses throughout the hospital. Many tend to regard ICU nurses with considerable ambivalence in which envy and projection play a part, and react to being treated as outsiders by retaliatory disregard, isolating the group further.

Group cohesiveness is a logical solution to the multiple practical problems on the job and provides essential emotional support. Being a part of a special group is a major advantage in bolstering the nurse's pride and strength. However, there are not so desirable consequences. The force of the group and the extent of its activities can become all-encompassing, taking over the roles of family and friends. Thus, it can interfere with personal autonomy and outside social relationships. The pressures of the job and group activities may limit healthy introspection. (This may have temporary adaptive value for the girl beset with life problems, or tangled in inner conflict, allowing her to retrench while thus losing herself. But obviously, this can be seriously maladaptive if pursued as a long-term escape.) Absence from the group due to a concurrent social activity may be seen unconsciously as disloyal by both the nurse and the group, though inevitably the familial and social aspect of the group will wear thin for the girl who has achieved maturity and seeks a life of her own. Yet the nurse who fails to use the group may find herself taking out the tensions of work on her family. She may let off steam to a boyfriend, a roommate, or a husband. But soon, she learns that this can strain the relationship since the person on the receiving end cannot know what it is like to work in the ICU.

Group loyalty reinforces work pressure in stimulating guilt about any absence. The nurse with a minor illness (or one suffering from "combat exhaustion") cannot, in good conscience, stay away as she should. This would increase the work load for her peers. If she does stay home, she cannot "rest easy." Nor, as described above, can she say no to a request to cover another girl's patients, even if she is already working at peak load. This would violate the group norms and threaten the shared fantasy of omnipotence linked to the concept of being special and to the defensive denial of anxiety about mistakes.

This same mechanism can work also to the collective detriment of the group. Like the individual nurse, the group self-destructively cannot say no to situations where its total work load is unrealistic. Paradoxically, the individual almost never can get the group to support protests about realistic problems or unfair exploitation so that changes can be made. Intragroup competitiveness and rivalry may play a part in this. The nurse who will not submerge constructive criticism to the group norm finds she must leave. Since many such nurses will be thoughtful, aggressive people with good ideas, leadership potential is drained away. The whole situation lends itself to perpetuating the status quo and to no recourse but permanent flight (i.e., resignation) when the pressures on an individual build to the point of intolerability.

Some Possible Solutions

From the foregoing, it seems obvious that a constructive approach will capitalize on the many positive aspects of the group process, while attenuating its pathological features. One excellent way to accomplish this is through regular group meetings devoted to exploring the work experience, especially its stressful aspects.[9] These discussions can provide: (a) an avenue for ventilating suppressed intragroup hostilities as well as shared gripes; (b) a recognition that fears, doubts, guilt, and uncertainty are shared, acceptable feelings; (c) the abreaction and working through of feelings aroused at times of stress but which cannot be expressed due to work demands; (d) the sharing of innovative ad hoc techniques which individuals have found helpful in dealing with problems arising on the job; (e) recognition of realistic superior abilities and their delineation from masochistic fantasies of omnipotence; (f) a realization that minor mistakes are ubiquitous and inevitable, leading to the detoxification of guilt and shame; and (g) the development of constructive solutions for problems and effective suggestions for communication to administration.

The person who leads these sessions must be experienced and psychologically sophisticated. Communication must be continually focused on the ICU situation rather than expanding into more general self-exploration; the interchange cannot be allowed to transcend limits that prevent comfortable working together between sessions. The leader cannot be a member of the ICU administrative hierarchy, nor of the staff group itself, yet he must have a genuine understanding of the work. In fact, he must spend some time regularly on the unit to retain his awareness of the ongoing situation and, thereby, be able to spot sources and signs of sudden increases in stress. Such a role may be filled by a "liaison psychiatrist," who can serve also as a consultant on individual patient management.[14] But it might appropriately be a selected nurse, now that there is a growing cadre within the profession of clinical specialists and others who have had advanced training in group and individual psychology. Or, such a nurse might serve as a co-leader, thereby helping to broaden perspectives and improve doctor–nurse relationships.

While this group process can enhance the appropriate sense of pride and "specialness," more can be done to bolster self-esteem. Here, we have something to learn from studies of morale in combat troups.[11] A distinctive uniform or an identifying patch may be helpful. A small pay differential, like that paid for special shifts, "hazardous duty pay," is an indication of special regard as well as a material reward. Periodic, brief, extra vacations (R and R—Rest and Recreation Leave) will do the same. Such periods might involve work on other nursing units rather than a true vacation, thereby providing education and communication for both staffs. One might consider also whether there should be a finite tour of duty on the ICU, with an enforced interval before a second tour. At the least, transfer to another unit should be made accessible and free from stigma; our experience suggests that often ICU nurses work past the point of "combat exhaustion" and then resign, sometimes with a sense of failure.

Another alternative might be to create a Unit Coordinator position through which the ICU nurses would periodically rotate. Freed from the regular nursing role and its duties, she could fulfill a number of important functions. In an emergency, she could help the head nurse organize the situation or provide an often crucial extra pair of hands. She could help orient new personnel. When consulting physicians arrive on the unit, she could familiarize them with its facilities and routine, thereby reducing their need for direct nursing assistance. She could serve as a major communication link with visitors, providing them with crucial emotional support, and keeping them "out of the hair" of others.

Competitive selection of nurses with superior skills appropriate for the job also will add to pride. In addition to technical expertise, applicants should be screened for psychological aptitude, perhaps by the liaison psychiatrist. In any event, an initial period of training and orientation[12] is essential, and should focus on job characteristics specific to the ICU. The group leader(s) should play a major role in this, so that the psychological aspects of the job experience are fully considered.

A sufficiently large nursing staff is necessary to allow coverage for vacations, weekends, and holidays without the use of outside "floating" assignees. The special characteristics of the unit should also be reflected in the assignment of other personnel. Insofar as the acuteness of its patients and the difficulty of their care are concerned, the ICU is highly specialized. In another sense, however, it is general: It provides care for almost every type of disease process. To provide the full range of treatment required, and to do so on a 24-hour, everyday basis, means that the ICU must be "a hospital within a hospital." Thus representatives of all relevant hospital services always must be at hand. Given a unit of sufficient size, a permanent pharmacist, inhalation therapist, X-ray technician, etc., may become a necessity as part of the regular ICU staff. At the very least, the person "on call" in each of these fields should be given the ICU as his regular assignment to ensure familiarity with the unit.

A *full-time* physician is an especial necessity, constantly and immediately available to examine patients, and as a source of information, advice, and support.[13] Whether a member of the attending or house staff, he must be delegated sufficient authority to be able to write new "orders" whenever indicated by the constantly changing condition of the patients, without necessarily consulting senior physicians of the specialty services to which the patients may be administratively assigned.

All must be familiar not only with their ICU and its patients, but with one another. Whatever their specialized delineation of function, all should act as, and identify themselves as, members of a single unified team. The group meetings, described earlier, should include all,[14] and efforts should be taken to ensure that difference of status and role are not allowed to block effective and open interchange.

The physical design of the ICU also deserves some comment. Consideration should be given to attenuation of the noise and visual bombardment, and some possibility for staff privacy. One potentially useful model is the circular one, in which patients occupy "spokes of a wheel."[15] (Each is separated by dividers providing some privacy, stimulus attenuation, and a barrier to contagion, while all remain in view of a central "hub" nursing station.) A nursing station enclosed in glass can permit the exchange of the "unthinkable" out of earshot of visitors and patients. A completely private lounge is also desirable. This can be used for breaks (which would have to be built into the work schedule—otherwise they would never occur!)[9] Also, there are times when the nurses may need the privacy to work out a dispute, to recover emotional stability connected with death, to "escape" from inescapable relatives, etc.

Conclusions

Perhaps it will seem as if we have been overly dramatic in our descriptions of the ICU as being so stressful. Most such units function very well. Other parts of the hospital (e.g., emergency and operating rooms) share many of the same stresses, and each deserves examination to understand its particular features. Moreover, nurses who work in the ICU do so by choice, suggesting that, for them, other assignments might be less gratifying or even more stressful. Yet, we believe that the seeming dramatization is, on careful scrutiny, an accurate portrayal and that the intensity and variety of the sources of stress in the ICU is unique. In any event, stress is there. Doubtless it is useful to an extent, enabling the nurses to maintain their critical alertness and ability to respond effectively to the needs of their patients. Yet there are many signs that its intensity goes well beyond this adaptive level. And since there are approaches to deal with this, it behooves us to utilize these for the benefit of both staff and patients.

Acknowledgment

The authors thank Mary Toomey, R.N., B.S.; Herbert Taylor, R.N., M.S.; David Robinson, M.D.; and Thomas Szasz, M.D., for their assistance and advice.

References

1. Abram, H. S. Adaptation to open heart surgery: A psychiatric study of responses to the threat of death. *American Journal of Psychiatry* **122**:659–667, 1965.
2. Bishop, L. F., & Reichert, P. The psychological impact of the coronary care unit. *Psychosomatics* **10**:189–92, 1969.
3. DeMeyer, J. The environment of the intensive care unit. *Nursing Forum* **6**:262–272, 1967.
4. Hackett, T. P., et al. Detection and treatment of anxiety in the coronary care unit. *American Heart Journal* **78**:727–730, 1969.

5. Margolis, G. J. Postoperative psychosis on the intensive care unit. *Comprehensive Psychiatry* **8:**227–232, 1967.

6. Vreeland, R., & Ellis, G. Stresses on the nurse in an intensive-care unit. *JAMA* **208:**332–334, 1969.

7. Gardam, J. F. Nursing stresses in the intensive care unit (Letters to the editor). *JAMA* **208:**2337–2338, 1969.

8. Salter, M. Nursing in an intensive therapy unit. *Nursing Times* **66:**486–487, 1970.

9. Kornfeld, D. S. Psychiatric view of the intensive care unit. *British Medical Journal* **1:**108–110, 1969.

10. Rome, H. The irony of the ICU. *Psychiatry Digest* **30:**10–14, 1969.

11. Grinker, R. R., & Spiegel, J. P. *Men under stress.* Philadelphia: Blakiston, 1945.

12. Boklage, M. G. ICU training program. *Hospitals* **44:**78–80, 1970.

13. Kornfeld, D. S. Psychiatric aspects of patient care in the operating suite and special areas. *Anesthesiology* **31:**166–171, 1969.

14. Koumans, A. J. Psychiatric consultation in an intensive care unit. *JAMA* **194:**633–637, 1965.

15. Armstrong, R. C. "Special care" unit for all intensive care needs. *Hospital Progress* **51:**40–42, 1970.

XI

The Final Crisis: Death and the Fear of Dying

Due in large part to advances in medical technology over the past few decades, fewer people die now of acute illnesses; however more and more face the prospect of a death preceded and prolonged by chronic illness and a slow decline. In this final section we are concerned with the patient who knows (or suspects) he is dying, and with the family members and health professionals who are closely involved with him. Some of the coping tasks are similar to those we have seen in earlier sections, but the stark irrefutable reality of death makes this confrontation a unique challenge.

When an individual becomes aware that he is probably dying, he realizes that certain fundamental aspects of his life will be determined by a force over which he has no control. He feels helpless as he faces the curtailment of his future (his goals unattained, his hopes and dreams abandoned), the necessary parting from cherished family and friends, and multiple threats to his self-esteem such as loss of productivity, increasing independence, and physical deterioration. The nature of this personal challenge is determined by several factors, including the characteristics of the disease involved (the degree of discomfort, disfigurement, and deterioration), the time span, and the quality of emotional, social, intellectual, financial, and other resources available to the individual.

How do people respond to these potent threats to their security and self-esteem? Normal reactions include feelings of anger at "cruel fate," sadness for what must be given up, inadequacy, helplessness, and anxiety. Fear of all kinds of the unknown, of being abandoned or rejected by loved ones, of physical degeneration, of dependency, of pain—crowd in on terminally ill patients. Some are overwhelmed by all this and live out their last days in unreachable depression or isolation, but many do manage to come to terms with their situation.

The fundamental coping tasks for the dying person include the management of anxiety, the maintenance of self-esteem, and the mourning of the people and objects he is losing. The mobilization of hope is one of the most significant coping mechanisms for the terminally ill. Even patients who have understood and accepted their prognosis can usually find some basis for hope, and doctors should be careful not to be so absolute as to eliminate this possibility.[1] A great source of anxiety is the patient's fear that because of changes in body appearance or function, the physical and economic burdens of his care, or simply his new status as a dying person, family, friends and physicians may reject or abandon him.[7,9] Warm and open communication with loved ones and trusting relationships with medical personnel provide invaluable emotional support. Patients who cannot acknowledge the prognosis or the related anxieties and rely heavily on denial, and those from whom the truth has been deliberately withheld, find themselves isolated and unable to share their concerns (see Glaser & Strauss[3] on mutual pretense and suspicious awareness contexts).

Maintenance of self-esteem and working through the loss of beloved people and things are the remaining tasks for the patient. Despite the dependent and helpless position in which they may find themselves, the terminally ill can still maintain their dignity, their value, and their individual identity by being responsible for decisions about their day-to-day lives and by setting realistic and realizable goals, which can provide a sense of achievement when the usual work and family functions have been relinquished. The mourning patient usually experiences feelings of anger and sadness for what is lost, and also guilt for the hurt his death will cause those who care about him.[5]

In our first article Claire Safran recounts the personal experience of Richard Kisonak and his family after they learn that he has a fatal illness. After an initial outburst of anger Dick began the difficult adjustment to the abrupt shortening of his future and his deteriorating physical condition. He set out to learn all he could about his illness, to dispel some of its mystery and have some idea of what to expect. The Kisonaks take it one day at a time with Dick functioning as normally as his fluctuating symptom level allows. As his symptoms became more visible and distressing he withdrew from social interaction, except with his family and close friends. Although the family was close and supportive, he sometimes withdrew even from them, a need they understood and respected. Between their hopes for the future and their determined efforts to make the present as meaningful as possible, Dick and his family were able to reach an acceptable adjustment for this early stage of the terminal process.

In our next selection, an excerpt from his book *Facing Death,* Robert Kavanaugh discusses the two phenomena which delimit the terminal process, the initial disclosure of the fatal prognosis and the final accommodation which must be reached in order to meet death with dignity. The debate about whether to tell a patient he has a fatal illness has gone on for decades, with some arguing that it is an unnecessary burden and others maintaining that people have a basic right to know as much of the truth as they wish in order to prepare themselves emotionally, as well as to take care of family responsibilities and settle practical arrangements. (For an interesting sociological study of the implications of withholding or disclosing a terminal prognosis see Glaser & Strauss[3].)

Kavanaugh focuses on two crucial elements involved in a person's coming to terms with approaching death: his need for permission from significant people in his life (including his care-givers) and his voluntary relinquishment of everyone and everything of value to him. Only when other people signify their readiness to accept his death are his feelings of guilt, inadequacy, and helplessness assuaged. Then he can begin his own grief work, mourning all that he must leave behind, so that in the end he feels ready and at peace.

As we have seen, family members, friends, and medical care-givers have a significant effect on the adaptation a dying patient makes, but they also need to make their own adjustments, to integrate into their own lives the impact of their involvement with the death of a human being. From their work with leukemic children Futterman and Hoffman[2] discerned a group of adaptive dilemmas for patients (which are applicable in part to other relatives and close friends of someone who is dying). A balance must be found within each pair of conflicting tasks: Accept the inevitable loss while maintaining some hope; attend to the immediate needs but begin to plan for the future; cherish the patient while allowing him to begin to separate; carry on daily activities (without letting upsetting feelings interfere) but find some safe outlet for expressing these disturbing feelings; offer the patient active personal care but recognize the need to sometimes delegate care to health professionals; place faith in medical personnel while recognizing their technical and human limitations; and maintain the level of attention and affection for the patient while beginning the gradual detachment which is part of anticipatory mourning.

Family members, like the patient, feel angry (at fate and at the patient), helpless, guilty (for their hostility, their sense of not doing enough, and even for their own good health), anxious, and sad. They may cope by denying, displacing, projecting, or isolating their distressing emotions or consciously controlling their mood, as in Beverly Kisonak's decision to be cheerful no matter what (chapter 27). Seeking information about the disease and its likely course and participating in the patient's care serve to bolster their sense of mastery and usefulness. Other strategies include keeping busy (whether productively or just for distraction), mobilizing hope, finding some meaning or purpose (for example, in religion) in the approaching death, and relying on available emotional support from medical personnel, clergy, social workers, and other family and friends.[4,8]

The effectiveness of the medical staff in dealing with terminal illness depends on their understanding of the needs and reactions of the patient and his family and their ability to recognize and cope with their own distress. Interpreting patient behavior accurately and responding in a way which facilitates appropriate coping is an important aspect of total patient care. A dying patient represents a personal threat to staff members—a reminder of their own mortality and an instance in which they have failed to fulfill their goal of healing (see also part X). A common way of managing this guilt and anxiety, especially for doctors, is to avoid the patient as much as possible and to deal only with concrete physical problems when with the patient. Redefining the meaning of the person's death ("He is in pain" or "She would be so disfigured") and regulating the tendency to identify with the patient or his family helps reduce the personal threat. Changing one's goal from curing the patient to making him comfortable, and, when little more can be done for the patient, to helping the family, is one of the most effective ways of managing the difficult professional and personal experience.[3]

When the patient dies, his struggle is over, but the survivors must go on. In the third article Stanley Goldberg discusses the adjustments the family must make when one of its members dies. Adaptive tasks for the family unit include allowing mourning to occur by encouraging the open expression of feelings, relinquishing the memory of the deceased as a force in family decisions, the realignment of intrafamilial roles (both practical and emotional), and the adjustment of extrafamilial roles to take into account status changes (for example, wife to widow). If there is general consensus on the direction of family reintegration, there is increased solidarity and greater support for individual members. (Individual coping with bereavement is another complex and interesting area; see Moos,[6] parts III and VIII, for a thorough discussion.) Terminal illness is a frightening thing because it forces one to face death (one's own or that of someone well loved) and come to terms with it. The challenge, like other developmental and situational crises, can be demoralizing or even overwhelming, but it also offers an opportunity for personal growth and development.

References

1. Alsop, S. *Stay of execution: A sort of memoir.* Philadelphia: J. B. Lippincott, 1973.
2. Futterman, E. H., & Hoffman, I. Crisis and adaptation in the families of fatally ill children. In E. J. Anthony & C. Koupernik (Eds.), *The child in his family: The impact of disease and death.* New York: Wiley, 1973.
3. Glaser, B. G., & Strauss, A. L. *Awareness of dying.* Chicago: Aldine, 1965.
4. Goldfogel, L. Working with the parents of a dying child. *American Journal of Nursing,* 1970, **70,** 1675–1679.
5. Kübler-Ross, E. *On death and dying.* New York: Macmillan, 1969.
6. Moos, R. H. (Ed.). *Human adaptation: Coping with life crises.* Lexington, Massachusetts: D.C. Heath, 1976.
7. Pattison, E. M. The experience of dying. *American Journal of Psychotherapy,* 1967, **21,** 32–43.
8. Pilsecker, C. Help for the dying. *Social Work,* 1975, **20,** 190–194.
9. Reynolds, D. K., & Kalish, R. A. The social ecology of dying: Observations of wards for the terminally ill. *Hospital and Community Psychiatry,* 1974, **25,** 147–152.

27

I Don't Intend To Die This Year

CLAIRE SAFRAN

For almost a year now, Beverly Kisonak has lived by the rhythm of a door that opens and closes. If the door to her husband's bedroom is open, it means that Richard is feeling well, that he'll be up and about, wanting to talk and share the day with her. If it's shut, it's his signal that he's having one of his bad days, that he feels a sharper tug than usual from the rare and fatal disease that is pulling him down.

"I used to resent that closed door," explains Beverly, a 41-year-old Maine housewife. "I felt he was shutting me out." Now she knows that Richard, 42, needs the privacy to renew his courage and be able to face the pronouncement of death made last November.

For several years Dick had been bothered with back trouble, then the symptoms had become more varied and obvious: He was losing weight, he felt tired, his words were slurred by his twitching tongue. He had his dentures realigned, but that didn't improve the speech problem. One doctor thought it was his nerves and referred the Kisonaks to a specialist.

"Your husband has a fatal disease," the young doctor told Mrs. Kisonak on November 11. He avoided Dick's eyes, talking only to her.

Beverly waited. "He's kidding, he's trying to scare us," she thought. She waited for him to say that he meant it could be that serious

---

Reprinted form *Today's Health,* September 1972. Published by the American Medical Association.

if Dick didn't follow the instructions and take the medicine he was going to give them. But the words never came. The doctor, inexperienced at breaking such news, continued. "It's called amyotrophic lateral sclerosis. It's also known as Lou Gehrig's disease."

She saw the shock of recognition on her husband's face. Lou Gehrig, the famous baseball player, died at the age of 38, two years after the diagnosis was made. The doctor explained that the disease attacks the nervous system and results in degeneration and weakening of the muscles. The victim faces extreme weakness, then paralysis, and finally death. "There is no cure. There is no medication for it," the doctor said.

Dick slammed his hand against the wall. "God damn," was all he could utter, the words slow and slurred by the very symptoms the doctor was describing.

There was still one question left and, in a small voice, Beverly asked it. "How long does he have to live?" The answer came quickly, bluntly: "One year, if he's lucky."

Numb, the Kisonaks left the doctor's office, not fully believing what they had heard. "I thought he was kidding. . . . I kept waiting for him to say he didn't mean it," Beverly said. What should they tell the children? Should they tell all three or only the eldest? Then, when they were almost home, the car had a flat tire. "A bad day all around," said Dick.

They realized the family was too closely knit to keep any secrets, and that night Beverly broke the news to the children, Richard, Jr., 16, Janis, 15, and Wayne, 11.

"I told them that we'd had bad news from the doctor, that Daddy had a disease whose name I couldn't even pronounce. I wrote it on a piece of paper and mentioned Lou Gehrig. They sat there shocked, not really believing. For a long time nobody said anything, and then Wayne, who watches all those medical shows, said, 'This doesn't happen in real life. This only happens on television.' After that, we all cried."

They had been high school sweethearts: Dick a top athlete and Beverly a pretty, five-foot-three blonde. They were married a year after graduation, and Beverly still remembers how his strong arms felt around her as they glided across the floor and promised each other, "We'll go dancing when we're 60."

Dick worked as a reporter for the Lewiston (Maine) *Daily Sun,* covering both politics and the police beat. They moved to a modest Cape Cod cottage on a tree-lined street and built a good life, making friends through Dick's newspaper work and Beverly's church activities.

Now a perverse fate, a quixotic disease, has erased their wedding promise and turned the rest of their life upside down.

Richard Kisonak does not want to leave his wife and children and he was angry when the doctor told him he was going to die. Like others faced with a great loss, Dick needed to express his rage before he could accept what lay ahead.

"Will I be able to die with dignity? God, I hope so," Dick says. "I hope I can hold my head high when it happens. I'm going to try like hell to do it."

Today, there are no hushed whispers, no red-rimmed eyes, no acts of pity allowed in the white-shingled house. Life is taken one day at a time. Dick wakes each morning, grateful if he can move his legs, fully aware that there is a wheelchair in his future. The Kisonaks believe that Dick will beat the doctor's one-year sentence, but they know that he will not have all the years that should have been his.

A second specialist and further tests confirmed the diagnosis, and the family has memorized what little is known of Dick's disease. Amyotrophic lateral sclerosis (ALS) occurs more often in men than in women, generally striking at ages 40 to 60. The National Multiple Sclerosis Foundation, under whose philanthropic umbrella the disease comes, estimates that there are from five to ten thousand cases in this country. Because there is no simple way of telling how long the patient has had the disease before it is detected, it is difficult to talk about life-span. In about half the cases, death comes within two or three years of diagnosis; for others the disease progresses more slowly, sometimes so imperceptibly that there seem to be long periods when it is arrested. Some patients remain active for 10 or 15 years or longer.

There are two forms of ALS. In the spinal variety, the legs and arms suffer the earliest, most severe weakening. In the bulbar variety, which Dick seems to have, loss of weight and the slurring of speech are the most dramatic first symptoms. Most patients eventually experience both sets of symptoms.

(Amyotrophic lateral sclerosis is not the same as multiple sclerosis. The latter is more common, more often affects younger people, including children, and is not fatal—death is usually the result of an intercurrent respiratory or genitourinary infection. Multiple sclerosis attacks the myelin sheathing of various nerves and produces a disabilitating effect on the muscles. More than half the cases remit following the initial attack, but there is no way of predicting further attacks.)

When the Kisonaks learned of Dick's disease, they tried to spend every possible moment with him. The children stayed at home, staring, watching. Wayne, a dedicated outdoorsman, rarely left the house, shadowing his father from room to room. Finally, Dick protested that he was being smothered. So the family forced themselves back to the more natural routines, trying to share their lives with Dick as much as possible.

"I worry most about Rick," Beverly says. "I thought he was going toward the ministry, but when this happened, he seemed to lose a little faith." At first, when physical medicine offered no help, Rick pored over his psychology books, hoping to find an answer there. He and his father talked for hours about what he'd read. During Dick's years on the newspaper night shift and then with his back troubles, they hadn't had much time together, and this seemed to bring them closer. "Then a social worker told him it wasn't healthy for him to be doing that, that he was taking the role of the father instead of the son," says Beverly. "I don't know why she had to say that, but Rick stopped. He felt that there was no way for him to help his father, and it really took the pins from under him." Now the young man, who dreams of going to art school, fills page after page with elongated, somewhat morbid faces instead of the playful mouse-people he used to draw. "I suppose they're his way of relieving tension," Beverly says.

The full impact of the situation hit Beverly one afternoon when she was giving Dick a back rub. His back felt hard in some spots and limp in others and the muscles were twitching involuntarily under the skin. "As if they were winking at me." Something malevolent and leering seemed to be alive under her husband's skin, and at that moment the terror and gravity of his illness overwhelmed her. She smothered a gasp, still forcing her fingers to keep rubbing. But she had to turn her head away and was grateful that, at that moment, Dick could not see her face.

To match her husband's courage, Beverly has developed her own way of coping. She is cheerful and optimistic—no matter what. "If I'm not smiling," she says, "how can I expect him to smile back?" But her tension shows in too many cigarettes. Still, she knows Dick cares, so she goes to the hairdresser, remembers her makeup, and dresses in bright, attractive clothes. During the long winter, when the walls seemed to be closing in on Dick, she invented reasons for him to accompany her on different errands, and she's developed a repertoire of casseroles and other soft-food dishes that are all he can manage now.

Medically, amyotrophic lateral sclerosis progresses in a steady line of deterioration. Few doctors, though, would discount the positive effects of optimism or the impact of a strong will to live. No textbook could have predicted that, after a long, dark winter, the Kisonaks would find unexpected reasons for a springtime of hope.

A few weeks after the doctor's fatal verdict, Beverly and Dick were alone, having the glass of port wine that has become a prelunch ritual. "It's important for Dick to keep his weight up, and this helps his appetite," Beverly says. "More than that, it's a companionable thing for us to do together. We've always enjoyed each other's company. When you're first married, there's the physical relationship as well as companionship. If there's illness, the physical element may not be possible. There has to be something more between a man and a woman, and we're lucky to have always had that."

They sat together at the kitchen table, with the pale winter sun coming dimly through the floral curtains. "There's something we have to talk about," Dick began. "Just this once. Then I don't want to mention it again." He explained that he needed her help to meet whatever was ahead with dignity. He talked about their financial situation now that he'd had to stop working. They owned little beside the house, but made plans to have a will drawn up. Months later, Beverly admitted to a visitor, "I know I have to arrange for a cemetery plot, but the final things are the hardest."

Dick was unconvinced by Beverly's strong belief in the hereafter, "something different but better than this life." "I'll have to see for myself," he told her. She found comfort in the prayer meetings at their Episcopal church, but Dick preferred to pray by himself at home. He was self-conscious about his speech and withdrew from public gatherings and from all but their closest friends and relatives.

One of the first persons Dick wanted to see after hearing the doctor's report was David Berent, a Lewiston rabbi. The two had both suffered from back troubles, and their initial association had long since developed into a deep friendship. It was the rabbi who told Dick, "All any of us can do, my friend, whether we're sick or well, is to live one day at a time."

The family took that as their motto, but they still found it impossible not to look at each event as something they would never share again. When Christmas came, they faced it as the last one they would have together. Dick, particularly, began feverish efforts to make it the best Christmas ever. His legs felt weak then, and often he'd have to hold on to the wall to take a few steps. But he oversaw the holiday preparations anxiously and, despite the shadow of illness, it was a good Christmas. Dick beamed with pleasure as gift after gift was opened. He joined in the holiday feasting, welcomed their friends, and visited his family. But at the end of Christmas day, when the children were asleep, Dick closed the bedroom door and wept.

The emotional strain and physical exertion of the holiday lowered Dick's resistance and, a few days later, a mild cold led to breathing problems. He was rushed to the hospital and given inhalation therapy to clear his lungs, as well as a warning not to overtire himself or neglect any cold symptoms.

Later in January, when Dick was feeling stronger, he and Beverly flew to Jamaica with money raised by members of their church. They escaped from the grim winter and the trip revived Dick's spirits—he'd been stationed in the Caribbean as a Navy man, and it brought back memories of a time when he was young and vigorous. But Beverly could not forget why they were there. "If there's a trip you've been wanting to take," the doctor had said, "take it now—while there's time."

In the middle of March there was another trip to the sun. The two Richards, senior and junior, went to Bermuda, where Dick hoped to reknit the father–son relationship. "I didn't accomplish everything I wanted to with Rick," he told Beverly afterward, "but it was more than I had thought possible."

At home, the Kisonaks lived quietly. They used to eat out occasionally, but now Dick was worried that one of his choking fits might occur in public and he was unwilling to face the awkward, pitying glances from others. Still, their good friends came to play cards on Saturday nights, joking and bantering over penny poker games around the kitchen table. Dick's old high school class even had a fund-raising drive to help them with expenses.

The winter lingered stubbornly. When Dick's door was closed, Beverly drove the children to school and came back home before doing the marketing. Once she returned to find him awake and dressed. "I just wanted a cup of tea before I went to the store," she told him. The children often hesitated to bother their father with their problems and came to Beverly instead. But whenever the door to his room was open, she sent the children to Dick, reaffirming his position as head of the household.

In April a newspaper in nearby Portland asked Dick to write his story for them. He declined at first, but then, for whatever help it might be to other people, he agreed. The story was picked up by one of the wire services and published in other newspapers around the country. The response to the story was overwhelming.

Letters and packages arrived by the sackful and Dick and Beverly spent their mornings poring over the hand-written prayers, encouraging messages, inspirational books, and carefully wrapped bottles of holy water from Lourdes and other shrines. They were profoundly moved that so many strangers from all over the country were reaching out to them.

Until then the Kisonaks had felt isolated in their anguish. Now they began to hear from other ALS victims and their families. "Don't settle for one year of life," they were told over and over. Letters spoke of husbands or sons who were alive for 9 years, 12 years, 17 years after the disease had struck.

The phone rang constantly with long-distance calls from the families of ALS patients. "I'm taking my husband out to dinner tonight," a California woman told them. "He's had ALS for 17 years. He's going in a wheelchair, but he's going out to dinner." Beverly Kisonak got a measure of comfort talking to other wives like herself, sharing symptoms, comparing notes, finding comfort in the common bond of tragedy.

Some of the callers asked if they could visit. An ALS victim from a nearby state came and talked to Dick. A young man told of his rebirth in Christ and they held hands in a circle and prayed together. At the young man's suggestion, Dick and Beverly began to read from the Bible together each day, and they hope that eventually their children will join them. But they cannot accept everything the visitor told them. "He said we should thank God for having sent us this test, and I cannot go that far," says Beverly. "I am not thankful for this disease and I do not believe that God sent it to us. But every day I do thank Him for the strength to bear it."

Along with the messages of encouragement came the long-awaited spring. Dick began to go out more, to run an errand with Beverly or visit a bookstore. On good days, he would drive the car, and even on bad days he eased his legs off the bed and tried to walk.

More letters came promising quick cures and miracles, and they tried to sift the real hopes from the false. One nutritionist urged massive doses of vitamins C and E. This was approved by their doctor and Dick began to take the vitamins, which he says make him feel stronger— although it is hard to tell if the improvement is physical or psychological.

Another letter told about an experimental program at the Pacific Medical Center in San Francisco, where Dr. Forbes Norris, Jr., has been trying to help ALS patients with guanidine, an old pharmaceutical that has fallen into disuse. Only a few patients have been treated so far with the drug, and its effects still remain to be proven. No patients have been "cured," but Dr. Norris says that about half have had "apparent benefits." As Dr. Norris is aware, the reaction to his experiments from other doctors ranges from skepticism to disbelief. There are serious questions about side effects and about whether the drug really acts as he describes it. Many doctors suspect that the improvements he sees are in cases where the disease progresses so slowly that there appears to be a recovery or remission. Dr. Norris is the first to emphasize that this treatment is still very much in the experimental stage, but he adds, "The traditional prognosis given to ALS patients should be modified to permit some hope."

Dick's doctor is reluctant to prescribe guanidine without further investigation, but at the Kisonaks' request, he has been in touch with Dr. Norris. To a family that has lived on deep faith and raw courage for almost a year, hope is in itself a powerful medicine.

The Kisonaks continue to live one day at a time, but that no longer means trying to share something today because their tomorrows are running out. "We no longer think in terms of his not being with us next Christmas," Beverly says. "Now we set little goals for ourselves and say that he's got to stay well so that he can do this or that. We're thankful for each day and we try to do the best we can for that day. When Dick worked nights and I worked part time during the day, we never had enough time together. Now we've got more time and we try to enjoy it."

For Beverly Kisonak, life still moves to the rhythm of an open and closed bedroom door, but the tempo has quickened and the door is rarely shut now. But there are still moments of depression. When information on the guanidine experiments was slow in coming, Dick complained, "They're wasting my time." More often, though, he joins in the plans for family excursions. A few weeks ago, Dick climbed the stairs to the boys' upstairs bedroom, the first time he's been able to do that in months, to see the new baby kittens. He has been up and down many times since then, stroking the furry promises of life. One morning he pulled out one of his golf clubs and a ball to putt around the back yard. "If you use a cart," Beverly encourages him, "there's no reason you can't get out on the course very soon."

When they believed that Dick had only a year to live, the family faced that. Now they are convinced that the best prescription is faith in the future. They talk about tomorrow, about next year when Rick graduates from high school, and the year after that when Janis graduates. "And then there's Wayne," Beverly tells him. "You have a lot to look forward to. A lot to live for."

ALS courses through its victims at different rates, but the Kisonaks talk about others who have stayed alive and how Dick will, too. Beverly thanks him for the red roses he sent for their 23rd anniversary. "That was fine," she says. "Now let me tell you what I want for my 25th. . . ."

Dick grins broadly. As he told a recent visitor, "I do not intend to die this year."

28

Humane Treatment of the Terminally Ill

ROBERT E. KAVANAUGH

Should patients who are doomed to die know their fate? This used to be a troublesome question, the most baffling in the entire issue of dying. Discussions were always theoretical. No scientific or clinical evidence existed for the comparison of the benefits in telling the patient with the benefits of remaining silent. Everybody guessed. Parlor talk and religion classes abounded with moral platitudes about man's right to know his condition or about our duty to keep the patient comfortable by silence. "Every man has the right to know so he can put his house in order!" "Happiness is an inalienable right and should not be destroyed when nothing is accomplished!" Doctors differed in theory. In practice they were nearly unanimous in not telling. Clergymen leaned toward telling, though they were easily convinced otherwise if they were asked to tell. The dying were seldom consulted, only left to suffer the results of the arguments outside their door.

At last we have abundant clinical evidence on what happens when dying patients are told their fate. And by deduction, we know what happens when they remain ignorant. Almost without exception, the case

ROBERT E. KAVANAUGH • Counseling Psychologist, University of California at San Diego, San Diego, California.

Reprinted in abridged form from Chap. 4 (pp. 59–79) of *Facing Death* (Los Angeles: Nash Publishing, 1972). Copyright 1972, by permission of Nash Publishing Corp.

histories reveal the value of an early and forthright disclosure. Dr. Elisabeth Kübler-Ross, the best known of the researchers, clearly documents the several stages which dying people pass through. From an original posture of denial and isolation, patients made aware of their terminal condition pass through stages of anger, bargaining, depression, and acceptance or resignation, without ever fully losing hope. Her documentation scuttles all our traditional arguments for reluctance. Patients who know their destiny can progress toward a peaceful and dignified death. Those left in ignorance of their diagnosis rarely make it past the fearful stage of denial and isolation.

In yesterday's speculation and confusion, the line of least resistance always became most attractive. Since patients were not asked, it was the teller's resistance that was measured. It was much simpler not to tell. Now we know it was not so easy for the untold patients.

Today, we can say with certainty that as a general rule, every patient should be made aware of his diagnosis. There may be exceptions, but I hesitate to mention a single one, because the fearful will find their own excuse in any exception I select. Instead of listing exceptional situations, I prefer to say that the only remaining questions are clear. When should the patient be told? How should he be told? And who should do the telling?

The terminal patient should know his prognosis as soon as it is medically certain. Any disclosure to any patient, most especially an early one, needs to be padded in hope. Doctors have been in error and predictions can be faulty. There have been sudden and near miraculous changes in conditions. New developments in medicine and in surgery are always around the corner.

Human beings have a magnificent filtering system built into their perceptual senses. When discussing any delicate subject, this system sifts out any data the mind is not ready to know. No matter how loud, how clear, or how often the speaker communicates an unwanted fact, the human mind resists acceptance until it is ready. You see this filtering system at work when lovers spat. The rejected lover always hears in hope, no matter how final the rejector makes his case. You can see this filter at its comic best in middle-aged marrieds who grow conveniently deaf to each other's bickering, while capable of hearing outsiders with ease. The dying make use of this remarkable system, filtering out what they will not know or are not ready to realize. Or, they listen now and hear later on, when facts can be digested at their individual pace and emotions are prepared to react to truth.

When death comes quickly and the dying person has only hours or days, it is still a general rule that the patient prospers by knowing what is taking place. In telescoped form, they endure the same problems and can move through the same stages as the lingering. They, too, will filter out what they would not know. The shock and tension around sudden deaths are usually so great that any rules I might offer would be pure folly. Bystanders need only try to do their best, not copping out to their personal fears and natural reluctance while the patient dies uninformed in hysteria and terror. Even a little talking, a little listening, coupled with loads of straightforward looking, eye to eye, will bring significant comfort and relief.

Heart patients, whose need to avoid additional stress is uppermost in every bystander's mind, need special consideration. The very act of telling about impending death is feared to cause it. Such victims need to talk, or if talking is no longer possible, they need to emote in any way they can, as long as consciousness lasts. They need human presence, with hands to hold and eyes that dare answer lovingly the questions their own eyes ask. They need loving listeners and lookers who understand that minimal talking, even wordless speech with eyes and hands, can alleviate much of the terror a sudden confrontation with death can bring.

There is no easy way to tell another human being that death is near. Awkwardness can be expected. Fear and uneasiness are always partners to the telling, unless we have lost our normalcy or have callousness for a mask. It is always better by far if there is no act of telling at all—only a two-way conversation that is open enough to allow the patient to announce his dying if he chooses. Once we ask a patient how he feels, indicating in our asking that we truly want to know, usually we have said enough. Patients themselves will almost always introduce the subject of dying to permission-giving listeners. Most of the time, telling a person that he or she is dying means no more than chatting about the self, without nervous Band-Aids being put over the mouth or eager protestations of artificial hope.

Television has taught all of us to recognize deathbed scenes, and when we find ourselves bedded down in one, we make all necessary deductions. Our biggest need when we realize that death is coming is for a confidant who will instigate and allow our honest talk. So often, when we hear of patients who did not want to know their terminal condition, we are actually hearing stories of relatives or bystanders who would not grant permission for candid conversation. A physician friend admitted that no patient of his had ever gone beyond the denial stage in dying, and he humbly knew that he was the major reason.

Patients who will not mention death when permitted to talk openly can be told in other ways. For literal folks, a medical diagnosis in straight terms might be the only way. For others, hints at being "terribly ill," of their being "sicker than ever before," or of our intense concern for their health may do the trick. Such implications plant a seed from which the patient can make appropriate deductions in due time.

There are patients who want nothing more than to deny until the end, and our only need is to respect their right to know. When tellers are novices, there are no right or wrong ways. There are never any sure ways. There is only the ethical need that each patient knows the truth, as much as he wants and in a manner he can accept. Pushing human beings to know what they sincerely and inalterably wish to deny can be as inhumane as the universal silence of yesterday.

Who is the best person to inform the patient about a terminal condition? The doctor in charge of total patient care has the moral and professional responsibility to see that his patient knows. Many people are better equipped than the doctor for the actual telling. A son or a wife, a kindly nurse or a respected crony. There is no proper person, only one brave and humble enough to try bringing the maximum of graciousness to a forbidding task. Doctors who take into account the mental health of patients as part of their healing concern will see that every patient knows the truth as desired.

Once it becomes clear to a person that death is inevitable, two important problems need facing if death is to occur with any degree of serenity for all concerned. First, the dying person needs to receive permission to pass away from every important person he will leave behind. Only then can the patient begin to deal with his second problem, the need to voluntarily let go of every person and possession he holds dear. Both problems deserve careful consideration, since therein lies the crux of dignified and peaceful dying.

At first it might seem strange to insist that the dying need permission to do the inevitable. Isolated patients will have no significant others from whom to seek permission. The unfeeling and those living in loveless situations will assume their right to die, covering themselves with self-pity while maintaining an outward denial of what is happening. But patients who feel any degree of human closeness or of responsibility to others, who had love in their lives and people near who needed them, require permission if death is to be peaceful. There is no other way to still feelings of guilt for going, for copping out on life, for becoming an emotional and financial burden, and for that feeling of horrible helplessness inside.

Reasonably sensitive persons know well and feel deeply the pain and sorrow their death will cause. They feel guiltily responsible even when they know logically they are not. Each tearstained face, each wringing hand, each look of futility pushes buttons of guilt inside a patient who cares. Always before there was a way out of guilt, an apology or explanation, a promise not to fail again, an act of special kindness in reparation. Because when dying there is only a single and unacceptable solution, permission becomes essential.

Before any dying patient can know that he wants or needs to accept permission, the head needs to be cleared. Jealousy and resentment toward the living need first to be stilled. Self-pity needs to be reduced if not removed, and the masks of denial need lifting. All of this takes time and requires at times the services of an enduring friend.

Permission to die need never be spoken aloud or written. The patient can read his permission in the ability of each visitor to cope with him as a person. The patient readily understands that friends and relatives who refuse to visit, or fail to confront him when they do, are blocking his death, refusing to let it become real. Visitors who grow hysterical or display an uncontrollable grief reveal to the patient strings of a dependency only someone harsh could violently sever.

Permission to die is granted in all open and honest confrontations where patient and visitor accept the reality and needs of each other. Together they willingly face the situation as it is. The patient reveals that he can die without displacing his feelings onto the living, blaming no one, demanding no beyond-the-grave commitments. The visitor, in turn, displays his ability to keep living without blaming the patient, without threatening irremediable anguish. Doctors and nurses grant their permission by continuing regular and devoted care when comfort replaces recovery as the plan of patient care. Occasional friends grant their permission by a continued availability without losing respect for the patient's recurring need for privacy.

Clinical studies record a visible relief in patients when loved ones accept their dying without blame or despair. Other patients seem to survive beyond usual expectations, suffering ineffable pain, as if waiting like beggars for a "yes" from important people. After administering the last rites, I frequently noted a new sense of relief in the patient. Naturally, I advertised the worth of the sacrament. Now, I wonder if the reception of the sacrament was not the patient's assurance that everyone important had given permission.

Once the permission to die is clearly granted, the dying patient can tackle the second major task, his personal work in voluntarily letting go. He can begin to release his hold on life, then gently, with growing decisiveness, unlock the chains that bind his heart to all earthly treasures, to valued persons, and to every possession. He begins with the outer circle of important acquaintances and business associates now rarely seen, extending to close friends and family. His individual freedom grows as he releases job and future plans, favorite scenes, golf clubs, yard, and home. If there is to be a tranquillity near death, all the dying can retain are what they truly own: their minds and loves, their memories and freedom, and their faith.

What does it mean to let go? Internally, the dying individual agrees to allow the world to go on without him. Positively put, he clings feverishly to all that is truly his own, learning to revel in himself and in his personal treasures. He learns to rejoice in what he is and has, ceasing to play Silas Marner with spouse and children, income and estate. At birth as at death, man is alone. At birth, our aloneness can only be felt in primitive feelings, while at death, our early feelings are resurrected and we know our isolation. The human struggle for the dying is not so much in letting go as in reaching out for revelry in what we hid from ourselves in life.

Once the terminal patient begins to unleash himself from ties and roles, he increasingly becomes a free spirit. His survivors also gain new freedom in his independence. This is a slow and halting process, overcoming decades of dependency, and interspersed with pauses for desperate clinging. Freedom one moment and almost despair the next. Sometimes the most difficult treasures for the expiring to release are foolish things like tennis rackets or an old fishing hat.

The task of totally letting go may be too much if we wait until death looms near. We begin to die well the first day we learn to cherish the world we know without crippling dependency on it. Many of the undiagnosed diseases in our daily lives will contribute to anguish near death unless a cure is found. Greed for material goods and leaning too heavily on those we love are diseases that decimate peace near death.

Patients denied permission to die will necessarily expire in a cruel isolation, struggling alone with burdens better shared. Rarely will they have their chance to let go of life if friends will not let go of them. Patients who cannot or will not release their hold on life's treasures, insisting upon hoarding to the end, will die in disappointment and near despair. Resentment and hostility will haunt them. Jealousy will gnaw at any peace. They deny themselves any outlet for the guilt and fearful impotence inside.

Throughout human history, recorders of deathbed scenes tell of a frequent and strange phenomenon. They note that the visage of the newly deceased is quite often wreathed in a gentle smile or in a look of uncommon peace. Interpreters offer many explanations, all of them guesses. Hagiographers report their saints and martyrs have seen their God. Nonbelievers claim that nature has her own mechanism for euphoria, an analgesic when all systems cease. My guess is that the smile or look of peace reflects a satisfaction limited to men of any creed who died in peace. They expired without earthly strings of any kind choking their hearts and they realized that they had bequeathed no strings to choke the hearts of those they left behind.

29

Family Tasks and Reactions in the Crisis of Death

STANLEY B. GOLDBERG

This article concerns death as a crisis for the family and the consequent reactions of the family as a unit to the loss of one of its members. The study of death has traditionally focused to a great extent upon the individual, attempting to elucidate the intrapsychic processes related to mourning by one who has suffered a loss, and the interactional focus is not usually considered. When a death has occurred, not only must each surviving individual bear the pain of grief and adjust to the loss; the surviving family must do so as well. There are specific family readjustment tasks, distinct from what we recognize as individual mourning tasks, that complement one another. Both need to be considered in understanding this aspect of human behavior, but the concern here is with the former; the intrapsychic aspects will be discussed only as they are relevant to this focus.

Crisis Concepts Applied to the Family

It is not difficult to understand why death is a crisis for the family. The basis of a family crisis is that "the situation cannot be easily han-

STANLEY B. GOLDBERG, A.C.S.W. ● Caseworker, Family Service of Detroit and Wayne County, Detroit, Michigan.

Reprinted from *Social Casework*, 1973, **54**, 398–405. Published by Family Service Association of America.

dled by the family's commonly used problem-solving mechanisms, but forces the employment of novel patterns. These are necessarily within the range of the family's capacities, but may be patterns never called into operation in the past."[1]

Not every stress that impinges upon a family precipitates a crisis. Why do we speak of death as such? According to Reuben Hill, three variables determine whether a stress event results in a crisis for the family: "(1) the hardships of the situation or event itself; (2) the resources of the family: its role structure, flexibility and previous history with crisis; and (3) the definition the family makes of the event; that is whether members treat the event *as if it were* or *as if it were not a threat* to their status, goals and objectives."[2]

Two characteristics of death as a stress event make it readily convertible into a crisis situation. One is its stark finality—the irretrievable loss of a human being. One can not replace the loss, but only adjust to it. The second characteristic is that because death is not a frequent occurrence one usually has little prior experience in dealing with it and, therefore, must seek a novel solution when it does occur. Thus, death is a severe hardship seen by the family as a threatening event and a crisis. A third variable—the family's resources—may mitigate the severity but will not necessarily prevent death from being perceived as a crisis.

The concept of a family crisis is a global one. Various kinds of crises may befall a family. Although death is not always unanticipated, as the family must sometimes bear witness to the dying process of a member, the death of a member is often an unanticipated crisis. Reuben Hill labels death as dismemberment.[3] A crisis event may be perceived differently by those whom it affects: as a threat, a loss, or a challenge.[4] Each is associated with a particular effect. The affect attending a crisis seen as a loss is, not surprisingly, mourning and depression.

In the resolution of a crisis, certain steps must be accomplished. These are designated as psychological tasks: "The essence of a struggle for mastery of stress can be specified by characteristic psychological tasks that each stress situation poses. It is possible to specify clearly what the person must do, psychologically and behaviorally, to achieve mastery."[5]

The family as a group must also accomplish certain tasks apart from what the individual must complete, although they proceed simultaneously. Thus, a major feature about death as a crisis-provoking event is that its effects can be discussed on two levels: intrapsychic as well as intrafamilial. Although the latter is of greater interest, we must be cognizant of intrapsychic adjustment as well, for in studying the family's reactions to death, we are observing a group of individuals who are working through their grief. It is a reciprocal interchange: Working through one's own grief facilitates the family's readjustment, which in turn further affects resolution of individual mourning.

Grief Work of the Individual

In a classic article, Erich Lindemann describes the course of grief as consisting of three phases: "emancipation from the bondage to the deceased, readjustment to the environment in which the deceased is missing, and the formation of new relationships."[6] Involved in this process are the two basic steps through which the ego progresses in mourning: introjection and the loosening of ties to the lost object.

> Under the influence of the reality that the object no longer exists, the ego gives up its libidinal ties to the object. This is a slow, piecemeal process in order that the ego will not be overwhelmed by a flood of feeling. The mourner pursues this task by introjecting the relationship with the lost object, and then loosening each tie to the now internalized object. . . . Thus introjection acts as a buffer by helping to preserve the relationship with the object while the gradual process of relinquishing is going on. . . . In this process, of course, the relationship to the lost person is not abandoned, but the libidinal ties are so modified that a new relationship can be established.[7]

When this process has occurred, the person has worked through his grief.

Family Tasks Following Death

What, then, are the family's psychological tasks? How do we know that a family is adequately achieving these tasks?

Allowing Mourning to Occur

The family in which a death has occurred must give permission for the grief process to proceed. There must be encouragement of mourning and expression of feelings. Often crying is represented as weakness;[8] the implication is that one should be strong. Lindemann observed: "One of the big obstacles to this work seems to be the fact that many patients try to avoid both the intense distress connected with the grief experience and the necessary expression of emotion."[9] Permitting family members to mourn in effect says, "We are all hurting. Let us suffer our pain together." Members can help one another.[10] The allowance of mourning might appear to be a preparatory step rather than an actual task, but it is basic. If the family is to successfully deal with the other tasks at this time, it must begin to work through the grief of individual members first. This is where one becomes cognizant of the psychological steps of the individual outlined above, but now more than one person is observed grieving.

A research project currently in progress at the Fort Logan Mental Health Center in Denver emphasizes the importance of this task. The project is studying the use of crisis intervention with bereaved families as a method of primary prevention of later psychiatric disorders or medical illnesses.[11] It has been observed that families with effective communication systems better meet the stress of a death: "The degree to which it is permissible to express feelings of sadness and loss, as well as the less acceptable reactions of anger, guilt, and relief, seems to play a large role in determining the success of the readjustment period."[12]

There are criteria by which to judge whether one has been able to do his grief work:

1.   Passing through the stages of normal grief as reviewed above.

2.   "Successful resolution of the mourning process implies that the deceased will remain a 'living memory' without the pain that originally accompanies the grief reaction."[13]

3.   Identifiable morbid grief reactions indicate unresolved mourning. Lindemann lists several morbid reactions: delay of mourning, overactivity without a sense of loss, appearance of symptoms of the deceased, a disease, change in relationships, hostility, decrease in social interaction, undertaking activities against one's best welfare, and agitated depression.[14]

Relinquishing the Memory of the Deceased

The memory of the deceased must be given up as a force in family activities. This activity is similar to the idea that the person must release himself from attachment to the dead individual. Thomas D. Eliot noted:

> An integrated family may resolve to live "as if" the lost member were still with them. If such motivation be kept on a high spiritual plane and not too specific, it may provide a valuable momentum—probably tapering off normally as it ceases to be a felt need. It may, however, become a "dead hand," the known habits or supposed wishes of the deceased being cited by a new family head as a device of supernatural sanction comparable to the "Thus spake the Lord" of the ancient prophets. Or the family may split over conflicting interpretations of "what mother would have said," each side quoting this authority to rationalize his own wishes.[15]

This task requires time. It is accomplished when the family, respecting and cherishing the memory of the departed, is able to make decisions based on what will best meet its present needs without continually invoking what the departed might have said or done. This task is also facilitated by the family's dealing successfully with its other tasks.

Realignment of Intrafamilial Roles

Death has created a change in the composition of the family group. A role has been left vacant. The family alters its relationships so that it can redistribute responsibilities and needs. Redistribution occurs in regard to instrumental and socioemotional functions. Instrumental functions as a broad category encompass specific tasks for every family: socialization of children, economic support, and maintenance of physical needs. Socioemotional functions are the complement of instrumental ones and might be variously referred to as the need-response or affectional system of the family. These functions are concerned with the giving and receiving of love.

Realignment of intrafamilial roles often refers to the problems of the one-parent family created by the death of a mother or father. We can not document fully the difficulties facing such a family other than to note two basic concerns, perhaps best summed up by the familiar statement, "I try to be both mother and father to my children." One concern is to provide continuing support for the family; this activity may involve living on various death benefits or seeking a substitute or additional means of support, such as the wife or oldest child going to work. Second, the surviving spouse is faced with providing the children with love previously given by two persons and satisfying his own emotional needs without a spouse. Increased family solidarity and support to one another would be indicative of dealing with this problem, or another person might be introduced into the role network either on a temporary (the spouse dating), facilitative (a Big Brother for the son), or permanent basis (remarriage).

Realignment of Extrafamilial Roles

Relationships with the organizations and institutions comprising the social system external to the family need realignment. Those relationships requiring change, if, for example, it was the husband-father who died, would be the wife's membership in the couples' club at the church or the son's participation on a father–son baseball team. Adaptive adjustment would mean either continuation in present activities or seeking activities better suited for one's new status: The widowed parent may withdraw from the couples' club and join Parents Without Partners or the fatherless boy may ask an uncle to participate in the Little League with him.

Some families are more successful than others in achieving these tasks. To examine how well the family copes, it is essential to understand the various reactions to the death of a member. Some reactions are indicative of more successful family readjustment, whereas others point toward dysfunctional interaction.

Reactions of Families to the Death of a Member

The intrapsychic process of mourning is paralleled on the family level by an interactional process generically labeled role change. Role change involves the reestablishment of a new equilibrium within the family.

Role Reorganization

The first reaction is role reorganization. This may seem synonymous with role change, but the concept of role reorganization is used more narrowly here. It is concerned with who will assume what responsibilities. The degree of role reorganization is a function of two variables: the number of roles held by the member who died and the type of role he fulfilled.[16] The process of readjustment is easier for the family which has lost an infant (as sad as that is) than for one which has lost a father; in the latter family, the father will have occupied not only more roles but more important ones than a baby.

Regarding role reorganization, the authors of the current bereavement research at the Fort Logan Mental Health Center stated:

> Our experience to date shows, however, that the single most important factor in the reorganization of a family as a continuing social system following a death is the role the decedent had been assigned, and which he assumed within the family system.
> The resumption of adaptive functioning, following a death, is facilitated in a family where vital roles and functions have been apportioned among members in a just and equitable manner . . . according to individual need, ability, and potential. In such a case, role assumption is usually explicit and well understood by all family members. When a member of this type of family dies, the critical period of reorganization is not likely to be experienced as a crisis because the family already has a built-in process which allows it to reallocate the role functions of the decedent with minimal difficulty.[17]

It would appear that families with a good communication system as well as prior equitable role allocation respond most adaptively to the crisis of death.

The literature on family crisis theory delineates three variables characterizing families that are better able to cope with crisis events. These variables are involvement, integration, and adaptation.[18] The above discussion on role reorganization actually refers to the process of adaptation, which is defined as "the ability of the family group and each of its members to change their responses to one another and the world around them as the situation demands—flexibility of the family in group structure and individual behavior"[19] and in essence spells out what the variable of adaptation means in a specific family crisis situation.

How does role reorganization proceed in families not characterized by a balanced apportionment of roles? Two results, quite diverse from one another, may occur based upon the roles of the scapegoated and the generator of conflict or tension.[20] If the member who died was a scapegoat in the family, readjustment following this loss must take into account his purpose within the interactional economy of the family. The scapegoating role may be reassigned. If roles cannot be realigned to incorporate a scapegoating function, the threat of collapse occurs. If, on the other hand, the death was of a member who produced conflict and tension within the family, such as a chronic alcoholic, the result may be increased family solidarity because of the removal of a divisive element.

A third variant of role reorganization occurs when the member who died occupied a position not seen as crucial by the rest of the family. Rita R. Vollman et al. see this person as the one who "was always a little different, never quite fit in." Readjustment is minimal and proceeds without difficulty. An example is the family in which the aged parent of one of the spouses had been living.

Increased Solidarity

Increased solidarity in the family is a second reaction to death. Two factors give rise to solidarity resulting from trouble. The principle is recognized that trouble brings individuals together, and so the family is united by its loss. Increased solidarity serves not only to ensure the successful functioning of the newly reconstituted unit but gives needed emotional support to all members at a crucial time. An example is the greater closeness which spouses are reported to achieve in facing the death of their child, provided their marriage is a solid one.[21] Second, solidarity can result when a member who caused conflict dies.

If solidarity is to occur, it presupposes the need for consensus regarding role reorganization. Family members must come to some understanding as to how the roles will be filled and by whom.[22] If agreement cannot be reached, roles are left unfulfilled or unnecessarily overlap and possibly conflict. The potential for disagreement increases with the family more advanced in its life cycle, because children have a greater voice in family matters by virtue of being older and by virtue of being future or present income producers who can be tapped for support. There may be several reasons for conflict: continuation of conflict regarding role definition prior to death of the member, several persons able and willing to assume the same role, and lack of clarity as to what the role entails. Another possibility, mentioned by Vollman et al., is that the member who died fulfilled a socioemotional role which kept hostilities and conflict dormant or at least under control. What was latent now becomes active. This reaction is seen in the family in which a child served to bind the parents into a tenuous relationship; with the child's death, difficulties previously held in check arise, and the spouses must confront a serious marital conflict.

Object Replacement

Death is even sadder when it is that of a child because we feel life has been cut so short for this human being. One way parents deal with this loss is by investing additional emotional energy in the remaining children. Or they may seek to have another child, especially if the deceased was an only child. This reaction is object replacement. It is not hard to understand the parents' wish for another child. The same wish is expressed when a parent remarries. In either case, the composition of the group has been restored to its original size. If parents have adequately worked through their grief, they are ready to accept a new child.

A danger arises when parents have not successfully completed their grief work; in that event, the new child may be forced to live in the image of the dead child. Albert and Barbara Cain studied this dynamic.[23] Because either one or both parents had not resolved their mourning, continual comparisons were made. "These parents grossly imposed the identity of the dead child upon his substitute and unconsciously identified the two."[24] The result was predictably sad: Children with no identities of their own were forced into the image of a sibling they never knew, with the conveyed message that they could not measure up; children were overprotected and restricted by parents whose fears that something might also happen to this child became unrealistically exaggerated; and children manifesting the dead sibling's physical symptoms in identification were filled with morbid preoccupations. The groundwork was laid for later personality difficulties for these children.

A somewhat similar process may occur in the spouse–spouse subsystem when one remarries and identifies the new partner with the deceased and tries to mold him into that image. However, personality damage would not result from object replacement on an adult–adult level; unlike the child who can not protest the molding of his personality according to the image of the deceased, an adult can.

Death calls forth many emotions, including loss, guilt, anger, a sense of relief, anxiety, a feeling of helplessness, hostility, and fear. These are, by and large, normal reactions during the course of bereavement. One individual may experience all of them, others only some. During bereavement one comes to grips with these feelings and, having worked the grief through, is no longer overcome by these emotions. A parent whose child has died may initially reproach himself for not having recognized sooner that his child was sick and gone to the doctor, possibly saving the child. If mourning proceeds successfully, the parent realizes he did all that was possible and the sense of guilt is relieved. For the parent who continues to accuse himself in an intense and bitter manner, we recognize that this emotion has become a severe mourning reaction. Lorraine Siggins wrote: "I myself regard mourning as pathological if any of the above reactions are excessively intense or violent, or if the process of mourning is unduly prolonged."[25]

Scapegoating

One effect of a pathological reaction is the possibility that the family may displace its guilt and anger over the death and create the role of a scapegoat. A common form of scapegoating may involve the relationship between both parents and a surviving child in the family. Parents may experience guilt for several reasons: an ambivalent relationship with the dead child marked by some hostility; a previous desire for him to die, experienced, perhaps, in a moment of anger but now recalled and unrealistically interpreted as leading to death; a feeling of anger at the deceased for dying; and the wish that more had been given of oneself while the deceased was living. Scapegoating a child serves to relieve and prevent parents from facing guilt. The scapegoating may occur, on one hand, with the parents' being annoyed at a surviving child and continually finding fault with whatever he does, or, on the other hand, with the parents' actively blaming him for the sibling's death. Unless the adults can come to grips with these feelings, the child is likely to remain a scapegoat.

In dealing with their anger over a death, parents may bitterly accuse the doctor of not giving proper treatment to the child, they may blame God, or they may even become angry toward a remaining child. The living child may become a temporary or permanent object toward which the parents may vent hostility without the child's knowing why he is being so treated.

Displaced guilt and hostility need not be directed only toward a child. Spouse may blame spouse, especially when the child's illness and death may be based upon genetic transmission.

Scapegoating may also occur in a family as a way of reachieving homeostasis when the previous family balance included a scapegoat. In this case, the scapegoat role may be reassigned, and if roles can not be realigned to incorporate the scapegoating function in the operational dynamics of the family, there occurs the threat of collapse.

Anticipatory Grief

Death has been discussed as an unanticipated crisis for the family. Sometimes, however, the death is anticipated for weeks, months, or even a year or two in advance. What does this fact imply in terms of a family's reaction? To answer we must first look at the nature of grief when a forthcoming death is known. This is anticipatory grief. In this situation the mourner is not spared the necessity of having to complete his grief work but "the shock and suddenness is lacking, and as a result the grief potential, at least for intensity, lowers."[26] In some instances, much of the grief work will have occurred by the time of death and the reaction may be one of relief, especially if the dying individual was suffering. In anticipatory grief, mourning is of longer duration but of lesser intensity; in grief precipitated by a sudden loss, mourning may not be as extended but is of greater intensity. Anticipatory grief enables a family to begin the aforementioned tasks. If it is an adult who is dying, anticipatory grief allows the family the benefit of his consultation regarding what they should do; a husband can advise his wife, for example, to sell his business and use the money to send the children to college. The dying individual can share in the preparatory mourning and facilitate it. It can be a powerful family-affective experience. For the family, mourning becomes a gradual, extended, and less intense process.

Conclusion

The attempt has been to examine the interrelational resolution of grief as the result of death, as worked out within the context of the family unit. Death is an anxiety-laden topic. In recognizing the personal and intense feelings of sorrow and grief a family experiences, we are reminded of our own mortality. The maladaptive mourning reaction, individual and familial, is not as frequent a reason for casework treatment as other psychosocial problems, but death is one of life's natural occurrences that brings pain to others, pain that social workers can share with their clients via the helping process.

References

1. Parad, H. J., & Caplan, G. A framework for studying families in crisis. In H. J. Parad (Ed.), *Crisis intervention: Selected readings.* New York: Family Service Association of America, 1965. P. 57.
2. Glasser, P. H., & Glasser, L. N.(Eds.), *Families in Crisis.* New York: Harper & Row, 1970. P. 7.
3. Hill, R. Generic features of families under stress. In H. J. Parad (Ed.), *Crisis intervention: Selected readings.* New York: Family Service Association of America, 1965. P. 37.
4. Golan, N. When is a client in crisis? *Social Casework* **50:**391 (July 1969).
5. Kaplan, D. M. Observations on crisis theory and practice. *Social Casework* **49:**152 (March 1968).
6. Lindemann, E. Symptomatology and management of acute grief. In H. J. Parad (Ed.), *Crisis intervention: Selected readings.* New York: Family Service Association of America, 1965. Pp. 10–11.
7. Siggins, L. D. Mourning: A critical review of the literature. *International Journal of Psychiatry* **3:**423 (May 1967).
8. Verwoerdt, A. Death and the family. *Medical Opinion and Review* **1:**43 (September 1966).
9. Lindemann, E. Symptomatology and management of acute grief. In H. J. Parad (Ed.), *Crisis intervention: Selected readings.* New York: Family Service Association of America, 1965. P. 11.
10. Eliot, T. D. The bereaved family. *Annals of the American Academy of Political and Social Science* **160:**188 (March 1932).
11. Vollman, R. R., Ganzert, A., Picher, L., & Williams, W. V. The reactions of family systems to sudden and unexpected death. *Omega* **2:**101–106 (May 1971); Williams, W. V., Polak, P., & Vollman, R. R. Crisis intervention in acute grief. *Omega* **3:**67–70 (February 1972).
12. Vollman, R. R., Ganzert, A., Picher, L., & Williams, W. V. Reactions of family systems to sudden and unexpected death. *Omega* **2:**104 (May 1971).
13. Shoor, M. & Speed, M. H. Death, delinquency, and the mourning process. In R. Fulton (Ed.), *Death and identity.* New York: John Wiley & Sons, 1965. P. 206.
14. Lindemann, E. Symptomatology and management of acute grief, pp. 13–16; Krupp, G. Maladaptive reactions to the death of a family member. *Social Casework* **53:**425–34 (July 1972).
15. Eliot, T. D. Bereavement: Inevitable but not insurmountable. In H. Becker & R. Hill (Eds.), *Family, marriage and parenthood.* Boston: D. C. Heath and Company, 1948. P. 661.
16. Vollman, R. R., Ganzert, A., Picher, L., & Williams, W. V. The reactions of family systems to sudden and unexpected death. *Omega* **2:**104 (May 1971).

17. Ibid.
18. Glasser, P. H., & Glasser, L. N. (Eds.). *Families in crisis.* New York: Harper & Row, 1970. P. 7.
19. Ibid, p. 8.
20. Williams, W. V., Polak, P., & Vollman, R. R. Crisis intervention in acute grief. *Omega* **3**:69–70 (February 1972).
21. Cobb, B. Psychological impact of long illness and death of a child on the family circle. *Journal of Pediatrics* **49**:748 (July–December 1956).
22. Eliot, T. D. The bereaved family. *Annals of the American Academy of Political and Social Sciences* **160**:188 (March 1932).
23. Cain, A. C., & Cain, B. S. On replacing a child. *Journal of the American Academy of Child Psychiatry* **3**:443–56 (July 1964).
24. Ibid., p. 446.
25. Siggins, L. D. Mourning: A critical review of the literature. *International Journal of Psychiatry* **3**:427 (May 1967).
26. Danto, B. L. Anticipatory grief (Paper presented at a meeting of the Foundation of Thanatology, Columbia Presbyterian Hospital, Columbia University, New York, N.Y., April 14, 1972).

Author Index

435

Subject Index

439

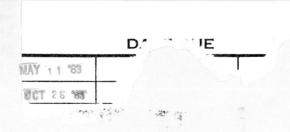